Compliments of
Rhône-Poulenc Rorer Canada

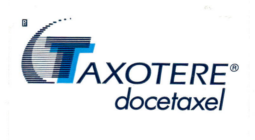

AXOTERE® *docetaxel*

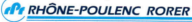

Oncology

RHÔNE-POULENC RORER

RHÔNE-POULENC RORER CANADA INC.
Saint-Laurent, Québec, H4R 2P9

TEXTBOOK OF BREAST CANCER

A Clinical Guide to Therapy

Edited by

GIANNI BONADONNA, MD
Professor of Medicine and Director
Division of Medical Oncology
Istituto Nazionale Tumori
Milan, Italy

GABRIEL N HORTOBAGYI, MD
Professor of Medicine and Chairman
Department of Breast Medical Oncology
The University of Texas
MD Anderson Cancer Center
Houston, USA

A MASSIMO GIANNI, MD
Professor of Medicine
Division of Medical Oncology
Istituto Nazionale Tumori
Milan, Italy

MARTIN DUNITZ

Although every effort has been made to ensure that drug doses and other information are presented accurately in this publication, the ultimate responsibility rests with the prescribing physician. Neither the publishers nor the authors can be held responsible for errors or for any consequences arising from the use of information contained herein.

© Martin Dunitz Ltd 1997

First published in the United Kingdom in 1997 by
Martin Dunitz Ltd
The Livery House
7–9 Pratt Street
London NW1 0AE

Reprinted 1998

A CIP catalogue record for this book is available from the British Library

ISBN 1-85317-348-7

Composition by Wearset, Boldon, Tyne and Wear
Printed and bound in the USA

Contents

The Editors and Publishers would like to dedicate the publication of this volume to Pinuccia Valagussa, without whose devotion and organizational skills they could never have achieved the finished book.

Contributors

Yutaka Ariyoshi, MD
Director
Prefectual Aichi Hospital
Okazaki 444
JAPAN

Jean Pierre Armand, MD
Chairman, Medical Oncology
Institut Gustave-Roussy
Rue Camille Desmoulins
94805 Villejuif Cedex
FRANCE

Gianni Bonadonna, MD
Director, Division of Medical Oncology
Istituto Nazionale Tumori
Via Venezian, 1
20133 Milan
ITALY

Aman U Buzdar, MD
Department of Breast Medical Oncology
The University of Texas
MD Anderson Cancer Center
Houston, TX 77030
USA

Giuseppe Capri, MD
Istituto Nazionale Tumori
Via Venezian, 1
20133 Milan
ITALY

Monica Castiglione-Gertsch, MD
Swiss Institute for Applied Cancer Research
CH 3008 Bern
SWITZERLAND

Jenny Chang, MRCP
The Royal Marsden NHS Trust
Downs Road
Sutton
Surrey SM2 5PT
UK

Lígia Bruno da Costa, MD
Oncologia Cascais
Travessa da Conceicão N° 1
2750 Cascais
PORTUGAL

Silvana Di Palma, MD
Istituto Nazionale Tumori
Via Venezian, 1
20133 Milan
ITALY

Heather S Feigelson, MD
University of Southern California
Department of Preventive Medicine
Los Angeles, CA 90033-0800
USA

Sebastian Fetscher, MD
Albert-Ludwigs-Universität Medical Center
Department of Medicine I
University of Freiburg
D 79106 Freiburg
GERMANY

John F Forbes, MS, FRACS, FRCS
Director, Surgical Oncology
Newcastle Mater Misericordiae Hospital
Waratah, NSW 2298
AUSTRALIA

A Massimo Gianni, MD
Istituto Nazionale Tumori
Via Venezian, 1
20133 Milan
ITALY

Luca Gianni, MD
Istituto Nazionale Tumori
Via Venezian, 1
20133 Milan
ITALY

Brian E Henderson, MD
Professor, Preventive Medicine
University of Southern California
Department of Preventive Medicine
Los Angeles, CA 90033-0800
USA

Gabriel N Hortobagyi, MD
Chairman
Department of Breast Medical Oncology
The University of Texas
MD Anderson Cancer Center
Houston, TX 77030
USA

Manfred Kaufmann, MD
Zentrum der Frauenheilkunde und
Gerburtshilfe
Klinikum der Johann Wolfgang
Goethe-Universität
D-60590 Frankfurt am Main
GERMANY

James Mackay, MD, MRCP
Consultant in Cancer Genetics
School of Clinical Medicine
Addenbrooke's Hospital
Cambridge   CB2 2QQ
UK

Paul N Mainwaring, FRACP
Breast Unit
The Royal Marsden NHS Trust
Fulham Road
London   SW3 6JJ
UK

Beryl McCormick, MD
Memorial Sloan-Kettering Cancer Center
1275 York Avenue
New York, NY 10021
USA

Roland Mertelsmann, MD, PhD
Medical Director, Oncology
Albert-Ludwigs-Universität Medical Center
Department of Medicine I
University of Freiburg
D 79106 Freiburg
GERMANY

Makoto Ogawa, MD
President
Aichi Cancer Center
Nagoya 464
JAPAN

Bruce A J Ponder, PhD, FRCP
Professor of Clinical Oncology
Oncology Centre
Addenbrooke's Hospital
Cambridge   CB2 2QQ
UK

Trevor Powles, PhD, FRCP
The Royal Marsden NHS Trust
Downs Road
Sutton
Surrey SM2 5PT
UK

Kathleen I Pritchard, MD, FRCPC
Professor, University of Toronto
Toronto-Sunnybrook Regional Cancer Centre
2075 Bayview Avenue
Toronto, Ontario   M4N 3M5
CANADA

Barbara F Rabinowitz, PhD, MSW, RN
Monmouth Medical Center
300 2nd Avenue
Long Branch, NJ 07740
USA

Peter M Ravdin, MD, PhD
University of Texas Health Science Center
7703 Floyd Curl Drive
San Antonio, TX 78284
USA

Franco Rilke, MD
Istituto Nazionale Tumori
Via Venezian, 1
20133 Milan
ITALY

Sjoerd Rodenhuis, MD
Chief of Medicine
The Netherlands Cancer Institute
1066 CX Amsterdam
THE NETHERLANDS

Robert D Rubens, MD, FRCP
Imperial Cancer Research Fund
Clinical Oncology Unit
Guy's Hospital
London Bridge
London SE1 9RT
UK

Ian E Smith, MD, FRCP, FRCPE
Breast Unit
The Royal Marsden NHS Trust
Fulham Road
London SW3 6JJ
UK

Pinuccia Valagussa
Istituto Nazionale Tumori
Via Venezian, 1
20133 Milan
ITALY

Gunter von Minckwitz, MD
Zentrum der Frauenheilkunde und
Geburtshilfe
Klinikum der Johann Wolfgang
Goethe-Universität
D-60590 Frankfurt am Main
GERMANY

1

Epidemiology and screening

Brian E Henderson, Heather S Feigelson

CONTENTS • **Descriptive factors** • **Analytic factors** • **Endogenous hormones** • **Exogenous hormones**
• **Genetic susceptibility** • **Other possible risk factors**

Breast cancer is the most common cancer of women world wide.[1] There have been sustained increases in the incidence of this cancer in developing countries in recent years. It has been estimated that, if these increasing rates persist, the annual worldwide incidence of breast cancer will be over one million by the year 2000.[2] Male breast cancer is rare compared with female breast cancer. Female : male incidence ratios vary from 70 to 130 around the world.

A substantial body of experimental, clinical and epidemiologic evidence indicates that hormones play a major role in the etiology of breast cancer.[3,4] The known risk factors for breast cancer (Table 1.1) can be understood as measures of the cumulative exposure of the breast to estrogen and, perhaps, progesterone. The actions of these ovarian hormones (and the hormones used in combination oral contraceptives [COCs] and hormone replacement therapy [HRT]) on the breast do not appear to be genotoxic, but they do affect the rate of cell division. Their effects on breast cancer rates are manifest in their effects on proliferation of the breast epithelial cell. Recent advances in molecular genetics of cancer have provided a molecular basis for the concept that cell division is essential

in the genesis of human cancer.

The activation of oncogenes and inactivation of tumor-suppressor genes (e.g. *BRCA*1, *TP*53) produce a sequence of genetic changes that lead to a malignant phenotype (Figure 1.1). The activation of oncogenes, whether by mutation, translocation or amplification, requires cell division. Genetic errors that precede the development of a fully malignant tumor also include

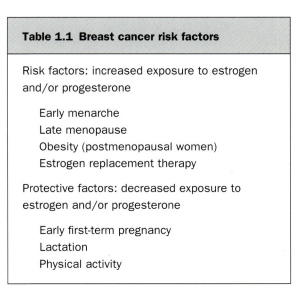

Table 1.1 Breast cancer risk factors
Risk factors: increased exposure to estrogen and/or progesterone

Early menarche
    Late menopause
    Obesity (postmenopausal women)
    Estrogen replacement therapy

Protective factors: decreased exposure to estrogen and/or progesterone

Early first-term pregnancy
    Lactation
    Physical activity

the loss or inactivation during mitosis of several tumor-suppressor genes which function to control normal cellular behavior.[5] Most of the models currently favored suggest that the first hit is the inactivation, by a mutational event, of one of the two alleles of a tumor-suppressor gene present in diploid cells, followed by a reduction to homozygosity of the faulty chromosome.[6] The initial mutagenic event and loss of the wild-type allele of the tumor-suppressor gene both require cell division. Thus, for expression of the full malignant phenotype, cells are absolutely required to divide.

As endogenous hormones directly affect the risk of breast cancer, there is reason for concern about the effects on breast cancer risk if the same or closely related hormones are administered for therapeutic purposes (e.g. as contraceptives or as HRT). It also follows that

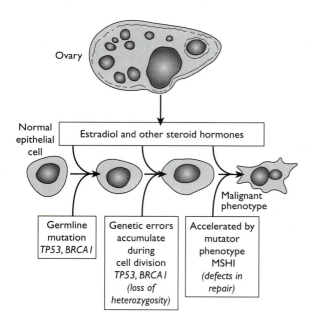

Figure 1.1 Estradiol and, to a lesser degree, other steroid hormones (e.g. progesterone) drive cell proliferation, which facilitates fixation of genetic errors by loss of heterozygosity or leads to genetic changes that facilitate mutation by defects in DNA repair enzymes. Germline mutations in relevant tumor-suppressor genes (e.g. *BRCA1*, *BRCA2*) accelerate the transformation into the malignant phenotype.

approaches to the prevention of breast cancer should focus on reducing the lifetime exposure of the breast to estrogen and progesterone, e.g. reducing the number of ovulations through exercise or perhaps lowering the levels of steroid hormone by increasing the fiber content of the diet or by pharmacological means.

DESCRIPTIVE FACTORS

As for other epithelial cancers, the most important demographic risk factor is increasing age. By the late teens the first cases of breast cancer occur, and thereafter there is a rapid risk in the age-specific rates. Up to the age of 50, the rate of increase is very high; after this, the rate of increase slows dramatically.[7]

There is substantial variation in breast cancer rates among different countries. Rates are some six times higher in the USA, Canada and northern Europe than in Asia or among black populations in Africa. These international differences in breast cancer rates do not appear to be determined primarily by variation in genetic susceptibility. Breast cancer rates for American black women are quite similar to rates for American white women, not to rates for African black women. Furthermore, Japanese migrants to Hawaii and California have increased rates of breast cancer compared with their counterparts in Japan.[8] Those Japanese women who are born in Japan and migrate to the USA as young adults experience only a modest increase in their breast cancer rates, approaching that of their white counterparts. Thus, the risk of breast cancer seems at least partly related to early life experiences. Nevertheless, Polish and Italian migrants to the USA and Australia appear to have substantial increases in breast cancer mortality within 20–25 years of migration.[9]

ANALYTIC FACTORS

Age at menarche

Early age at menarche has been demonstrated as a risk factor for breast cancer in most case-control studies (see Table 1.1). In general, a decrease of about 20% in breast cancer risk results from each year that menarche is delayed. For a fixed age at menarche, women who establish regular menstrual cycles within 1 year of the first menstrual period have more than double the risk of breast cancer of women with a 5-year or more delay in onset of regular cycles.[4] Women with early menarche (age 12 or younger) and rapid establishment of regular cycles had an almost fourfold increased risk of breast cancer when compared with women with later menarche (age 13 or older) and long duration of irregular cycles.

These observations suggested that regular ovulatory cycles increase a woman's risk of breast cancer[4] and supported results from an earlier study of circulating hormone levels in daughters of breast cancer patients and age-matched daughters of controls. The daughters of the breast cancer patients, who as a group have at least twice the breast cancer risk of the general population, had higher levels of circulating estrogen and progesterone on day 22 of the menstrual cycle than did the controls.[10] As cumulative estrogen levels are greater during the normal luteal phase than during a comparable period of a non-ovulatory cycle, cumulative frequency of ovulatory cycles is an index of cumulative estrogen exposure (and of progesterone exposure as well). Apter and Vihko,[11] in a longitudinal study of 200 schoolgirls, also found that those with early menarche establish ovulatory cycles more quickly than girls with later onset of menstruation.

Physical activity

Strenuous physical activity may delay menarche. Girls who engage in regular ballet dancing, swimming or running have a considerable delay in the onset of menses. In one study, ballet dancers had a mean age at menarche of 15.4 years compared with 12.5 years for controls.[11] Breast development was also delayed in the dancers, and they experienced intermittent amenorrhea through their teenage years, as long as they remained active dancers. Even

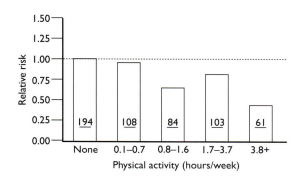

Figure 1.2 Average hours of intense physical activity per week, breast cancer cases aged 40 and under and controls.[14] $p = 0.0004$ (trend).

moderate physical activity during adolescence can lead to anovular cycles.[12] Girls who engaged in regular, moderate physical activity (averaging at least 600 kcal (2.52 MJ) of energy expended per week) were 2.9 times more likely to be anovular than girls who engaged in lesser amounts of physical activity.[13] More recently, we reported that adolescent and adult physical activity significantly reduces the risk of breast cancer in young women (≤40 years of age).[14] The risk of breast cancer among women who averaged four or more hours per week of exercise activity during their reproductive years was nearly 60% lower than that of inactive women (Figure 1.2).

Age at menopause

The relationship between menopause and breast cancer risk has been known for some time. The rate of increase in the age-specific incidence rate of breast cancer slows markedly at the time of the menopause, and the rate of increase in the postmenopausal period is only about one-sixth the rate of increase in the premenopausal period.

It has been estimated that women who experience natural menopause (defined as cessation of periods) before the age of 45 have only one-half the breast cancer risk of those whose menopause occurs after the age of 55.[15] Another way of expressing this result is that women with 40 or more years of active menstruation have twice the breast cancer risk of those with fewer than 30 years of menstrual activity. Artificial menopause, by either bilateral oophorectomy or pelvic irradiation, also markedly reduces breast cancer risk. The effect appears to be just slightly greater than that of natural menopause, probably because surgical removal of the ovaries causes an abrupt cessation of hormone production whereas some hormone production continues for a few months or years after the natural cessation of menses at the menopause.

Pregnancy

Two of the earliest known and most reproducible features of breast cancer epidemiology are the decreased risk associated with increased parity and the increased risk of childless women.

MacMahon et al[16] made a major advance in our understanding of the role of pregnancy in altering breast cancer risk through their analysis of an international collaborative case-control study. Single and nulliparous married women were found to have the same increased risk of breast cancer – about 1.4 times the risk of parous married women. Among married women in each country, parous cases had fewer children than parous controls. These authors clearly demonstrated, however, that this protective effect of parity resulted from a protective effect of early age at first birth. Those women with a first birth under the age of 20 had about one-half the risk of nulliparous women. Controlling for age at first birth, subsequent births had no influence on the risk of developing breast cancer. More recent studies in other populations have observed a small residual protective effect of an increasing number of births, suggesting that, under certain circumstances, multiparity does offer some further protection. In a study in Shanghai, we observed a protective effect of multiple pregnancies, which was most notable after the fifth pregnancy.[17] The main protective effect is, however,

undoubtedly associated with the first full-term pregnancy.

Married women who have a late first full-term pregnancy are actually at an elevated risk of breast cancer compared with nulliparous women. This paradoxical effect has been confirmed repeatedly; a possible explanation is suggested by several related observations. In a hospital-based case-control study, the risk of breast cancer was substantially higher among women who had given birth during the 3 years before the interview than among comparable women whose last birth occurred 10 years earlier (relative risk = 2.66).[18] We found that a first trimester abortion, whether spontaneous or induced, before the first full-term pregnancy, was associated with an increased risk of breast cancer.[19]

It appears that pregnancy has two contradictory effects on breast cancer risk which are particularly notable in the first pregnancy. This apparent paradox actually has a physiologic explanation that is based on estrogen and prolactin secretion and metabolism during pregnancy. During the first trimester of pregnancy, there is a rapid rise in the level of 'free' estradiol, an effect that is more apparent in the first, compared with subsequent, pregnancies.[20] The net effect of this early part of pregnancy, in terms of estrogen exposure to the breast, is equivalent to several ovulatory cycles over a relatively short time.

However, in the long run, this negative effect of early pregnancy on breast cancer risk can be overridden by two beneficial consequences of a completed pregnancy. Several years ago it was reported that prolactin levels were substantially lower in parous compared with nulliparous women.[4] In addition, we found that parous women had higher levels of sex hormone-binding globulin (SHBG) and lower levels of free (non-protein bound) estradiol than their nulliparous counterparts.[4]

Lactation

Lactation has been increasingly reported to provide protection against breast cancer development. If the cumulative number of ovulatory cycles is directly related to breast cancer risk, a beneficial effect of long duration of nursing would be expected, because nursing results in a substantial delay in re-establishing ovulation following a completed pregnancy. With only a small proportion of mothers having a large cumulative number of nursing months, most previous epidemiologic studies have been unable to provide precise estimates of the effects of lactation on breast cancer risk. In a population-based case-control study in China, a progressive reduction in breast cancer risk was observed with an increasing number of years of nursing experience (Figure 1.3).[17]

Weight

In addition to the menstrual and reproductive risk factors described in the foregoing, there is a strong relationship between weight and breast cancer risk. The relationship is critically dependent on age. For women under the age of 50, there is little or no increased risk associated with increased weight, but by the age of 60, a 10-kg increment in weight results in approximately an 80% increase in breast cancer risk.[21]

Whether this weight effect is one of excess weight (body fat) or weight as such is unclear. Contradictory results have been reported, for

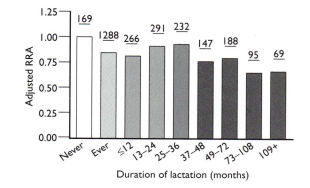

Figure 1.3 Duration of lactation among parous breast cancer cases and controls in China.[17]
*Case/controls; test for trend: two-sided $p < 0.01$.

example, on whether Quetelet's index (a measure of body mass) is correlated with breast cancer risk. Unadjusted weight appears to be as good an indicator of risk as any function of weight and height. In the postmenopausal period, the major source of estrogen is from extraglandular (largely adipose tissue) conversion of the adrenal androgen, androstenedione, to estrone so plasma levels of estradiol are higher in obese women.[4]

ENDOGENOUS HORMONES

Estrogens

The association of breast cancer with cyclic ovarian activity implies that estrogen is important in the pathogenesis of this disease. We have discussed the rationale that hormones and, in particular, estradiol can directly increase the incidence of breast cancer.[4] A substantial amount of experimental work demonstrates the critical role of estrogens in breast cancer in experimental animals. Exogenous estrone, estradiol and, under some conditions, estriol increase the incidence of mammary tumors and decrease the time to induction after administration of dimethylbenzanthracine.

Attempts to understand and quantify the role of estrogen in breast cancer development have been limited to some extent by our technical capability for measuring steroid hormones in human blood. A few studies of estrogen levels in premenopausal patients and controls have been reported. England and co-workers[22] found a 15% average elevation of plasma total estrogens in patients with breast cancer, compared with similar increases reported by others for total urinary estrogens.[22,23]

The first substantial study of plasma estrogen levels in postmenopausal breast cancer cases and controls was reported by England et al.[22] They studied the estradiol levels of 25 cases and 25 controls and found that, on average, the levels were 30% higher in the cases. There have been at least 12 additional studies on plasma estrogens and seven on urinary estrogens in postmenopausal breast cancer cases and controls. Taken together, these studies support the finding of increased levels of estrogen and, in particular, estradiol, as found by England and associates.[22]

Recent findings emphasize the possible importance of bioavailable estradiol fractions in the etiology of breast cancer. Siiteri and colleagues[24] studied a small group of breast cancer patients and controls matched on age, weight, height and menopausal status; they found the known interrelationship of obesity, SHBG and increased free estradiol in both patients and controls. They also found that some 'normal weight' breast cancer patients with normal SHBG levels had an elevated percentage of free estradiol. These results suggest that, in breast cancer patients, free estradiol in serum may be elevated by factors unrelated to the SHBG concentration.

The most carefully done international studies comparing estrogen levels in populations at differing risks of breast cancer also support a role of estrogens, particular estradiol, in the pathogenesis of breast cancer. In the early 1970s, MacMahon et al[25] conducted a series of studies on teenagers and young women to investigate whether some aspect of estrogen metabolism was responsible for the large differences in breast cancer rates between Asia and North America. They found that, in overnight urine samples collected on the morning of day 21 of the menstrual cycle, total urinary estrogen levels were 36% higher in the North American teenagers. In nulliparous women aged 20–24, total urinary estrogen levels were 49% higher on day 21 and 38% higher on day 10; similar differences were found among parous women aged 30–39. In two more recent studies, we have characterized the relationship between serum estradiol levels and the international differences in breast cancer risk.[26,27] Geometric mean estradiol levels were higher in breast cancer cases than in controls in Shanghai and Los

Table 1.2 Geometric mean values (with 95%CI) for serum estradiol and SHBG on premenopausal women with breast cancer and individually matched control women in Shanghai, China (39 pairs) and Los Angeles, California (42 pairs)*

Variable	Study group	Cases	Controls	p value[†] Case vs control
Estradiol (pmol/l)	Shanghai Chinese	584 (509–671)	501 (444–565)	0.089
	Los Angeles whites	669 (586–761)	604 (530–687)	0.23
	p value[†] (control comparison)		0.036	
SHBG (nmol/l)	Shanghai Chinese	59.4 (50.3–70.2)	61.6 (55.4–68.6)	0.71
	Los Angeles whites	54.1 (46.4–63.0)	59.1 (51.5–68.0)	0.28
	p value[†] (control comparison)		0.63	

* From Bernstein et al.[26]

† Two-sided p value; paired t-test for matched case-control comparisons and Student's t-test for comparison of controls.

Angeles, and higher in Los Angeles controls compared with Shanghai controls (Table 1.2). In a comparison of postmenopausal women, the differences were even more striking, with estradiol levels 36% higher in Los Angeles women than their age-matched Japanese counterparts.[27] There are at least two possible explanations for these differences in estradiol levels: (1) physical activity, e.g. greater physical activity among Asians, which might alter the frequency or length of ovulatory cycles; and (2) higher dietary fiber intake among Asians, which might alter fecal excretion of enterohepatic steroids and thereby lower plasma estradiol levels.

Progesterone

Evidence that elevated levels of the other major ovarian hormone, progesterone, may also be an important factor in increasing breast cancer risk has been summarized in the literature.[28] The mitotic activity of breast epithelium varies markedly during the normal menstrual cycle, with peak activity occurring late in the luteal phase.[29] This suggests that progesterone, at least in the presence of estrogen, induces mitotic activity in breast epithelium. This effect of progesterone would be in sharp contrast to its effect on endometrial tissue, in which the peak mitotic activity occurs in the estrogen-dominated follicular phase of the cycle. It strongly agrees, however, with the experimental findings that progesterone induces ductal growth in rodent breast tissue.[30] If progesterone does increase breast cancer risk, then regular ovulatory cycles should be more common in breast cancer patients than in controls. Breast cancer patients would be expected to have shorter cycles on average than controls, because differences in cycle length result almost completely from differences caused by the length of the follicular phase. In ovulatory menstrual cycles, the shorter the cycle length the greater the proportion of time a woman spends in the luteal phase with its associated high progesterone level. Although few studies have addressed these issues, they all provide support for this role for progesterone.[10]

Several studies have measured progesterone, or its major urinary metabolite pregnanediol, in premenopausal women. All four studies of pregnanediol, and five of six studies of progesterone, found lower levels in breast cancer cases than in controls.[28] There is reason to suspect, however, that early in the clinical course of breast cancer, the regularity of ovulation is disrupted, so that such case-control comparisons may be misleading. Furthermore, luteal phase progesterone levels are difficult to quantitate with spot samples, because the amount of progesterone detected in plasma or the amount of progesterone metabolites in urine depends specifically on the day of sampling in relation to the luteal phase peak. Three prospective studies have examined breast cancer incidence in women with clinical evidence of progesterone deficiency and all report elevated risks.[28] Overall, there is little objective evidence supporting the role of progesterone in the pathogenesis of breast cancer. More direct evidence to support or refute the role of progesterone should come from surveillance of women receiving medroxyprogesterone as a form of contraception or HRT.

EXOGENOUS HORMONES

Oral contraceptives

Pike et al[31] summarized the population-based studies of COC use and breast cancer that had been published during 1990 and derived a weighted average for the relative risk (RR) for 10 years of COC use among women under 45 years of age. This RR estimate was 1.36 which is equivalent to a 3.1% (95% confidence interval [CI] = 1.7–4.6) in breast cancer risk, per year of COC use. The weighted RR for young women who took COCs for 10 years before their first full-term pregnancy was 1.45 compared with women who never took COCs. For women aged 45 years or over, there is no evidence of any increase in breast cancer risk with COC use.

A 1993 review by Malone et al[32] provided a comprehensive overview of the literature on

COCs since 1990. The authors concluded that, overall, there was no apparent relationship between ever-use of COCs and breast cancer risk, but that ever-use is probably too crude a measure of exposure to be accurate. The most consistently observed positive associations were from studies of women under the age of 45. Possible associations with duration of use before first full-term pregnancy, use before the age of 25 or overall long duration of use, while not consistent across all studies, was suggestive of an increased risk for breast cancer in younger women.

Since this review appeared, five additional studies have been published evaluating COC use and breast cancer risk.[33-37] Two of these studies[33,34] are population based, whereas the remaining three are hospital-based studies.[35-37] The two population-based studies give somewhat conflicting results. Primic-Zakelj et al[34] evaluated breast cancer risk and COC use in Slovenian women aged 25–54. There was no association in ever-users of COCs. For women who had used COCs for 8 years or more, the adjusted RR for breast cancer was 1.16 (95%CI = 0.76–1.73) compared with never-users. There was no increase in risk with interval since first use, age at first use, use before first full-term pregnancy, or time between menarche and age at first use.

Brinton et al[33] examined COC use and breast cancer risk among younger women residing in three geographic areas of the USA. The RR associated with use of COCs was significantly elevated among women younger than 35 years of age (RR = 1.7, 95%CI = 1.2–2.6). The risk was less marked among women aged 35–39 years (RR = 1.4, 95%CI = 1.0–1.8), whereas there was no significant elevation in women aged 40–45. The RR for breast cancer for those whose COC use began early (before age 18) and continued long term (10 or more years of use) was even higher (RR = 3.1, 95%CI = 1.4–6.7). As for Primic-Zakelj et al,[34] risk was elevated among women with more recent use. The RRs observed for those who used COCs within 5 years of cancer diagnosis were higher than for those who had not, with the effect being most marked for those under the age of 35 (RR = 2.0,

95%CI = 1.3–3.1). However, this did not emerge as a more important determinant of risk than duration of use.

As COC use was very common among both cases (85%) and controls (82%) younger than 45 years of age, the referent group of 'non-users' actually comprised women who had either never used COCs or used them for less than 6 months.[33] This is probably a better referent group than one defining never-users as one month of COC use or less. Many women who experience side effects from COCs will try different formulations in an attempt to find a COC formula that they can tolerate for a few months, before turning to a different method of contraception. The common side effects, such as nausea, breast tenderness and water retention, are believed to result from the estrogen component. These women who cannot tolerate the side effects of COCs probably have a different endogenous estrogen profile from women who take COCs with minimal or no side effects and should, therefore, probably not be combined with longer-term users. However, this may also make them non-comparable to true 'never-users' who may or may not have experienced COC side effects if they had been exposed. Thus, inclusion in either the 'exposed' or 'unexposed' group could introduce bias. Where possible, analyses should be conducted excluding these short-term users to observe whether the RR changes.

Estrogen replacement therapy

More than 30 million postmenopausal women live in the USA. The advisability of long-term use of estrogen replacement therapy (ERT) for such women remains controversial. Nevertheless, by the mid-1970s, over 28 million prescriptions of non-contraceptive estrogens were being filled annually in the USA. Concerns about the carcinogenic potential of ERT on the endometrium, however, led to a 50% decline in the number of estrogen prescriptions by 1980. Hence, a cyclic estrogen– progestogen regimen became widely recommended and prescribed. By 1983, prescriptions of estrogen had increased once again.

The most commonly prescribed ERT for menopausal women in the USA includes conjugated equine estrogens (CEEs), with a preferred dose of 0.625 mg/day for 25 days in a 28-day treatment cycle. This dose is lower than those commonly prescribed during the 1970s. When progestins are added to estrogen, the resulting combination is referred to as HRT. The usual dose is medroxyprogesterone acetate 5–10 mg/day added during days 14–25.

Pike et al.[31] summarized the population-based epidemiologic studies that had been published during 1990 and derived a weighted average of the RR for the effect of ERT use on breast cancer risk. Of the ten studies included, nine showed a positive association and the results of five were statistically significant. Based on these studies, the average annual increase in breast cancer risk was 3.1% per year of ERT. For women with 10 years of ERT, the risk of breast cancer was 1.36 times that of women who had never used these preparations. The studies conducted in the USA allow the estimation of breast cancer risk associated with use of a standard CEE dose of 0.625 mg/day; on this basis, the increase in breast cancer risk is estimated to be 2.2% per year of ERT. The estimated 2.2% increase in breast cancer risk associated with a CEE regimen of 0.625 mg/day translates into RR values for breast cancer of 1.1 after 5 years of use, 1.2 after 10 years of use and 1.4 after 15 years of use. In fact, this figure may be an under-estimation because some of these studies made inadequate adjustment for age at menopause. This would tend to produce estimates of breast cancer risk that are too low because the use of ERT is associated with early menopause, which is a protective factor for breast cancer.

Of five other recent meta-analyses published, three found a small increased risk associated with long-term use, whereas two found no increased risk.[38] Those with positive findings had results of similar magnitude to those of Pike et al.[31] Subsequently, three large population-based studies conducted in the USA have been published.[39–41]

The Nurse's Health Study,[39] a large cohort established in 1976, found an increased risk for breast cancer with ever-use of ERT (RR = 1.32, 95%CI = 1.14–1.54), HRT (RR = 1.41, 95%CI = 1.15–1.74) and progestin-only use (RR = 2.24, 95%CI = 1.26–3.98). When evaluating current compared with past use, no association was seen with past use, not even for long duration ($\geq$10 years) of past use. Among current users, risk of invasive breast cancer was increased for all categories of duration, with increasing duration associated with increased risk; however, only use for 5 years or more showed statistically significant increased risk: 5–9 years of use, RR = 1.46 (95%CI = 1.22–1.74); 10 or more years of use, RR = 1.46 (95%CI = 1.20–1.76). Women aged 60–64 who had used hormones for 5 or more years were at greatest risk: RR = 1.71 (95%CI = 1.34–2.18). These results included all hormone users; the type of hormone(s) used is not specified in the analysis.

In a population-based case-control study by Newcomb et al[40] that included 3130 cases and 3698 controls, ERT did not increase the risk of breast cancer. There was no association with ERT and breast cancer in ever, former or recent users of ERT, or in women who had used ERT for long durations, even for 15 or more years. The authors found similar results among users of combination HRT. When all types of HRT users were considered together, there was a suggestion of a small increased risk of breast cancer associated with 15 or more years of use, although the estimate is statistically imprecise (RR = 1.11, 95%CI = 0.87–1.43).

Stanford et al[41] found no association between ERT use and breast cancer in a population-based case-control study, even when considering long-term use of 20 or more years. No association was seen between all types of HRT and breast cancer (RR = 0.9, 95%CI = 0.7–1.3 for ever-users). If anything, women who used estrogen–progestin HRT for 8 or more years had a reduced risk of breast cancer (RR = 0.4, 95%CI = 0.2–1.0), although data on use for more than 8 years were few.

Although these studies vary by design, they are all large, well designed and population based. Unfortunately, they do not bring us any closer to resolving the concerns about the risk of breast cancer attributed to ERT or HRT use. It does appear that short duration of ERT does not substantially increase the risk of breast cancer. Long-term use of ERT, i.e. 10 years or more, appears to increase risk for breast cancer by about 20–30%.[31] There are insufficient data on HRT use to draw meaningful conclusions about its possible association with breast cancer.

GENETIC SUSCEPTIBILITY

Remarkable advances in molecular biology and careful study of cancer-prone families have recently led to the identification of two breast cancer susceptibility genes – BRCA1 and BRCA2. These genes may cause as much as 90% of breast and ovarian cancer in some families, but probably no more than 5% of all breast cancers in the USA is attributable to these two loci.[42] Clearly, additional genes probably contribute to breast cancer risk. Much more common are multiple susceptibility genes which have low absolute risk, but potentially high population-attributable risk. One such class of genes is the one that codes for enzymes or receptors which control the metabolism and intracellular transport of estrogens.

The paradigms that have been developed from studies of bladder cancer have been used to propose a model for individual susceptibility to breast cancer.[43] We have assumed that, within and between ethnic groups, genetic differences exist which affect steroid hormone metabolism and transport. Markers (i.e. genetic polymorphisms) of these differences are likely to provide a more precise measure of risk than circulating levels of steroid hormones. The polygenic model that we have developed for breast cancer assumes that there are functionally important polymorphisms in genes encoding enzymes involved in steroid hormone biosynthesis and metabolism, which lead to differences in individual susceptibility to breast cancer and may interact with exogenous hormone exposures.

The schematic presentation of estrogen metabolism in the ovaries and breast epithelium and

the three candidate genes which may play a role in breast cancer etiology[43] are shown in Figure 1.4. The genes of interest are the 17β-hydroxysteroid dehydrogenase 2 (EDH17B2) gene, the cytochrome P450c17α (CYP17) gene, and the estrogen receptor (ER) gene. The EDH17B2 gene codes for the enzyme 17β-hydroxysteroid dehydrogenase type 1 (17HSD1) which catalyzes the final step of estradiol biosynthesis, namely the interconversion of estrone (E1) into the more biologically active estrogen fraction, estradiol (E2). 17HSD1 acts in the theca cells of the ovary and is expressed in both normal and malignant breast epithelium.[39] CYP17 codes for the cytochrome P450c17α enzyme which mediates both steroid 17α-hydroxylase and 17–20 lyase activities and functions at key branch points in human steroidogenesis. 17α-Hydroxylase activity converts steroids to precursors of the glucocorticoid cortisol, and 17–20 lyase activity yields precursors to estradiol and testosterone. The primary role of steroid receptors, such as ER, is to regulate the rate of transcription of certain genes by binding as a hormone receptor complex to specific sequences of DNA called hormone response elements (HREs). Interaction between the receptor and HREs can result in either up- or down-regulation of transcription, depending upon binding and action of auxiliary factors specific to the target gene and the

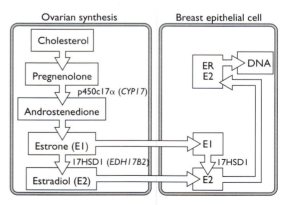

Figure 1.4 Schematic presentation of CYP17, EDH17B2 and ER in estrogen metabolism in the ovaries and breast epithelium.[43]

tissue. Polymorphisms in the *ER* gene may affect estrogen binding and subsequent transcription in target genes.

Metabolic genes and their role in carcinogenesis are a relatively new area of research with scant information at present. Studying mutations and polymorphisms in these and other genes involved in estrogen metabolism will further our understanding of breast cancer. Individual differences in estrogen metabolism attributed to genetic polymorphisms and mutations should help us define women who may be at greater risk of breast cancer for certain exposures, such as exogenous estrogens, compared with other women who may be relatively genetically 'insensitive' to the same exposure.

OTHER POSSIBLE RISK FACTORS

Dietary factors

Much attention has been focused on dietary differences, particularly fat consumption, to explain both the international pattern of breast cancer occurrence and the changes in rates of breast cancer with migration.[44] International breast cancer mortality rates are highly correlated with per capita consumption of fat ($r = 0.93$).[45] There is a wealth of evidence that nutrition profoundly influences breast cancer occurrence by modifying age at menarche and weight, but the correlation of fat with international breast cancer mortality remains highly significant after statistical adjustment for those factors. Hirayama[46] reported that breast cancer mortality rates in various regions of Japan are highly correlated with fat consumption. When international breast cancer incidence rates rather than mortality rates are considered, the magnitude of the correlation coefficient is still very high ($r = 0.84$).[45]

Many case-control studies of fat consumption and breast cancer have found only small differences between cases and controls – generally no larger than the differences in total calorie consumption. However, Howe and colleagues[47] recently conducted a combined analysis of dietary risk factors for breast cancer from 12 large case-control studies, representing populations with a wide range of dietary habits and underlying breast cancer rates. They found a positive association between both total fat and saturated fat intake and breast cancer risk among postmenopausal women (about a 50% difference in risk among individuals in the highest versus the lowest quintile of intake). Nevertheless, the five cohort studies that have used food-frequency questionnaires to study the relationship of diet and breast cancer have found no clear or consistent relationship with total fat, saturated fat or vegetable fat.[48]

Diets high in fiber may protect against breast cancer, perhaps because fiber may reduce the intestinal reabsorption of estrogens excreted via the biliary system.[49] Assessment of fiber intake in epidemiologic studies has been problematic because of a paucity of data on the fiber content of individual foods and disagreement about the most appropriate methods of biochemical analysis to determine different types of fiber. In their meta-analysis of 10 case-control studies, which included data on dietary fiber intake, Howe et al[47] reported a statistically significant 15% reduction in risk for a 20 g/day increase in dietary fiber. The relationship between total dietary fiber intake and subsequent breast cancer incidence in a large prospective investigation was very close to null,[50] which suggests that any protective effect of dietary fiber is likely to be small.

Micronutrient intake and breast cancer risk have been the subject of several studies, but no consistent relationship has emerged. Perhaps the most interesting results suggest a protective effect of vitamin A.[51] Randomized clinical trials utilizing various micronutrients are under way and should provide more definitive information on this issue.

Finally, foods rich in phytoestrogens, in particular soy protein, have been found in a study in Singapore to be protective.[52] However, two case-control studies in the People's Republic of China show no evidence of such protection.[53]

Alcohol consumption

A positive association between alcohol consumption and breast cancer has been reported in a large series of recent studies. These have been extensively reviewed and summarized in meta-analyses conducted by Howe et al.[54] Summarized data suggest that women who consume three or more alcoholic drinks per day have about a 50–70% increase in breast cancer risk compared with non-drinkers. This association is not caused by confounding by other dietary factors, including total caloric or fat consumption. For lower levels of consumption, the risks are correspondingly lower and confidence intervals generally include 1.0. It is presumed that self-reporting of alcohol consumption is not entirely reliable and that the actual risks of breast cancer could be higher than have been observed. Several possible explanations for the association between alcohol and breast cancer have been suggested. These include altered hepatic function which could increase estrogen levels or a direct mitogenic effect of alcohol on breast epithelium. More recently, Reichman et al[55] provided evidence that twice daily alcohol intake increases estrogen levels.

Table 1.3 Selection criteria and estimates of breast cancer mortality from eight randomized trials of mammography

Study (year started)	Age at entry (years)	Screening frequency (months)	Sample size Study	Control	Duration of follow-up (years)	Relative risk* All ages	>50 years
Canada NBSS1 (1980)	40–49	12	30 239	30 756	7	1.36 (0.84–2.21)	
Canada NBSS2 (1980)	50–59	12	19 711	19 694	7		0.97 (0.62–1.52)
Edinburgh (1976)	45–64	12–24	23 226	21 904	10	0.84 (0.63–1.12)	0.86 (0.41–1.80)
HIP (1963)	40–64	12	30 239	30 756	10	0.71 (0.55–0.93)	0.77 (0.50–1.16)
Sweden							
Two County (1977)	40–74	24–33	78 085	56 782	12	†0.68 (0.52–0.89) 0.82 (0.64–1.05)	0.75 (0.41–1.36) 1.28 (0.76–2.33)
Göteborg (1982)	40–59	18	20 724	28 809	7	0.86 (0.54–1.37)	0.73 (0.27–1.97)
Malmö (1976)	45–69	18–24	21 088	21 195	12	0.81 (0.62–1.07)	0.51 (0.22–1.17)
Stockholm (1981)	40–64	28	39 164	19 943	8	0.80 (0.53–1.22)	1.04 (0.53–2.05)

*Values in parentheses are 95% confidence intervals. †Results for Kopparberg and Ostergotland reported separately.

Breast cancer screening

Systematic study of breast cancer screening, including self-examination, physician examination and mammography, began with the randomized trial of the Health Insurance Plan of New York (HIP) in 1963. There have been seven additional randomized trials plus numerous smaller analytical studies. Selected characteristics of these eight trials are shown in Table 1.3 along with the most recent outcome data for the use of mammography in women of all ages and those less than 50 years of age.[56–64]

As is evident from Table 1.3, these trials varied in interval, and they also varied in whether one-view or two-view mammograms were used. Some of the trials included clinical breast examination (e.g. the HIP, Canadian and Edinburgh trials) along with mammography. Compliance rates varied but were generally high.

For women of all ages combined, every trial demonstrated some degree of benefit from screening, although in some of the studies (e.g. NB552), the confidence intervals included 1.0 and thus were not statistically significant. In the HIP trial, the relative risk was 0.71 for women of all age groups with a similar value (0.68) when restricting the analysis to those aged 50–64 years. Combining the results of all eight trials in a joint analysis, the summary benefit is a 30% reduction in mortality for women aged 50–69 at 10–12 years of follow-up.[56]

For women less than 50 years of age, the results for these randomized trials do not demonstrate a consistent or overall benefit in reduced mortality. Only the HIP study showed any benefit and this was modest (a 25% reduction in mortality) and observed only after 10–18 years in the study. The combined Swedish trials showed a 13% decrease in mortality which was not statistically significant. A combined meta-analysis of the trials at 5–7 years of follow-up produced a summary relative risk of 1.08 (95%CI = 0.85–1.39).

One explanation for the discrepancy in the results of mammographic screening in women aged 40–47 compared with those aged 50–69 years is that there is decreased sensitivity in the younger age group as a result of a greater frequency of both false-positive and false-negative results. The amount of fibrous and epithelial density is greater in premenopausal women and the presence of such densities can produce 'apparent' abnormal masses while obscuring 'true' masses. A recent study by Laya et al[65] has demonstrated that the use of ERT produces a decrease in mammographic screening specificity for such reasons. It is possible that the current widespread use of ERT could mitigate against some of the beneficial effects of mammographic screening.

Implications for cancer prevention

For women, breast cancer risk appears to be determined in large part by the cumulative exposure of breast epithelium to estrogen and progesterone. Most of this exposure is accumulated over the years of active ovarian function. Possible approaches to primary prevention require a detailed understanding of the factors that influence the onset, regularity and quality of ovarian activity.

Differences in childhood nutrition patterns and energy balance seem to be reasonable explanations for much of the international differences in breast cancer risk, but require further exploration. Regular participation in moderate physical activity, reducing the frequency of ovulatory cycles, may provide an opportunity for the primary prevention of breast cancer. Using the breast cancer incidence model discussed above, it is possible to demonstrate the considerable impact of modest changes in the ovulatory frequency at a young age. Reducing the number of ovulatory cycles between menarche at age 12 and first full-term pregnancy at age 22 by one-half could lower a woman's lifetime risk of breast cancer by more than 50%.

Chemoprevention of breast cancer via hormonal manipulation has recently received much attention.[66] One such formulation using a luteinizing hormone-releasing hormone agonist for total suppression of endogenous estrogen and progesterone production, coupled with a low-dose conjugated equine estrogen, has been proposed.[66] The potential benefits of such a regimen, particularly in women at increased risk of breast cancer, should spur efficacy studies.

Tamoxifen, a synthetic non-steroidal 'anti-estrogen' that is a widely used chemotherapeutic agent for postmenopausal breast cancer, has been advocated for chemoprevention.[66] When used for chemotherapy of postmenopausal breast cancer, there is strong evidence of a lower incidence of breast cancer in the contralateral breast. Tamoxifen-treated versus control patients show a 38% reduction in risk of the contralateral breast. Tamoxifen treatment, despite being anti-estrogenic for the breast, results in substantial increases in circulating estrogen levels in premenopausal women. This effect has spurred concerns about possible adverse consequences of tamoxifen therapy on other organs, especially the endometrium. Nevertheless, recruitment has started for a large national trial of the hormonal chemoprevention of breast cancer in healthy young women using tamoxifen.

There has been considerable discussion about the usefulness and feasibility of dietary fat reduction in middle-aged women as a method of reducing the incidence of breast cancer. Prentice et al[67] have argued that the international variation in breast cancer rates is probably mainly the result of variations in dietary fat consumption. They have proposed a large, 10-year intervention trial with a goal of reducing dietary fat from 40% to 20% of the number of calories consumed. They believe that such a reduction would achieve a 17% reduction in breast cancer incidence. The accuracy of this figure has been questioned because it assumes that the postmenopausal rate of breast cancer would actually decline to a level below that of a woman passing through menopause. The time interval required to achieve such reduction has also been seriously questioned. Given that a fat reduction diet results in weight loss or maintenance of an ideal body weight, such a diet could be expected to reduce breast cancer incidence.

Until suitable avenues for primary prevention of breast cancer are established, the most viable approach to reducing breast cancer mortality for the postmenopausal patient is through regular mammography and physician breast examination. The benefit of mammography in reducing breast cancer mortality in premenopausal women remains controversial.

The characterization of mutations in BRCA1 and other candidate breast cancer susceptibility genes opens the door to the real possibility that individual susceptibility can be more precisely determined. Potential polymorphisms in genes that control estradiol metabolism and cellular transport can further define the polygenic nature of breast cancer and lead to genetic counseling, earlier diagnosis and, perhaps, genetic therapeutic manipulation.

REFERENCES

1. Parkin DM, Stjernsward J, et al. Estimates of worldwide frequency of twelve major cancers. *Bull World Health Organ* 1984; **62:**163–82.
2. Miller AB, Bulbrook RD. UICC multidisciplinary project on breast cancer: the epidemiology, aetiology and prevention of breast cancer. *Int J Cancer* 1986; **37:**173–7.
3. Henderson BE, Ross RK, et al. Endogenous hormones as a major factor in human cancer. *Cancer Res* 1982; **42:**3232–9.
4. Henderson BE, Ross RK, et al. Estrogens as a cause of human cancer: The Richard and Hinda Rosenthal Foundation Award Lecture. *Cancer Res* 1988; **48:**246–53.
5. Stanbridge E. Identifying tumor-suppressor genes in human colorectal cancer. *Science* 1990; **247:**12–13.
6. Knudson A. Mutation and cancer: statistical study of retinoblastoma. *Proc Natl Acad Sci USA* 1971; **68:**820–3.
7. Pike MC. Age-related factors in cancer of the breast, ovary, and endometrium. *J Chron Dis* 1987; **40** (suppl 2):595–695.
8. Buell P. Changing incidence of breast cancer in Japanese–American women. *J Natl Cancer Inst* 1973; **51:**1479–83.
9. Prentice RL, Kakar F, et al. Aspects of the rationale for the women's health trial. *J Natl Cancer Inst* 1988; **80:**802–14.
10. Henderson BE, Gerkins VR, et al. Elevated serum levels of estrogen and prolactin in

daughters of patients with breast cancer. *N Engl J Med* 1975; **293**:790–5.

11. Apter D, Vihko R. Early menarche, a risk factor for breast cancer, indicates early onset of ovulatory cycles. *J Clin Endocrinol Metab* 1983; **57**:82.

12. Frisch R, Gotz-Welbergen A, et al. Delayed menarche and amenorrhea of college athletes in relation to age at onset of training. *JAMA* 1981; **246**:1559.

13. Bernstein L, Ross RK, et al. Effects of moderate physical activity on menstrual cycle patterns in adolescence: implications for breast cancer prevention. *Br J Cancer* 1987; **55**:681–5.

14. Bernstein L, Henderson BE, et al. Physical exercise activity reduces the risk of breast cancer in young women. *J Natl Cancer Inst* 1994; **86**:1403–8.

15. Trichopoulos D, MacMahon B, et al. The menopause and breast cancer risk. *J Natl Cancer Inst* 1972; **48**:605.

16. MacMahon B, Cole P, et al. Age at first birth and cancer of the breast. A summary of an international study. *Bull World Health Organ* 1970; **43**:209.

17. Yuan JM, Yu MC, et al. Risk factors for breast cancer in Chinese women in Shanghai. *Cancer Res* 1988; **48**:1949–53.

18. Bruzzi P, Negri E, et al. Short term increase in risk of breast cancer after full term pregnancy. *BMJ* 1988; **197**:1096.

19. Pike MC, Henderson BE, et al. Oral contraceptive use and early abortion as risk factors for breast cancer in young women. *Br J Cancer* 1981; **43**:72–6.

20. Bernstein L, Depue RH, et al. Higher maternal levels of free estradiol in first compared to second pregnancy: a study of early gestational differences. *J Natl Cancer Inst* 1986; **76**:1035–9.

21. de Waard FJ, Cornelis J, et al. Breast cancer incidence according to weight and height in two cities of the Netherlands and in Aichi Prefecture, Japan. *Cancer* 1977; **40**:1269.

22. England P, Skinner L, et al. Serum oestradiol-17β in women with benign and malignant breast disease. *Br J Cancer* 1974; **30**:571.

23. MacMahon B, Trichopoulos D, et al. Age at menarche, probability of ovulation and breast cancer risk. *Int J Cancer* 1982; **29**:13.

24. Siiteri P, Hammond G, et al. Increased availability of serum estrogens in breast cancer: a new hypothesis. In: *Hormones and Breast Cancer* (Pike M, Siiteri P, Welsh C, eds). Cold Spring Harbor, NY: Cold Spring Harbor Laboratories, 1981: 87–106.

25. MacMahon B, Cole P, et al. Urine oestrogen profiles of Asian and North American women. *Int J Cancer* 1974; **14**:161–7.

26. Bernstein L, Yuan JM, et al. Serum hormone levels in premenopausal Chinese women in Shanghai and white women in Los Angeles: results from two breast cancer case-control studies. *Cancer Causes Control* 1990; **1**:51–8.

27. Shimizu H, Ross RK, et al. Serum oestrogen levels in post-menopausal women: comparison of American whites and Japanese in Japan. *Br J Cancer* 1990; **62**:451–3.

28. Key T, Pike M. The role of oestrogens and progestogens in the epidemiology and prevention of breast disease. *Eur J Cancer Clin Oncol* 1988; **24**:29.

29. Ferguson D, Anderson T. Morphological evaluation of cell turnover in relation to the menstrual cycle in the 'resting' human breast. *Br J Cancer* 1981; **44**:177.

30. Dulbecco R, Hwenahan M, et al. Cell types of morphogenesis in the mammary gland. *Proc Natl Acad Sci USA* 1982; **79**:7346.

31. Pike M, Bernstein L, et al. Exogenous hormones and breast cancer risk. In: *Current Therapy in Oncology* (Neiderhuber J, ed.). St Louis: BC Decker, 1993.

32. Malone K, Daling J, et al. Oral contraceptives and breast cancer risk. *Epidemiol Rev* 1993; **15**:30.

33. Brinton LA, Daling JR, et al. Oral contraceptives and breast cancer risk among younger women. *Natl Cancer Inst* 1995; **87**:827–35.

34. Primic-Zakelj M, Evstifeeva T, et al. Breast cancer risk and oral contraceptive use in Slovenian women aged 25 to 54. *In J Cancer* 1995; **62**:414–20.

35. Rosenberg L, Palmer JR, et al. Case-control study of oral contraceptive use and risk of breast cancer. *Am J Epidemiol* 1996; **143**:25–37.

36. La Vecchia C, Negri E, et al. Oral contraceptives and breast cancer: a cooperative Italian study. *Int J Cancer* 1995; **60**:163–7.

37. Lipworth L, Katsouyanni K, et al. Oral contraceptives, menopausal estrogens, and the risk of breast cancer: a case-control study in Greece. *Int J Cancer* 1995; **62**:548–51.

38. Colditz GA, Egan KM, et al. Hormone replacement therapy and risk of breast cancer: results from epidemiologic studies. *Am J Obstet Gynecol* 1993; **168**:1473–80.

39. Colditz GA, Hankinson SE, et al. The use of estrogens and progestins and the risk of breast cancer in postmenopausal women. *N Engl J Med* 1995; **332**:1589–93.

40. Newcomb PA, Longnecker MP, et al. Long-term hormone replacement therapy and risk of breast cancer in postmenopausal women. *Am J Epidemiol* 1995; **142**:788–95.

41. Stanford JL, Weiss NS, et al. Combined estrogen and progestin hormone replacement therapy in relation to risk of breast cancer in middle-aged women. *JAMA* 1995; **274**:137–42.

42. Easton D, Ford D. Breast and ovarian cancer incidence in BRCA-1 mutation carriers. *Am J Hum Genet* 1995; **56**:265–71.

43. Feigelson H, Ross R, et al. Genetic susceptibility to cancer from exogenous and endogenous exposures. *J Cell Biochem* 1996; in press.

44. Armstrong B, Doll R. Environmental factors and cancer incidence and mortality in different countries, with special reference to dietary practices. *Int J Cancer* 1975; **15**:617–31.

45. Gray GE, Pike MC, et al. Breast cancer incidence and mortality rates in different countries in relation to known risk factors and dietary practices. *Br J Cancer* 1979; **39**:1–7.

46. Hirayama T. Epidemiology of breast cancer with special reference to the role of diet. *Prev Med* 1978; **7**:173–95.

47. Howe GR, Hirohata T, et al. Dietary factors and risk of breast cancer: combined analysis of 12 case-control studies. *J Natl Cancer Inst* 1990; **82**:561–9.

48. Hunter DJ, Spiegelman D, et al. Cohort studies of fat intake and the risk of breast cancer – a pooled analysis. *N Engl J Med* 1996; **334**:356–61.

49. Aldercreutz H, Hockerstedt K, et al. Effect of dietary components, including ligands and phytoestrogens, on enterohepatic circulation and liver metabolism of estrogens and on sex hormone binding globulin (SHBG). *J Steroid Biochem* 1987; **27**:1135–44.

50. Willett WC, Hunter DJ, et al. Dietary fat and fiber in relation to risk of breast cancer. *JAMA* 1992; **268**:2037–44.

51. Hunter D, Manson J, et al. A prospective study of the intake of vitamins C, E, and A and the risk of breast cancer. *N Engl J Med* 1993; **329**:234–40.

52. Lee HP, Gourley L, et al. Dietary effects on breast cancer risk in Singapore. *Lancet* 1991; **337**:1197–200.

53. Yuan JC, Wang Q, et al. Diet and breast cancer in Shanghai and Tianjin, China. *Br J Cancer* 1995; **71**:1353–8.

54. Howe G, Rohan T, et al. The association between alcohol and breast cancer risk: evidence from the combined analysis of six dietary case-control studies. *Int J Cancer* 1991; **47**:707–10.

55. Reichman M, Judd J, et al. Effects of alcohol consumption on plasma and urinary hormone concentrations in premenopausal women. *J Natl Cancer Inst* 1993; **85**:722–7.

56. Fletcher S, Black W, et al. Report of the International Workshop on Screening for Breast Cancer. *J Natl Cancer Inst* 1993; **85**:1644–56.

57. Chu KC, Smart CR, et al. Analysis of breast cancer mortality and stage distribution by age for the Health Insurance Plan clinical trial. *J Natl Cancer Inst* 1988; **80**:1125–32.

58. Miller AB, Baines CJ, et al. Canadian National Breast Screening Study. 1. Breast cancer detection and death rates among women ages 40 to 49 years. *Cancer Med Assoc J* 1992; **147**:1459–76.

59. Miller AB, Baines CJ, et al. Canadian National Breast Screening Study. 2. Breast cancer detection and death rates among women ages 50 to 59 years. *Cancer Med Assoc J* 1992; **147**:1477–88.

60. Roberts MM, Alexander FE, et al. Edinburgh trial of screening for breast cancer: mortality at seven years. *Lancet* 1990; **335**:241–6.

61. Nyström L, Rutqvist LE, et al. Breast cancer screening with mammography: an overview of the Swedish randomized trials. *Lancet* 1993; **341**:973–8.

62. Tabar L, Fagerberg G, et al. Update of the Swedish two-county program of mammographic screening for breast cancer. *Radiol Clin North Am* 1992; **30**:187–210.

63. Andersson I, Aspegren K, et al. Mammographic screening and mortality from breast cancer: the Malmö mammographic screening trial. *BMJ* 1988; **297**:943–8.

64. Frisell J, Eklund G, et al. Randomized study of mammography screening – preliminary report on mortality in the Stockholm trial. *Breast Cancer Res Treat* 1991; **18**:49–56.

65. Laya MB, Larson EB, et al. Effect of estrogen replacement therapy on the specificity and sensitivity of screening mammography. *J Natl Cancer Inst* 1996; **88**:643–9.

66. Henderson BE, Ross R, et al. Hormonal chemoprevention of cancer in women. *Science* 1993; **259**: 663–8.

67. Prentice RL, Kakar F, et al. Aspects of the rationale for the Women's Health Trial. *J Natl Cancer Inst* 1988; **80**:802–14.

2

Pathology

Franco Rilke, Silvana Di Palma

CONTENTS • **Benign lesions mimicking carcinoma** • **Tumours of the breast**

A substantial number of lesions of the breast are surgically excised and come to the attention of the pathologist. In pathology laboratories, breast biopsies represent a conspicuous amount of the routine activity which is currently increasing as a result of the widespread application of mammography. The final distinction between benign and malignant lesions still relies on cytological and/or histological examination of smears and tissue samples, respectively. In the context of benign breast lesions, *fibrocystic disease*, a complex mixture of alterations, such as adenosis, sclerosing adenosis, cysts, apocrine metaplasia and epithelial hyperplasia, is commonly observed. Contrary to traditional belief, most of these findings are not associated with carcinoma of the breast, although some of them may closely mimic malignancy, such as radial scar, microglandular adenosis and epithelial hyperplasia of varying degree; these deserve a brief description.

BENIGN LESIONS MIMICKING CARCINOMA

Radial scar

On gross and mammographic examination, radial scar may closely resemble infiltrating carcinoma as a result of its stellate appearance. Histologically, it consists of an interplay of adenosis, epithelial hyperplasia and occasional small cysts, with a central area of scleroelastosis.

Microglandular adenosis

Microglandular adenosis is composed of tubules bordered by a monolayer of benign-looking ductal cells without a myoepithelial component. Contrary to tubular carcinoma, the tubules show no angulation, the lumina being round and uniformly small.

Epithelial hyperplasia

The proliferating cells in epithelial hyperplasia may show both ductal and lobular features, even though they all derive from the terminal duct lobular unit. The spectrum of epithelial hyperplasia ranges from benign to atypical ductal and lobular hyperplasia, and ends short of ductal and lobular carcinoma in situ. The separation of the various entities is often a controversial matter, as shown by the low rate of diagnostic reproducibility among pathologists.[1]

Epithelial hyperplasia is currently the most debated area of breast pathology, particularly as a result of its presence in most breast biopsies taken from mammographic abnormalities.

Pseudoangiomatous hyperplasia

Pseudoangiomatous hyperplasia is a benign lesion of the mammary stroma which can mimic a grade I angiosarcoma. It is made up of slit-like spaces lined by endothelial-like cells which show no immunoreactivity for the usual vascular markers. Contrary to the first reports, it is no longer considered to be a distinct entity as pseudoangiomatous changes are observed in association with other breast lesions.[2]

Diabetic mastopathy

Diabetic mastopathy, also known as sclerosing lymphocytic lobulitis, is associated with long-standing type I diabetes mellitus in young patients, and rarely with autoimmune thyroiditis. Histologically, the mammary stroma has a dense fibrous appearance with a few atrophic lobules partly obscured by a heavy lymphocytic infiltrate. The lesion has no neoplastic implication and a possible autoimmune aetiology is suggested.[3]

TUMOURS OF THE BREAST

Most tumours of the breast are malignant. Of these, the majority are carcinomas and the minority sarcomas. Benign pure epithelial and pure connective tissue tumours are rare, whereas benign mixed epithelial and connective tissue tumours are common.

A wide range of histological types is found among carcinomas and only about half a dozen are clinically relevant. The most significant effort in the classification of tumours of the breast was that produced by the World Health Organization.[4] Other more recently identified subentities have been added and are listed in the classification reported in the current edition

of the fascicle 'Tumors of the mammary gland' issued by the US Armed Forces Institute of Pathology.[5]

Benign epithelial tumours

Intraductal papillomas may be single or multiple. Solitary or central papillomas usually grow within the terminal portion of major ducts, which may be dilated or transformed into cysts (intracystic papilloma). The arborescent fronds are lined by layers of epithelial and myoepithelial cells. Malignant transformation and recurrence after removal are unusual. Multiple papillomas are rare, usually peripheral in the breast, occasionally bilateral, and may be associated with epithelial proliferation in some ducts showing clinging, micropapillary and cribriform patterns. Histological transition from benign papilloma to atypical intraductal proliferations, including ductal carcinoma in situ (DCIS), can be observed.[6]

Adenoma of the nipple is also termed 'florid or subareolar (erosive) papillary adenoma'. It consists of a nodule of papillary hyperplasia that is usually ill defined, intermixed with fibrous stroma and occasionally moderate cellular abnormalities. A rare entity is the infiltrating syringomatous adenoma, which closely mimics malignancy.[7] Adenoma of the breast is a rare benign epithelial mammary tumour and may be made up of either regular tubules (tubular adenoma) or acinar structures, with signs of milk secretion (lactating adenoma).[8] Ductal adenoma arises from mammary ducts and is characterized by significant sclerosis. Pleomorphic adenomas of the salivary gland type, along with adenomyoepithelioma and myoepithelioma, are exceptional in the human breast.[9] Other rare adenomas are homologous to sweat gland tumours.

Malignant epithelial tumours

All carcinomas of the breast, both invasive and non-invasive, are classified on the basis of the histological and/or cytological appearance. The histogenetic connotation of the adjectives ductal and lobular is, to a major extent, conventional and inaccurate because it is generally accepted that most carcinomas actually arise from epithelial cells lining the terminal duct (ductule) lobular unit.[10] Irrespective of the type of carcinoma, a number of gross findings should always be recorded including site, size, shape, consistency, colour, gross appearance of margins, relationship to adjacent mammary (skin, nipple) and extramammary structures (fascia, muscle), and the number of foci that appear malignant.

Non-invasive mammary carcinoma

The separation of *lobular carcinoma in situ* (LCIS) from atypical lobular hyperplasia relies on subtle criteria, such as cellular crowding in the absence of any luminal cracks, distension by atypical cells of most acini of a lobular unit, and on the evidence of the involvement of more than 50% of one lobule (Figure 2.1a). For lesser involvement, the diagnosis of atypical lobular hyperplasia is warranted.[11] LCIS is an incidental histological finding which is not uncommonly seen in biopsies of mammographic abnormalities; it reveals no special gross features, is often multicentric (50%) and bilateral (40%), self-regressing and tends to recur.[12] There may be anterograde spread along the extralobular ducts in a pagetoid fashion (Figure 2.1b). The differential diagnosis of well-differentiated LCIS, showing a solid pattern and extended along the lobules, may be difficult if not impossible. Some data suggest that the two lesions could be interrelated.[13] The cells are round with a high nuclear : cytoplasmic ratio; the cytoplasm is clear and nucleoli are inconspicuous. Occasionally, the cells reveal cytoplasmic vacuoles which contain Alcian blue-positive mucinous material.[14] The term 'signet ring cell variant of LCIS' is applied in cases of massive and diffuse vacuolization of all cells. Sclerosing adenosis and other benign lesions such as fibroadenoma and intraductal papilloma may be colonized by LCIS, and yield a pseudoinfiltrative pattern. It has recently been re-emphasized that LCIS hardly deserves the connotation of carcinoma, as it is a risk marker for possible future breast cancer.[15]

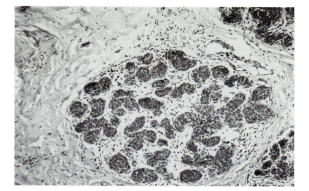

(a)

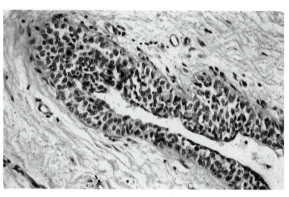

(b)

Figure 2.1 (a) Lobular carcinoma in situ: a terminal duct lobular unit is filled with monomorphous tumour cells (b) extending along a large duct.

Ductal carcinoma in situ

Before mammography ductal carcinoma in situ (DCIS) represented less than 5% of malignant breast lesions. As a result of its relative rarity, DCIS was considered a homogeneous entity on both pathological and clinical grounds. With the advent of mammography, for both screening and clinical diagnostic purposes, DCIS has a three- to four-fold increased frequency. In addition, a number of reports have shown clinical differences between various subtypes of DCIS based on their diverse cytohistological features. Several attempts have been made to classify DCIS into subgroups. Traditional classifications were mainly based on architectural patterns, although some studies had stressed the relevance of cell type and nuclear grade.[16]

Table 2.1 Histological classification of DCIS*
Well differentiated
Moderately differentiated
Poorly differentiated

*DCIS: ductal carcinoma in situ.

An early and simple approach subdivided DCIS into large and non-large cell subtypes. Subsequently, an integrated classification based on cytological features as well as histological architecture was proposed (Table 2.1).[13]

Poorly differentiated DCIS shows marked cellular atypia and absence of architectural differentiation, resulting in a solid growth pattern often showing central necrosis and producing the so-called comedo pattern. In well-differentiated DCIS, the tumour cells are uniform, display little atypia, and are arranged in an orderly architecture. Intermediately differentiated DCIS shares the features of both extremes. The architectural patterns cover solid, with or without central necrosis, cribriform and micropapillary, as well as the clinging type (Figure 2.2).[17] The last type of DCIS consists of one or a few layers of atypical ductal cells firmly attached to the duct wall. As a result of its non-obtrusive histological pattern, the lesion may therefore be easily over-

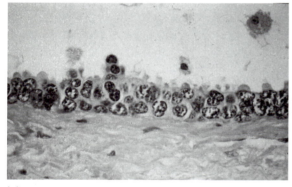

(a)

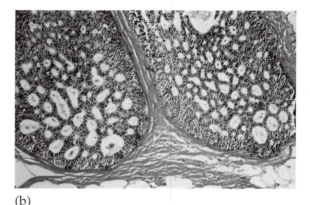

(b)

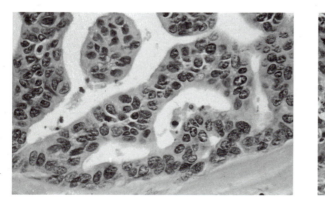

(c)

(d)

Figure 2.2 Ductal carcinoma in situ showing: (a) clinging, (b) cribriform, (c) papillary and (d) solid patterns with variable degrees of cellular atypia.

looked. Clinging DCIS probably represents the minimal unequivocally atypical lesion of the breast.[18] In a recent proposal of DCIS classification, only two morphological features, namely presence/absence of comedo-type necrosis and presence/absence of high-grade nuclear atypia, are considered for the subdivision of DCIS into three prognostically relevant groups.[19] Group 3 is characterized by high nuclear grade, whereas all other lesions that are non-high nuclear grade are classified as group 2 if comedo-type necrosis is present, and as group 1 if necrosis is absent.

Separation of poorly differentiated/high-grade DCIS from well-differentiated/low-grade DCIS is critical because of the higher likelihood of the former developing an infiltrating carcinoma.[11,20] A recent study,[21] based on a long-term follow-up of DCIS, with particular reference to the well-differentiated clinging type, allowed the identification of at least two different clinicopathological profiles. Poorly differentiated DCIS is more frequently associated with subsequent infiltrating carcinoma which develops after a short time interval. Well-differentiated DCIS, on the other hand, is rarely followed by infiltrating carcinoma, and only after a long time interval. Quantitatively, DCIS may be subdivided into microfocal (<0.5 cm in diameter), tumour-forming and diffuse types.[22] The high-grade DCIS cells are characterized by an abnormal DNA content,[23] and peculiar kinetic and biological features.[24] Overexpression of c-erbB-2 identifies cases of DCIS with extensive intraductal disease.[25]

The main differential criteria for distinguishing DCIS from atypical ductal hyperplasia reportedly include cytological features that are not necessarily related to cellular atypia, peculiar structural patterns and anatomical extent of the lesion.[26]

Cancerization of adjacent lobules may simulate early invasion. Bona fide early invasion is rarely detectable, and has been called 'micro-invasive carcinoma' of the breast when it measures less than 1 mm.[27] The myoepithelial cell component has usually been disrupted at this stage. Signet ring,[28] cystic hypersecretory[29] and argyrophilic endocrine DCIS are uncommon,

but well-recognized, histological variants.[30] Non-invasive intracystic papillary carcinoma is usually a discrete single nodule made up of slender, branching papillae lined by atypical cells. The outer fibrous covering is usually not infiltrated by the neoplastic growth.

Inadequate sampling and non-detection of invasive foci are probably the major reasons for the detection of axillary nodal metastases in 1–2% of DCIS cases. Multicentricity (up to 30%) and occult invasion (up to 20%) are found with increasing frequency the larger the lesion.[31] Multicentricity also accounts for the high recurrence rate (15%) of large lesions excised by tumourectomy only.[32]

Infiltrating carcinoma

The term 'infiltrating ductal carcinoma' (IDC) covers and replaces scirrhous carcinoma, carcinoma simplex, infiltrating carcinoma not otherwise specified (or of no special type) and adenocarcinoma of the breast with or without productive fibrosis. It makes up 50–60% of all breast cancer cases. The considerable histological and cytological variability of IDC makes this entity an ideal target for several available grading systems which are essentially based on the degree of organoid differentiation (tubule formation), nuclear atypia and mitotic rate. The original Bloom and Richardson histopathological grading system[33] was recently modified in Nottingham, and the data derived therefrom show that grade 1 (well-differentiated) carcinomas constitute the smallest fraction (18%) of IDC, whereas grade 2 carcinomas constitute 37%, and grade 3, 45%.[34] Although the interobserver agreement is very high for tubule formation only and moderate for both mitotic count and nuclear pleomorphism, it is nevertheless recommended as a simple method for grading infiltrating carcinoma of the breast in routine practice (Tables 2.2 and 2.3).[35] Infiltrating ductal carcinoma may show minor foci of mucinous carcinoma or medullary carcinoma-like areas (also termed 'atypical medullary carcinoma') which should be disregarded for final diagnosis.

In most cases of IDC, variably sized foci of DCIS and/or LCIS surround the dominant

Table 2.2 Histological grading of breast carcinoma

Feature	Score
Tubule formation	
Majority of tumour (>75%)	1
Moderate degree (10–75%)	2
Little or none (<10%)	3
Nuclear pleomorphism	
Small, regular uniform cells	1
Moderate increase in size and variability	2
Marked variation	3
Mitotic counts	
Dependent on microscope field area	1–3

Table 2.3 Histological grading of breast carcinoma

Points	Grade	Feature
3–5	I	Well differentiated
6–7	II	Moderately differentiated
8–9	III	Poorly differentiated

invasive area. After the introduction of mammography, the combination of IDC with varying proportions of solid-type, high nuclear grade DCIS is seen even more frequently.[36] A time-honoured subentity of IDC is 'invasive ductal carcinoma with a predominant intraductal component'[4] in which the intraductal component should cover four times the size of the invasive area. The introduction of new techniques for conservative surgical management of breast cancer stressed the importance of the findings of DCIS within and/or adjacent to the excised invasive carcinoma. A subgroup of patients has been identified who, after local excision and radiotherapy, are at high risk for local recurrences. This group is characterized by invasive ductal carcinoma of the breast with extensive intraductal component.[37]

Tumour emboli are often found in blood and lymphatic vessels within and outside invasive ductal carcinomas (Figure 2.3). Intratumoral vascular invasion can be found in most IDCs, whereas peritumoral lymphatic invasion by tumour emboli is found in 8–10% of node-negative patients with invasive ductal mammary carcinoma and is a predictor of recurrence and metastatic spread.[38] The non-comedo type of ischaemic necrosis of variable extent in the centre of invasive carcinomas may be found in a variable percentage of cases, and has been related to a worse prognosis independently of other adverse factors. Necrosis is also directly related to tumour grade and tumour size;[39] in combination with other histopathological features, such as elastosis, fibrosis and inflammatory cell reaction in IDC, it has prognostic significance because these four variables tend to be associated with high tumour grade, large tumour size and nodal metastases. In the last few years close attention has been paid to the angiogenic response of breast tissue that harbours carcinomas of various histological type. In particular, the number of microvessels has been correlated with prognosis, although conflicting results have been produced. More recently, the presence and distribution of microvessels surrounding foci of DCIS have been studied. Poorly differentiated comedo-type DCIS shows a higher microvessel density than more differentiated DCIS.[40] Multifocality (multiple foci of IDC and DCIS adjacent to each other) and multicentricity (multiple foci of both non-invasive and invasive growth in quadrants distant from that containing the primary cancer) of breast cancer are evident in 25–30% of cases.[41] Histological distinction of a contralateral primary from metastatic spread of the first primary of the same histological type may be difficult or impossible. The latter event is reportedly much rarer than the former.

Invasive lobular carcinoma (ILC): To gain diagnostic recognition, ILC should be 90% pure. Its

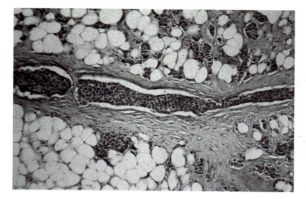

Figure 2.3 Infiltrating duct carcinoma: a tumour embolus filling an intramammary vessel.

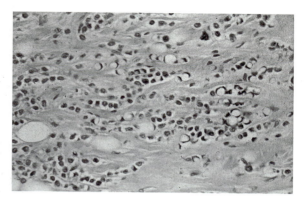

Figure 2.4 Infiltrating lobular carcinoma showing the so-called Indian file growth pattern and occasional signet ring cells.

most common histological appearance is the classic, multifocal, single-file, linear arrangement composed of uniform cells (Fig. 2.4). If these cytohistological criteria are applied strictly, the frequency of ILC is less than 5%. However, the same uniform small-size cell type may display other growth patterns, such as solid, tubulolobular, alveolar and mixed features in the so-called 'variant' forms of ILC (Table 2.4). On the other hand, breast tumours showing the classic growth pattern may be composed of bizarre cells, such as pleomorphic lobular carcinoma, in which the cells manifest apocrine features.[42] Hence, by combining all these variants ILC accounts for 10–15% of epithelial malignancies of the breast. Classic ILC and variants do not differ in terms of tumour size, nodal status, recurrences and survival, with the exception of the more aggressive pleomorphic variant.[42]

Signet-ring carcinoma: This is rare, has a poor prognosis, and may possibly represent a special variant of mucus-producing ILC. The variant of ILC with neuroendocrine features is made up of a considerable number of Grimelius-positive cells also containing dense core granules at electron microscopy.

The mixed ductal and lobular type of infiltrating carcinoma is implicated in 5–7% of breast cancers, and deserves the status of a

Table 2.4 Histological variants of invasive lobular carcinoma
Alveolar
Tubulolobular
Pleomorphic
Mixed

Modified from Holland et al[13]

separate histological entity; this illustrates the possible transition between IDC and ILC.

Cytological differences between IDC and ILC are sufficiently distinct to identify the histological type of the primary, even when metastatic sites are found before the primary, e.g. lymph nodes, cerebrospinal fluid, peritoneal and retroperitoneal tissues, ovaries, bone marrow, stomach, uterus and adnexa. The distribution pattern of the metastatic spread for patients with classic ILC and variants thereof does not vary.

There are histological types of breast cancer with a more favourable prognosis in node-negative patients.

Mucinous (colloid) carcinoma (Figure 2.5): This represents about 2% of breast cancers. To be designated as mucinous the tumour must be

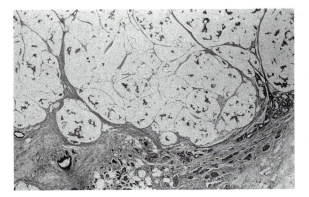

Figure 2.5 Mucinous carcinoma of the breast showing abundant gelatinous material in which small tumour cell clusters are freely floating.

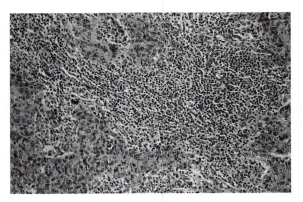

Figure 2.6 Medullary carcinoma of the mammary gland showing solid strands of malignant cells admixed with a marked lymphocytic infiltrate.

pure without other components. It has been shown that, with comparable tumour size and in the absence of an IDC component, mucinous carcinoma develops a lower number of nodal metastases and has a better prognosis than IDC.[43] The cellularity of mucinous carcinomas often represents only a fraction of the tumour mass; the cell aggregates lack pleomorphism; the stroma is scanty and necrosis absent. A number of mucinous carcinomas reveal a component of argyrophilic cells containing dense-core, neuroendocrine granules. An in situ component is usually absent.

Medullary carcinoma nowadays represents less than 2% of breast cancers because in the past it has frequently been over-diagnosed.[44] Gross characterization is by well-defined pushing margins. Microscopically, the cells are arranged in irregular sheets which are separated by lymphoid stroma (Figure 2.6). The large tumour cells show high-grade nuclear atypia, large nucleoli and high mitotic rate, with no organoid differentiation. An in situ component is usually absent. Medullary variant ('atypical medullary') carcinoma (3%)[45] shows some, but not all, of the features of pure medullary carcinoma and is best classified as IDC. Various histopathological criteria have been proposed to diagnose medullary carcinoma; however, the clear-cut distinction of medullary carcinoma

from atypical medullary carcinoma and infiltrating ductal carcinoma not otherwise specified (NOS) is often difficult.

Infiltrating papillary carcinoma:[46] This represents less than 2% of breast cancers and is the outcome of neither a pre-existing papilloma nor a micropapillary DCIS. It consists of papillary fronds lined by atypical cells. As a result of the subtle cytological and architectural criteria which segregate benign from well-differentiated malignant papillary lesions, frozen section diagnoses are better deferred until permanent sections become available. Invasive papillary carcinoma should be kept separate from invasive micropapillary carcinoma – a more recently described entity resembling papillary carcinoma of the ovary, which is characterized by micropapillary structures growing into empty spaces.[47]

Tubular carcinoma of the breast accounts for about 2% of clinically identified breast cancers, whereas it is more frequent (up to 20%) in case series detected by mammography. It is usually a small desmoplastic tumour. The tubular spaces are small, triangular or oval, and lined by a single layer of bland-looking cells the nuclei of which are similar to those of LCIS. Differential diagnosis with radial scar may be challenging. An in situ component often coexists. Associated non-tubular components should not exceed 10–15%. The *mixed tubular*

Table 2.5 Uncommon types of breast carcinoma
Adenoid cystic
Mucoepidermoid
Secretory
Cystic hypersecretory
Small-cell neuroendocrine

and ductal subtypes of breast cancer (10%) usually show a central core of tubular type and a ductal-type structure at the periphery. *Invasive cribriform carcinoma* is fairly rare (<1%), and cytologically and prognostically similar to tubular carcinoma.[48] The structure of the cell aggregates resembles that of cribriform DCIS.

Uncommon types of carcinoma of the breast (Table 2.5) comprise:

- *Adenoid cystic carcinoma*, which is histologically (Figure 2.7) identical to that of salivary glands
- *Mucoepidermoid carcinoma*, mostly of low-grade malignancy

- *Secretory carcinoma*, which is the only well-documented type of carcinoma of the breast that may arise in children and adults of both sexes[49]
- *Cystic hypersecretory carcinoma* which may be both in situ and infiltrating, and histologically consists of cystic spaces filled by a dense secretion similar to colloid.

Apocrine carcinoma has recently gained the attention of pathologists, as a result of the similarity between a protein characteristic of apocrine epithelium (Figure 2.8) and the prolactin-inducible protein.[50] The cells of in situ and infiltrating apocrine carcinoma show eosinophilic granular to foamy cytoplasm with clear features, as in histiocytoid carcinoma, which was considered a distinct subtype of breast carcinoma, but is currently considered an ILC in which apocrine differentiation has taken place.[42] Rare types are also the *lipid-secreting carcinoma* (Figure 2.9) and the *glycogen-rich clear-cell carcinoma*. Glycogen-rich carcinoma accounts for less than 3% of all breast carcinomas,[51] and can be either in situ (intraductal) or invasive. Differential diagnosis with other clear-cell tumours of the breast without glycogen content include myoepithelioma, adenomyoepithelioma and other rare primary carcinomas, such as lipid-rich, secretory and histiocytoid lobular carcinoma.[51]

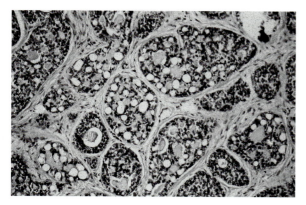

Figure 2.7 Adenoid cystic carcinoma of the breast displaying the characteristic cribriform pattern. Intraluminal basement membrane-like material is surrounded by hyperchromatic neoplastic cells.

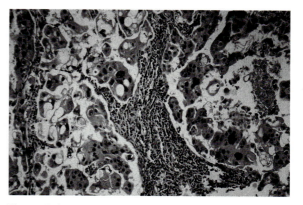

Figure 2.8 Axillary nodal metastasis of an apocrine carcinoma. The tumour cells display a dense eosinophilic cytoplasm.

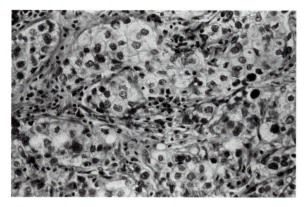

Figure 2.9 Lipid-secreting carcinoma: the clear appearance of the cytoplasm results from the presence of lipids.

In fact, contrary to common belief, no correlation of argyrophilia with overall survival appears to exist.[52] Pure carcinoids of the breast, similar to those of other sites, have been described, but they are not considered a specific histological category, having a better prognosis. *Small-cell neuroendocrine carcinoma* is a rare high-grade malignant tumour which is cytologically identical to similar malignancies of other sites. Uncommon clinicopathological presentation of breast carcinoma is given in Table 2.6.

Inflammatory carcinoma of the breast is a T4 clinical presentation of breast cancer displayed by less than 1% of IDCs with the main, but inconstant, histopathological feature of a variable degree of intralymphatic spread within the dermis. Another histological nonentity is *carcinoma of the male breast.*

Carcinoma with endocrine differentiation: Some carcinomas of the breast contain peptide hormones detectable by electron microscopy, and histochemical and immunohistochemical stainings of the tumour tissue (Figure 2.10). Both IDC and DCIS may contain argyrophilic granules, as do invasive and in situ lobular carcinoma. In the context of other tumour types, such as papillary, tubular and mucinous carcinoma, argyrophilic cells may be detected.

Table 2.6 Uncommon clinicopathological presentation of carcinoma of the breast

Inflammatory carcinoma
Mammary Paget's disease
Occult breast carcinoma presenting with axillary lymph-node metastasis

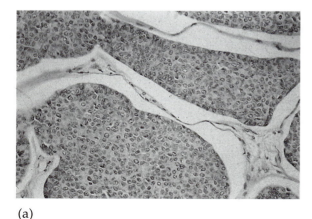

(a)

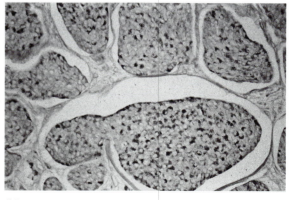

(b)

Figure 2.10 (a) Carcinoma with neuroendocrine differentiation, (b) demonstrating intense argyrophilia with the Grimelius stain.

Mammary Paget's disease of the nipple and areola is a non-invasive intraepithelial proliferation (Figure 2.11) of atypical cells with large, pale-staining cytoplasm which contains acidic mucinous material, occasionally melanin pigment and cytokeratins of simple epithelia. Paget's disease is often accompanied by intraductal mammary carcinoma or, less commonly, by invasive ductal carcinoma without continuity, and occasionally by no malignancy.

Occult breast carcinoma presenting with axillary lymph node metastases: In this unusual condition there is no clinicomammographic evidence of breast carcinoma, the first clinical sign being a lump in the axilla. Less than 1% of patients have a subclinical carcinoma presenting with axillary metastases only.[53] One lymph node may be involved as well as virtually all axillary nodes. The origin of the primary is often found in the axillary tail of the breast or, less commonly, in axillary breast tissue. Usually the primary shows IDC features with or without predominant intraductal component where the intraductal foci are surrounded by a marked lymphocytic infiltrate.[53] Axillary nodal metastases in the absence of an obvious primary usually show the same features of the primary, although three different patterns can be recognized. Most cases show single cells with abundant apocrine cytoplasm diffusely infiltrating the lymph node (Figure 2.12a). These melanoma-like cells do not form glands but show mucinous secretion and positive immunoreactivity for cytokeratins (Figure 2.12b). When glandular formation is more obvious, the diagnosis of metastatic breast carcinoma can be straightforward. Mixed pattern secondaries are the third type of metastatic involvement. In spite of the unusual presentation, patients with occult carcinoma presenting with axillary metastases have a similar, if not better, prognosis than those patients with primary carcinoma of the breast plus axillary metastases.[54]

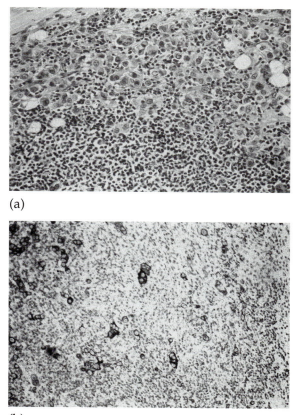

(a)

(b)

Figure 2.12 Occult carcinoma of the breast presenting with axillary lymph node metastases. (a) Tumour cells with abundant cytoplasm are present within the marginal sinus and the lymphoid tissue. (b) The immunostain for cytokeratins confirms the epithelial phenotype.

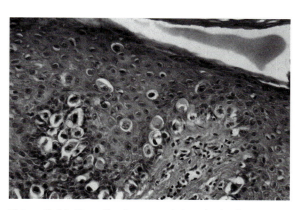

Figure 2.11 Paget's disease of the nipple: large tumour cells infiltrate the epidermis.

Drug-induced changes of breast carcinoma. When carcinoma of the breast is treated preoperatively with chemoradiotherapy, definite histopathological changes of the normal breast tissue, the primary carcinoma and the axillary metastases take place. Apart from a variable degree of tumour cell reduction, some stromal fibrosis and an inflammatory infiltrate, marked abnormalities of residual tumour cells can be seen. The epithelial tumour cells acquire a histiocyte-like appearance showing abundant foamy cytoplasm with vacuoles and/or eosinophilic granules. The nuclei tend to be enlarged, hyperchromatic and occasionally multiple; there are abnormal mitotic figures and large nucleoli. The differential diagnosis of histiocytes and residual tumour cells may be difficult, especially on frozen sections. Immunocytochemistry may be of great help in revealing positive immunoreaction of tumour cells for antibodies against cytokeratins.[55]

Metaplastic carcinoma, pseudosarcomatous carcinoma, sarcomatoid carcinoma: Focal squamous metaplasia can be seen in trivial IDC of the breast where the metaplastic component usually constitutes less than 10% of the tumour. In sarcomatoid carcinoma most of the tumour is composed of carcinomatous cells showing a variety of sarcoma-like changes which obscure the epithelial nature of the neoplasm, simulating a breast sarcoma. Classification of sarcomatoid carcinoma is controversial because different histological types have been suggested. Currently, five different types of metaplastic carcinoma are recognized, namely: matrix-producing, spindle cell, carcinosarcoma, squamous cell carcinoma of ductal origin and osteoclastic giant cells (Table 2.7).[56–60] Histologically, the sarcomatoid component includes 'homologous' and 'heterologous' components. Usually squamous metaplasia (Figure 2.13a) is associated with spindle-cell and fibrosarcomalike sarcomatoid elements, whereas in adenocarcinomas a 'heterologous' osseous and/or cartilaginous (Figure 2.13b) component may be observed.[61] The diagnosis of sarcomatoid carcinoma may be difficult to recognize by haematoxylin and eosin stain, when the epithelial component is very limited. Only then can

Table 2.7 Histological classification of metaplastic carcinoma of the breast
Matrix producing
Spindle cell
Carcinosarcoma
Squamous cell carcinoma of ductal origin
With osteoclastic giant cells

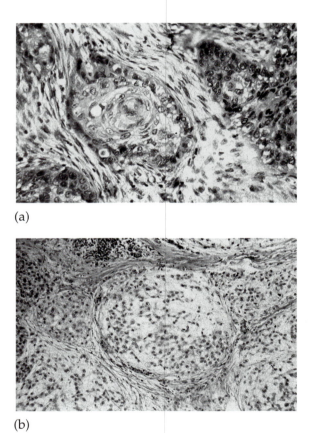

(a)

(b)

Figure 2.13 Metaplastic (sarcomatoid) carcinoma showing (a) squamous and (b) cartilaginous metaplasia.

immunocytochemistry demonstrate reactivity for cytokeratins of carcinomatous foci. Moreover, along with the immunocytochemical investigation, extensive tissue sampling may be necessary to detect the epithelial component in order to exclude a diagnosis of true mammary sarcoma. A prognostically more favourable variant of metaplastic carcinoma is *adenosquamous carcinoma*, with equally represented glandular and squamous features.

Mixed connective tissue and epithelial tumours (Table 2.8)

These comprise the trivial *fibroadenoma*, the giant fibroadenoma, the variably sized fibroadenoma of adolescent girls (juvenile fibroadenoma) which has a cellular stroma and shows ductal epithelial hyperplasia, and the *phyllodes tumour*, formerly termed 'cystosarcoma phyllodes'. Phyllodes tumour may histologically be benign (60%), potentially malignant (15%) or malignant (25%), even though, from the personal experience of the author, the truly malignant cases are less than 10%. It has also been suggested that the potentially malignant group should be considered malignant even though they are of low-grade malignancy.[62] Currently, there are no reliable histological features that can predict the clinical behaviour of phyllodes tumour. Diagnostic criteria in this respect are the degree of cellularity, the pleomorphism of the stromal cells and the mitotic index (Figure 2.14). The presence of stromal overgrowth, defined as the absence of ductal component in a low power field, was suggested as a strong indicator of potential recurrence in phyllodes tumour.[63] Local recurrences of malignant phyllodes tumours are frequent, but not necessarily evidence of malignancy. Occasionally, the sarcomatous growth attains the features of a specific type of sarcoma, e.g. malignant fibrous histiocytoma, liposarcoma and fibrosarcoma.

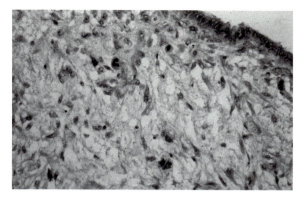

Figure 2.14 Phyllodes tumour: atypia, pleomorphism and mitotic activity of stromal cells. The epithelial lining is composed of bland cells.

The recognition of carcinomas with various types of connective tissue metaplasia leaves very little space for the existence of true carcinosarcoma.

Non-epithelial tumours

Primary stromal sarcoma of the breast is histologically indistinguishable from a malignant phyllodes tumour without epithelial component, and is exceedingly rare. Many sarcomas in the past were probably incompletely sampled phyllodes tumour or metaplastic carcinomas with an extensive pseudosarcomatous pattern. Even though, in the breast, all types of soft tissue tumours may arise, and are probably unrelated to the mammary gland as such, a few of them more commonly originate in the breast than at other sites and may be considered to be related to the mammary stroma. These neoplasms account for about 1% of mammary tumours and include *aggressive fibromatosis* (extra-abdominal desmoid tumour),[64] the spectrum fibrosarcoma–*malignant fibrous histiocytoma*,[65] and *angiosarcoma* which represents less than 10% of breast sarcomas. An attempt to identify various degrees of differentiation in the context of mammary angiosarcomas succeeded in separating out three groups of lesions which correlate with prognosis and survival.[66]

Table 2.8 Mixed connective tissue and epithelial tumours	
1. Fibroadenoma	4. Phyllodes tumour
2. Giant fibroadenoma	Benign
3. Juvenile fibroadenoma	Potentially malignant
	Malignant

Primary angiosarcoma is also a well-known complication of chronic lymphoedema of one upper limb, and shows the clinical features of the post-mastectomy Stewart–Treves syndrome. Usually, this type of angiosarcoma develops 5–9 years after breast surgery.[67] Angiosarcoma of the chest wall after post-mastectomy radiotherapy is another well-recognized lesion arising within a 10-year postradiation interval.[65]

In the last 5 years, there have been about 20 case reports of angiosarcoma arising on the skin or in breast tissue after conservative surgery plus radiotherapy for breast carcinoma. The average interval of a few years is much shorter than that reported for angiosarcoma after radiotherapy or chronic lymphoedema. The possible role of radiotherapy in the pathogenesis of these angiosarcomas is still unclear, although atypical vascular lesions[68] have been observed in the field of radiotherapy for breast cancer, and chromosomal analysis of angiosarcoma after radiotherapy has revealed multiple clonal rearrangements on various chromosomes.[69] The occurrence of angiosarcoma in the irradiated breast after conservative treatment for carcinoma is actually very rare. In a series of 3295 patients observed at the Istituto Nazionale per lo Studio e la Cura dei Tumori of Milan, only two similar cases were identified.[70] This incidence is too low to justify changes in the current conservative treatment for breast cancer. Grade III sarcomas NOS also appear to be associated with radiotherapy after breast-conserving treatment. The diagnosis of primary osteosarcoma, chondrosarcoma and rhabdomyosarcoma of the breast has to be made with caution, and only after extensive sampling and immunostaining for cytokeratins can the presence of an epithelial component be ruled out.

Hodgkin's disease of the breast is exceptional, whereas non-Hodgkin's lymphomas are slightly more common, representing less than 0.2% of all breast malignancies and less than 5% of mammary sarcomas. The absolute majority (over 90%) of non-Hodgkin's lymphomas are of B-cell lineage and 50% are centroblastic and hence of high-grade malignancy.[71] Low-grade B-cell non-Hodgkin's lymphomas of the breast are cytologically reminiscent of mucosa-associated lymphoid tissue lymphomas. Bilaterality is found in about 10% of cases.

REFERENCES

1. Rosai J. Borderline epithelial lesions of the breast. *Am J Surg Pathol* 1991; **15**:209–21.
2. Ibrahim RE, Sciotto CG, Weidner N. Pseudo-angiomatous hyperplasia of mammary stroma. Some observations regarding its clinicopathologic spectrum. *Cancer* 1989; **63**:1154–67.
3. Schwartz IS, Strauchen JA. Lymphocytic mastopathy. An autoimmune disease? *Am J Clin Pathol* 1990; **93**:725–30.
4. Hartmann WH, Ozzello L, Sobin LH, Stalsberg H. Histological typing of breast tumours. In: *International Histological Classification of Tumours*, No. 2, 2nd edn. Geneva: World Health Organization, 1981.
5. Rosen PP, Oberman HA. Tumors of the mammary gland. *Armed Forces Institute of Pathology (AFIP) Fascicle 7*, third series, 1993.
6. Ohuchi H, Abe R, Kasai M. Possible cancerous change of intraductal papillomas of the breast. A 3-D reconstruction of 25 cases. *Cancer* 1984; **54**:605–19.
7. Jones MW, Norris HJ, Snyder SC. Infiltrating syringomatous adenoma of the nipple. A clinical and pathological study of 11 cases. *Am J Surg Pathol* 1989; **13**:197–201.
8. James K, Bridger J, Anthony PP. Breast tumour in pregnancy ('lactating' adenoma). *J Pathol* 1988; **156**:37–44.
9. Tavassoli FA. Myoepithelial lesions of the breast. *Am J Surg Pathol* 1991; **15**:554–68.
10. Wellings SR, Jensen HM, Marcum RG. An atlas of subgross pathology of the human breast with special reference to possible precancerous lesions. *J Natl Cancer Inst* 1975; **55**:231–73.
11. Page DL, Anderson TJ. *Diagnostic Histopathology of the Breast*. Edinburgh: Churchill Livingstone, 1987.
12. Ottesen GL, Graversen HP, Blichert-Toft M, Zedeler K, Andersen JA. Lobular carcinoma in situ of the female breast. Short-term results of a prospective nationwide study. The Danish Breast Cancer Cooperative Group. *Am J Surg Pathol* 1993; **17**:14–21.
13. Holland H, Peterse JL, Millis RR, et al. Ductal

carcinoma in situ: a proposal for a new classification. *Semin Diagn Pathol* 1994; **11**:167–80.

14. Andersen JA, Vendelboe ML. Cytoplasmic mucous globules in lobular carcinoma in situ. Diagnosis and prognosis. *Am J Surg Pathol* 1981; **5**:251–5.

15. Carson W, Sanchez-Forgach E, Stomper P, et al. Lobular carcinoma in situ: observation without surgery as an appropriate therapy. *Ann Surg Oncol* 1994; **1**:141–6.

16. Lagios MD, Margolin FR, Wesdahl PR, Rose MR. Mammographically detected duct carcinoma in situ. Frequency of local recurrence following tylectomy and prognostic effect of nuclear grade on local recurrence. *Cancer* 1989; **63**:618–24.

17. Azzopardi J. *Problems in Breast Pathology.* Philadelphia: Saunders, 1979.

18. Eusebi V, Foschini MP, Cook MG, et al. Long-term follow-up of in situ carcinoma of the breast with special emphasis on clinging carcinoma. *Semin Diagn Pathol* 1989; **6**:165–73.

19. Silverstein MJ, Poller DN, Waisman JR, et al. Prognostic classification of breast ductal carcinoma-in-situ. *Lancet* 1995; **345**:1154–7.

20. Lagios MD. Heterogeneity of duct carcinoma in situ (DCIS): relationship of grade and subtype analysis to local recurrence and risk of invasive transformation. *Cancer Letters* 1995; **90**:97–102.

21. Eusebi V, Feudale E, Foschini MP, et al. Long-term follow-up of in situ carcinoma of the breast. *Semin Diagn Pathol* 1994; **11**:223–35.

22. Andersen J, Blicher-Toft M, Dyreborg U. In situ carcinomas of the breast. Types, growth pattern, diagnosis, and treatment. *Eur J Surg Oncol* 1987; **13**:105–11.

23. Leal CB, Schmitt FC, Bento MJ, Maia NC, Lopes CS. Ductal carcinoma in situ of the breast. Histologic categorization and its relationship to ploidy and immunohistochemical expression of hormone receptors, p53, and c-erbB-2 protein. *Cancer* 1995; **75**:2123–31.

24. Zafrani B, Leroyer A, Fourquet A, et al. Mammographically-detected ductal carcinoma in situ of the breast analyzed with a new classification. A study of 127 cases: correlation with estrogen and progesterone receptors, p53 and c-erbB-2 proteins, and proliferative activity. *Semin Diagn Pathol* 1994; **11**:208–14.

25. De Potter CR, Schelfhout AM, Verbeeck P, et al. Neu overexpression correlates with extent of disease in large cell ductal carcinoma in situ of the breast. *Hum Pathol* 1995; **26**:601–6.

26. Page DL, Rogers LW. Combined histologic and cytologic criteria for the diagnosis of mammary atypical ductal hyperplasia. *Hum Pathol* 1992; **23**:1095–7.

27. Royal College of Pathologists Working Group. Pathology reporting in breast cancer screening. *J Clin Pathol* 1991; **44**:710–25.

28. Fisher ER, Brown R. Intraductal signet ring carcinoma: a hitherto undescribed form of intraductal carcinoma of the breast. *Cancer* 1985; **55**:2533–7.

29. Rosen PP, Scott M. Cystic hypersecretory duct carcinoma of the breast. *Am J Surg Pathol* 1984; **8**:31–41.

30. Maluf HM, Koerner FC. Solid papillary carcinoma of the breast. A form of intraductal carcinoma with endocrine differentiation frequently associated with mucinous carcinoma. *Am J Surg Pathol* 1995; **19**:1237–44.

31. Lagios MD, Westdahl PR, Margolin FR, Rose MR. Duct carcinoma in situ: relationship of extent of non invasive disease to the frequency of occult invasion, multicentricity, lymph node metastases, and short-term treatment failures. *Cancer* 1982; **50**:1309–14.

32. Fisher ER, Sass R, Fisher B, et al. Pathologic findings from the National Surgical Adjuvant Breast Project (Protocol no. 6). II. Relation of local breast recurrence to multicentricity. *Cancer* 1986; **57**:1717–24.

33. Bloom HJG, Richardson WW. Histological grading and prognosis in breast cancer. *Br J Cancer* 1957; **11**:359–77.

34. Elston CW, Ellis IO. Pathological prognostic factors in breast cancer. I. The value of histological grade in breast cancer: experience from a large study with long-term follow-up. *Histopathology* 1991; **20**:479–89.

35. Frierson HF Jr, Wolber RA, Berean KW, et al. Interobserver reproducibility of the Nottingham modification of the Bloom and Richardson histologic grading scheme for infiltrating ductal carcinoma. *Am J Clin Pathol* 1995; **103**:195–8.

36. Moriya T, Silverberg SG. Intraductal carcinoma (ductal carcinoma in situ) of the breast. A comparison of pure noninvasive tumors with those including different proportions of infiltrating carcinoma. *Cancer* 1994; **74**:2972–8.

37. Holland R, Connolly JL, Gelman R, et al. The presence of an extensive intraductal component following a limited excision correlates with prominent residual disease in the remainder of the breast. *J Clin Oncol* 1990; **8**:113–18.

38. Clemente C, Boracchi P, Andreola S, et al.

Peritumoral lymphatic invasion in patients with node negative mammary duct carcinoma. *Cancer* 1992; **69**:1396–403.

39. Carlomagno C, Perrone F, Lauria R, et al. Prognostic significance of necrosis, elastosis, fibrosis and inflammatory cell reaction in operable breast cancer. *Oncology* 1995; **52**:272–7.

40. Guidi AJ, Fischer L, Harris JR, Schnitt SJ. Microvessel density and distribution in ductal carcinoma in situ of the breast. *J Natl Cancer Ins* 1994; **86**:614–9.

41. Carter D. Margins of 'lumpectomy' for breast cancer. *Hum Pathol* 1986; **17**:330–2.

42. Eusebi V, Magalhaes F, Azzopardi JG. Pleomorphic lobular carcinoma of the breast: an aggressive tumor showing apocrine differentiation. *Hum Pathol* 1992; **23**:655–62.

43. Andre S, Cunha F, Bernardo M, Meneses e Sousa J, Cortez F, Soares J. Mucinous carcinoma of the breast: a pathologic study of 82 cases. *J Surg Oncol* 1995; **58**:162–7.

44. Gaffey MJ, Mills SE, Frierson HF Jr, et al. Medullary carcinoma of the breast: interobserver variability in histopathologic diagnosis. *Mod Pathol* 1995; **8**:31–8.

45. Fisher ER, Gregorio RM, Fischer B, Redmond C, Vellios F, Sommers SC. The pathology of invasive breast cancer. A syllabus derived from findings of the National Surgical Adjuvant Breast Project (Protocol no. 4). *Cancer* 1975; **36**:1–84.

46. Fisher ER, Palekar AS, Redmond C, et al. Pathologic findings from the National Surgical Adjuvant Breast Project (Protocol no. 4). VI. Invasive papillary cancer. *Am J Pathol* 1980; **73**:313–22.

47. Siriaunkgul S, Tavassoli FA. Invasive micropapillary carcinoma of the breast. *Mod Pathol* 1993; **6**:660–2.

48. Venable JG, Schwartz AM, Silverberg SG. Infiltrating cribriform carcinoma of the breast: a distinctive clinicopathologic entity. *Hum Pathol* 1990; **21**:333–8.

49. Krausz T, Jenkins D, Grontoft O, et al. Secretory carcinoma of the breast in adults: emphasis on late recurrence and metastasis. *Histopathology* 1989; **14**:25–36.

50. Pagani A, Eusebi V, Bussolati G. Detection of PIP-GCDFP-15 gene expression in apocrine epthelium of the breast and salivary glands. *Appl Immunol* 1994; **21**:29–35.

51. Hayes MM, Seidman JD, Ashton MA. Glycogen-rich clear cell carcinoma of the breast. A clinico-pathologic study of 21 cases. *Am J Surg Pathol* 1995; **19**:904–11.

52. Scopsi L, Andreola S, Pilotti S, et al. Argyrophilia and granin (chromogranin/secretogranin) expression in female breast carcinomas. Their relationship to survival and other disease parameters. *Am J Surg Pathol* 1992; **16**:561–76.

53. Haupt HM, Rosen PP, Kinne DW. Breast carcinoma presenting with axillary lymphnode metastases. An analysis of specific histopathologic features. *Am J Surg Pathol* 1985; **9**:165–75.

54. Merson M, Andreola S, Galimberti V. Breast carcinoma presenting as axillary metastases without evidence of a primary tumor. *Cancer* 1992; **70**:504–8.

55. Kennedy S, Merino MJ, Swain SM, Lippman ME. The effect of hormonal chemotherapy on tumoral and nonneoplastic breast tissue. *Hum Pathol* 1990; **21**:192–8.

56. Wargotz ES, Norris HJ. Metaplastic carcinomas of the breast. I. Matrix-producing carcinoma. *Hum Pathol* 1989; **20**:628–35.

57. Wargotz ES, Deos PH, Norris HJ. Metaplastic carcinomas of the breast. II. Spindle cell carcinoma. *Hum Pathol* 1989; **20**:732–40.

58. Wargotz ES, Norris HJ. Metaplastic carcinomas of the breast. III. Carcinosarcoma. *Cancer* 1989; **64**:1490–9.

59. Wargotz ES, Norris HJ. Metaplastic carcinomas of the breast. IV. Squamous cell carcinoma of ductal origin. *Cancer* 1990; **65**:272–6.

60. Wargotz ES, Norris HJ. Metaplastic carcinomas of the breast. V. Metaplastic carcinoma with osteoclastic giant cells. *Hum Pathol* 1990; **21**:1142–50.

61. Foschini MP, Dina RE, Eusebi V. Sarcomatoid neoplasms of the breast: proposed definitions for biphasic and monophasic sarcomatoid mammary carcinomas. *Semin Diagn Pathol* 1993; **10**:128–36.

62. Hart WR, Bauer RC, Oberman HA. Cystosarcoma phylloides: a clinicopathologic study of twenty-six hypercellular periductal stromal tumors of the breast. *Am J Clin Pathol* 1978; **70**:211–16.

63. Ward RM, Evans HL. Cystosarcoma phyllodes a clinicopathologic study of 26 cases. *Cancer* 1986; **58**:2282–9.

64. Wargotz ES, Norris HJ, Austin RM, Enzinger FM. Fibromatosis of the breast. A clinical and pathological study of 28 cases. *Am J Surg Pathol* 1987; **11**:38–45.

65. Jones MW, Norris HN, Wargotz ES, Weiss SW. Fibrosarcoma-malignant fibrous histiocytoma of

the breast. A clinicopathologic study of 32 cases. *Am J Surg Pathol* 1992; **16:**667–74.

66. Rosen PP, Kimmel M, Ernsberger D. Mammary angiosarcoma. The prognostic significance of tumor differentiation. *Cancer* 1988; **62:**2145–51.

67. Capo V, Ozzello L, Fenoglio CM, Lombardi L, Rilke F. Angiosarcomas arising in edematous extremities: immunostaining for Factor VIII-related antigen and ultrastructural features. *Hum Pathol* 1985; **16:**144–50.

68. Fineberg S, Rosen PP. Cutaneous angiosarcoma and atypical vascular lesions of the skin and breast after radiation therapy for breast carci-noma. *Am J Clin Pathol* 1994; **102:**757–63.

69. Gil-Benso R, Lopez-Gines C, Soriano P, Almenar S, Vazquez C, Llombart-Bosch. A cytogenetic study of angiosarcoma of the breast. *Genes, Chromosomes Cancer* 1994; **10:**210–2.

70. Zucali R, Merson M, Placucci M, Di Palma S, Veronesi U. Soft tissue sarcoma of the breast after conservative surgery and irradiation for early mammary cancer. *Radiother Oncol* 1994; **30:**271–3.

71. Giardini R, Piccolo C, Rilke F. Primary non Hodgkin's lymphomas of the female breast. *Cancer* 1992; **69:**725–35.

3

Prognostic factors in breast cancer

Peter M Ravdin

Studies of prognostic factors are undertaken with two major goals: one is to provide information to help guide clinical decision-making; the other is to understand the basic mechanisms that are central to breast cancer biology, controlling breast cancer occurrence and properties.

The most commonly addressed clinical question is that relating to the risk of systemic recurrence and/or death after definitive primary therapy. This information is useful in guiding patient counseling about adjuvant therapy, and is aimed at defining patient prognosis. A second major class of questions relates to the selection among therapeutic options. Can information be obtained from the tumor to predict which therapy might be particularly advantageous? Thus, most clinical studies are aimed at defining prognosis or predicting treatment response.

Most of the prognostic and predictive factor literature can be viewed as an extension of the early major successes in the field. In the definition of risk of relapse, classic TNM staging was shown to have powerful prognostic implications for breast cancer patients, as it does for patients with other major adenocarcinomas. The second major conceptual advance was the demonstration that expression of the estrogen receptor was predictive of response to endocrine therapy.[1] These early successes have led to a large number of studies using classic pathologic techniques, immunohistochemical methods,

classic biochemical measurements, and new approaches dependent on molecular biology methodologies. The purpose of this chapter is to review the current status of these studies in terms of where their current applications lie, and what their future prospects may be.

A PERSPECTIVE BASED ON CURRENT CONSENSUS RECOMMENDATIONS

The past decade has seen major advances in the basic sciences, with the development of many new investigational techniques and the discovery of a large number of macromolecules that are important in biologic processes. Many investigators have applied these advances to the problem of identifying prognostic and predictive variables in breast cancer. This has presented a special challenge to the clinician, because often it is not immediately apparent when the research results are ready for clinical application or whether they are still to be viewed as preliminary. This problem has been addressed by several committees that reviewed available evidence to help define what variables should be applied to prognostic and predictive questions. Table 3.1 shows the views of four consensus groups addressing these issues.

All groups have endorsed classical staging (the American Society of Clinical Oncology guidelines only addressed what laboratory derived information might be used in addition

Table 3.1 Recommendations of four groups about what information might be used in prognostic/predictive assessment of breast cancer patients

Source	Prognostic factors	Predictive factors
NIH (1990)[2]	Nodal status Tumor size ER, PR Nuclear grade Histologic type Proliferation S phase Cathepsin D	Not addressed
St Gallen's (1995)[3]	Nodal status Tumor size Histologic grade Age ER	Menopausal status ER

ACP (1995)[4]	TNM
	Histologic type
	Histologic grade
	Of possible value
	  Proliferation
	    Mitotic count
	    S phase
	    Ki67 MIB1
	  c-erbB–2
	  p53
	  Angiogenesis
	  Vascular invasion
		Not addressed

ASCO (1996)[5]	No laboratory-based measures	ER, PR

ACP, American College of Pathologists.
ASCO, American Society of Clinical Oncology.
NIH, National Institutes of Health.

to classical staging), and all groups endorsed the use of estrogen receptor (ER) and progesterone receptor (PgR) determinations at least for prediction of reponse. Beyond these variables, there was a lack of clear general consensus, and in general a cautious approach to acceptance of nearly all the new markers. Clearly, even for expert panels the available data can lead to different interpretations of the value of available information.

CAVEATS ABOUT THE PROGNOSTIC FACTOR LITERATURE

A number of reviews of the prognostic factors have pointed out some inherent weaknesses in the prognostic factor literature.[6,7] These weaknesses lie in clinical, technical and statistical categories; some of these potential problems are listed in Table 3.2. These weaknesses complicate the interpretation of the prognostic and predictive factor literature. Prognostic factor studies are not amenable to techniques such as meta-analysis which has been used so successfully in the analysis of adjuvant treatment

effects,[8] because studies of individual prognostic factors often differ in techniques used for measurement (e.g. antibodies etc.), interpretations of results (what is interpreted as high versus low values) and study end-points (definition of relapse and death). In addition, most prognostic factor studies are not undertaken by large cooperative consortia, but rather by single institutions, making it difficult to account for the possible bias of underreporting of negative results and overreporting of positive results.

Taken together, these weaknesses have slowed the broad international acceptance of many of the mechanistically interesting new prognostic factors. This is reflected in the uncertainty as to their use, the very cautious endorsement of few prognostic variables by guideline committees, and the lack of their widespread adoption by cooperative trial organizations for patient selection and stratification. In addition, reports by commercial laboratories to the clinician of this information are often vague and cautiously ambiguous. That a factor conveys a 'favorable' outcome begs the questions of for which subsets of patients it is favorable, and how favorable compared with the average patient (which requires statements as to the relative risk conferred and the prevalence of positive tests). Thus a review of the recent prognostic literature, by the nature of the literature itself, cannot easily come to precise recommendations, but may be useful in providing better definitions of where the uncertainties and special potentials seem to be.

The clinician's approach to evaluation during adjuvant therapy decision-making for a patient with a newly diagnosed carcinoma of the breast includes the following questions:

1. Is this cancer invasive?
2. If invasive, does it have a special histologic subtype?
3. What is its anatomical extent as defined by TNM variables?
4. What is the patient's age, menopausal status and hormone receptor status?
5. What additional prognostic and predictive information is known?

Most of these questions are involved in the

Table 3.2 Elements complicating interpretation of studies of prognostic factors

Clinical
  Confounding effects of treatment
    Treated vs untreated
  Definition of relapse and death
    Local vs systemic relapse
    Overall vs breast cancer-specific mortality

Technical
  Assay reproducibility
    Reagents
    Variance (by instrument or observer)
  Tissue type used
    Fresh/Frozen/Fixed

Statistical
  False-positive studies
    Exploratory definitions of factors
    Subset analysis
  False-negative studies
    Size too small to find effect
    Too many co-variates
  Reporting results
    Multivariate?
    Relative risk given?
  Validation vs exploratory?

prognostic assessment of the patient, but some help guide the selection among treatment options.

In this review of the literature the use of prognostic information is examined in the following general groupings:

1. Classic prognostic variables
2. Patient-related information
3. Steroid hormone receptors
4. Proliferation markers
5. Proteases
6. Peptide hormone receptors
7. p53 and apoptosis-related proteins
8. Angiogenesis.

Classic prognostic variables

Histologic type

Most cancers of the breast are invasive adeno-carcinomas, but an increasing percentage are non-invasive forms. These non-invasive cancers ((ductal and lobular carcinoma in situ DCIS and LCIS)) have essentially no metastatic potential. They require definitive local therapy, but because they are associated with a very low risk of systemic relapse (<1%), they do not require systemic therapy or axillary staging. Prognostic factor evaluation of these lesions has no role at this time, although for DCIS pathologic variables, such as high histologic grade or comedo subtype, may be associated with increased risk of local recurrence after conservative local therapy.

In general, histologic subtype of invasive breast cancer is not a major predictor of outcome, but there are some histologic subtypes of invasive ductal adenocarcinomas that do appear to be associated with very low risk of systemic dissemination. These include pure tubular carcinomas, pure papillary forms and mucinous carcinomas. These are discussed elsewhere in this book. In most series these tumors are associated with favorable features such as low histologic grade and low rates of axillary nodal involvement, and it is not absolutely clear that these histologic subtypes are independent predictors of favorable outcome (see Pereira et al[9]); however, these histologic subtypes

Table 3.3 Five-year breast cancer-specific mortality rates from SEER analysis

Size (cm)	5-year mortality rate (%) for number of positive nodes		
	0	**1–3**	**>3**
<0.5	0.8	4.7	41.0
0.5–0.9	1.7	6.0	45.8
1.0–1.9	4.2	13.4	32.8
2.0–2.9	7.7	16.6	36.6
3.0–3.9	13.8	21.0	43.1
4.0–4.9	15.4	30.2	47.4
>5.0	17.8	27.0	54.5

Adapted from Table 4 of Carter et al.[11]

are excluded from some adjuvant trials as being at too low a risk for recurrence to benefit from therapy.

TNM staging

Classic staging of all visceral adenocarcinomas including breast cancer depends on assessment of tumor size and regional lymph node involvement.[10] Nearly all large studies have shown that both tumor size and number of involved axillary lymph nodes are independent predictors of both disease-free survival and overall survival for breast cancer patients.

Perhaps this is best illustrated in Table 3.3, which shows the breast cancer-specific mortality rates at 5 years of follow-up for 24 740 women with early invasive breast cancer, as assessed by the American National Registry, the Surveillance, Epidemiology, and End Results (SEER) Program.[11] This analysis shows the excellent prognosis of patients with node-negative disease, the worsened prognosis of patients with one to three nodes, and the poor prognosis of patients with more than three involved axillary nodes. It also shows that, within each of these nodal categories, increasing size of the primary is associated with increased breast cancer-specific mortality. This analysis has several strengths: it is large and it is population based. It also has weaknesses, with an undefined minority of the women having adjuvant therapy (the cases were from 1977 to 1982). Another potential weakness is the fact that breast cancer-specific mortality was calculated from the observed total mortality by indirect adjustment for expected, age-adjusted, non-breast cancer mortality, obtained from national actuarial tables. Nevertheless the estimates from the SEER analysis are very useful starting points for examining the relative strength of the estimates that can be made on the basis of tumor size and number of nodes alone. The SEER estimates are consistent with those from other sources[12-14] showing the excellent prognosis of patients with T1N0 tumors and the importance of tumor size and number of nodes for patients with larger tumors.

There are features used in classic TNM staging, such as the presence of fixation to the skin or underlying muscle, matting or fixation of the axillary nodes, and inflammatory component,[15] which also define the subset of patients with poor prognosis. Although these features have not been included in the large recent multivariate analyses, they are widely accepted as placing patients in poor risk categories where adjuvant therapy is mandated.

There are several special issues that not infrequently come up. One is whether, in a tumor with both intraductal and invasive components, the size used in estimates should be that of the entire tumor or only of the invasive component. The data from the SEER registry are based on the size of the invasive component. For patients with small areas of microinvasive disease (<1 mm) within larger non-invasive tumors, the risk of recurrence and nodal involvement is very low.[16,17] However, when less stringent definitions of microinvasion are used, an incidence of axillary nodal involvement up to 10% has been reported.[18,19] In large part, the disagreements about the prognostic significance of microinvasive disease may result from differing definitions of what microinvasive carcinoma is. A second issue in the evaluation of nodal status

is the prognostic significance of aggregates of cancer cells within the lymph nodes that are missed on initial sectioning, but identified later on resectioning or with special immunochemical stains. It appears that discovery of nodal involvement on standard histopathologic review does imply that the patient has a worse prognosis,[20,21] although this is less clear for such nodal metastases identified by immunohistochemical[22-24] or molecular biology techniques.[25]

Classic TNM staging is thus the basis of prognostic evaluation of breast cancer patients. It supplies information that is crucial to the prognostic assessment of breast cancer patients. All other prognostic variables are useful only if they add prognostic information and if this addition of statistically independent information is confirmed by multivariate analysis.

TNM-related information does not seem to allow prediction of response to therapy. The meta-analysis of adjuvant therapy trials shows similar proportional risk reductions for axillary node-negative (NN) and node-positive (NP) patients.[8] When TNM-based information is used to select patients not to receive adjuvant therapy, the rationale is that, for low-risk patients, the absolute reduction in their risk of relapse or breast cancer-related death is too low to justify adjuvant therapy.

Histologic grading

Histologic grading has long been recognized to have potential value in evaluating prognosis of adenocarcinoma of the breast. Classic studies such as those of Bloom and Richardson[26] suggested that histologic grading might improve prognostic assessment beyond that of simple nodal staging. Histologic grading is usually based on combined scores for nuclear grade, mitotic rate and architectural differentiation. A number of large studies have confirmed the association between histologic grade and outcome, and have suggested minor variations in the grading schemes to make grading more quantitative, reproducible, or to increase its prognostic power.[27] An area of controversy about histologic grading is whether it can be done with acceptable interobserver reproducibility. A study by Gilchrist et al[28] found

Table 3.4 Breast cancer-specific mortality at 5 years in patients by TNM and histologic grade (based on 22 616 cases of breast cancer in the SEER database[31])

TNM	Mortality rate (%) at histologic grade of				
	1	2	3	4	All
NN T < 2 cm	1	2	6	11	4
NN T 2–5 cm	3	9	16	14	12
NN T < 2 cm	1	11	21	19	16
NP T 2–5 cm	15	21	35	37	30

NN, node-negative; NP, node-positive; T, tumour,

unacceptably low reproducibility, but more recent studies done in the USA[29] and Australia[30] suggest that interobserver agreement can be excellent when pathologists follow well-defined guidelines.

Powerful evidence has been provided that the average pathologist can produce estimates of histologic grade that are predictive, in a study by Henson and Ries[31] using the SEER American tumor registry. Even though the histologic grading was being done in an unsupervised, non-standardized way, histologic grading clearly was a powerful predictor when added to tumor size and nodal status (Table 3.4). They reported 5-year breast cancer-related mortality rates of 1%, 2% 6% and 11% for NN tumors less than 2.0 cm in size of histologic grades 1–4 (averaging 4% for these tumors). For patients with NN tumors 2–5 cm in size, the average mortality rate was 12%, but again the use of histologic grading allowed tumors to be divided into subsets with 3%, 9%, 16% and 14% risks of relapse, respectively.

There are strong proponents for nuclear grading and, as done by some pathologists, it is clearly strongly predictive. There are also other pathologic features that have been studied as potential prognostic markers. Perhaps the most widely studied is lymphatic vessel invasion (LVI). In some[32,33] but not all[34] studies presence of LVI is predictive of poor outcome. The independent relative risk (RR) conferred by LVI is poorly defined, and thus it is unclear how to use it in the prognostic assessment of breast cancer patients.

Histologic grading clearly has clinical value, and should be used.[35] Quality control programs to assess the ability of individual pathologists to perform grading may lead to its broader application.

Patient-related information
Age
Of the patient characteristics that are important in decision-making about adjuvant therapy, patient age is clearly the most important. Patient age is not only important for predicting response to adjuvant chemotherapy (where a major part of this effect is the result of menopausal status),[8] and influences estimates of net years gained from use of adjuvant therapy,[36] it also seems to be a prognostic variable. Nearly all studies suggest that younger age, particularly age under 35, is associated with a higher incidence of a number of poor prognostic features, and with generally poorer outcome.

The more valuable investigations of this topic have performed multivariate analysis to see if age is an independent predictor. Albain et al[37] found that age under 35 years conveyed an additional RR of 1.8 when tumor size and number of nodes were accounted for (but that the inclusion of S phase eliminated the young age at diagnosis as a predictive variable). De la Rochefordiere et al[38] who showed that age under 33 years was a predictor of poor outcome, compared with other premenopausal patients, even when adjustments were made for tumor size, nodal status and histologic grade, conferring an additional relative risk of about 1.8. Similar results were reported by Bonnier et al[39] and Nixon et al[40] who found that age under 35 was a predictor of poorer outcome, with higher recurrence rates and shortened survival even after adjustment for lymph node status, tumor size, histopathologic grade and ER status, conferring an additional risk of about 1.6.

Another special aspect of prognostic factors in younger women is the issue of second primary breast cancers in this population. This was observed in some early studies.[41] With the description of the *BRCA*1 and *BRCA*2 genes, it is clear that very young women are at higher risk of having the hereditary rather than the sporadic form of the disease. Whether this association has prognostic implications and whether it should lead to different interpretation of prognostic tests is a matter addressed by ongoing studies, although an initial report suggests that patients with hereditary *BRCA*1- and *BRCA*2-related breast cancer actually seem to have a better prognosis, despite having such negative features as a higher proliferative rate on average.[42]

It is a matter of clinical debate whether very young breast cancer patients with otherwise favorable tumor prognostic features should always receive adjuvant therapy. No study includes enough patients in this category to address this question definitively, but using data from all patients (both NN and NP) the additional risk conferred by young age appears modest (<2.0), although it may be enough to affect some decisions.

Steroid hormone receptor-related proteins
ER and PR

Most large studies have not shown the estrogen receptor and/or progesterone receptor to distinguish strongly between patients with favorable and unfavorable outcomes, although studies consistently show a trend for better disease-free survival and overall survival for patients who are ER or PR positive. Nevertheless some sources (e.g. the St Gallen consensus conference) recommend stratifying NN patients into prognostic subsets, partly on the basis of steroid hormone receptor status. It is therefore important to re-examine whether ER or PR determinations are of particular prognostic value in NN patients.

There are several large studies that address this issue in NN patients who received no adjuvant therapy. In the National Surgical Adjuvant Breast and Bowel Project (NSABP) B-06 there were 825 NN patients with known ERs (obtained with the ligand binding assay).[43] The risk of systemic relapse at 5 years was 28% in the ER-negative subset and 20% in the ER-positive subset. Risk of death at 5 years was 18% in the ER-negative subset and 8% in the ER-positive subset. Although in univariate analysis these differences were statistically significant, no independent contribution to defining risk was found after multivariate analysis, although the contribution of ER may have been eliminated by the inclusion of strongly predictive nuclear grading in the multivariate analysis.

Similar results have been reported by Silvestrini et al[44] in a study of 1800 NN patients with known ERs and PRs (by ligand binding assay), 8 years of follow-up, and not receiving adjuvant therapy. In this patient population ERs and PRs were only very modest univariate predictors of systemic relapse (RR of 1.4 and 1.3, respectively), but this predictive power was not maintained on multivariate analysis when thymidine labeling index (TLI) was included. For overall survival, ERs and PRs were highly significant univariate predictors (RR = 1.9, 2.2), but only PRs were a predictor in multivariate analysis, conferring a statistically significant RR of 1.6. A third large study by Arriagada et al,[45] reporting the results of 1906 NN patients who did not receive adjuvant therapy, also reported that ERs and PRs were weakly prognostic for disease-free survival, conferring an additional RR of 1.2.

There are a number of complications in the interpretation of the literature about the prognostic value of ERs and PRs. One is the multiplicity of assay techniques. Classically, ERs and PRs have been measured by ligand binding assays, but more recently a number of assays have been developed that use immunologic techniques to measure ERs and PRs on cytosols or on sectioned tissue. These assays generally correlate well with each other,[46–48] but for some of the assays there is uncertainty as to where the appropriate cut-offs for defining ER- and PR-positive subsets are.

A second aspect complicating the assessment of the prognostic value of ERs and PRs is an apparent time dependence of the contribution of ERs and PRs to the annual hazard of relapse and breast cancer-related death.[49] In the first years after the diagnosis of breast cancer, the difference in the annual hazard of relapse between ER-positive and ER-negative cases is large, but after 5 years there is little difference in annual hazard rates. This makes the Kaplan–Meier curves diverge rapidly in the first years after diagnosis, but then become parallel to each other or even begin to converge. This leads to estimates of the RR conferred by ERs being large for studies with short follow-up, but then decreasing or disappearing in studies with more follow-up.

Thus, a review of these studies suggests that ERs and PRs are not strong predictors of prognosis, but may confer a relatively modest (RR < 1.5) effect on outcome, independent of tumor size and nodal status. This contribution may be lost with long follow-up or if other prognostic variables are included in the analysis.

For predicting responsiveness to endocrine therapy for patients with metastatic breast cancer (MBC), the value of ERs and PRs defined by the ligand binding assay is well established.[50] The meta-analysis of adjuvant therapy trials also shows that this assay can be used to select patients with a particularly high degree of benefit from adjuvant endocrine therapy.[8] Patients with MBC who are ER positive can be expected to have about a 50% response rate to front-line endocrine therapy. PRs can be used to refine this estimate further, splitting the ER-positive patients into subsets with about 40% and 60% response rates.[51] Patients who are ER and PR negative have a less than 5% response rate to endocrine therapy. The other ER and PR assays are also widely accepted as being predictive of endocrine response but the use of specific cut-off points for defining subsets with different response rates is not as well defined.

pS2

pS2 is an estrogen-inducible peptide whose exact physiologic role remains obscure.[52] However, because it is estrogen inducible, it might, like PRs, be used to define cancers with a more favorable prognosis, or more responsive to endocrine therapies.[53] pS2 has been a disappointment with respect to a possible role as a prognostic factor with none of the four studies on cytosols,[54–57] and none of the four studies using IHC (immunohisto-chemistry),[58–61] finding pS2 determinations to be a prognostic variable retained on multivariate analysis. There is conflicting evidence as to the value of pS2 for predicting response to endocrine therapy.[60–62] Thus although in theory pS2 determinations might be used to select patients for endocrine therapy, on a practical basis there is no information that it adds to ERs and PRs which are far more established for this purpose.

Proliferation markers

Measures of proliferation rates of neoplastic tissue are strongly prognostic for a number of cancer types, including breast cancer. There are a number of techniques that have been used to measure breast cancer cell proliferation. These include direct measures of proliferation such as thymidine labeling index, and more indirect measures such as measures of cell cycle compartments by DNA flow cytometry or image cytometry, measures of proteins expressed

Table 3.5 Studies of the prognostic value of TLI as a prognostic factor in breast cancer

Study	Subset	n	Follow-up (months)	Assay	Cut-off point (%)	High (%)	Univariate		Multivariate (RR)	
							DFS	OS	DFS	OS
Silvestrini[63]	NN	1800	96	TLI	3	62	+	+	1.5	1.6
Cooke[64]	All	185	96	TLI	7.3	50	ND	NS	ND	NS
Courdi[65]	NN	162	~60?	TLI	2.1	50	+	ND	+(2.2)	ND
Tubiana[66]	All	128	180	TLI	<0.25	19, 61	+	+	+	+
					>3.8	20			1/2.8/ 3.6	1/2.5/ 2.9

+, $p < 0.05$; NS, $p > 0.05$; ND, not done; NN, node negative; NP, node positive; All, both NN and NP; DFS, disease-free survival; OS, overall survival; RR, relative risk.

during specific parts of the cell cycle (Ki67, MIB1, Ki-S1, PCNA), and measures of cells in mitosis, such as mitotic index either alone or as incorporated into histologic grading.

Thymidine labeling index
The most direct way of measuring mitotic rate is to measure the incorporation of tritiated thymidine into nuclei of tumor tissue. Autoradiography is then used to assess the percentage of tumor nuclei that are in the active process of cell division. This assay must be done in vitro on minced fresh tumor. Most, but not all, studies suggest that TLI is an independent predictor of outcome. Table 3.5 shows the results of four studies. In three of the four studies TLI was an independent predictor. In the one negative study there may have been technical problems with the assay as the authors commented that they did not get good reproducibility with this technique; they found a median value for the assay that was considerably higher than the other studies. One major study found good reproducibility of this technique between centers at least as far as the interpretation of the autoradiographs.[62] As it requires special tissue handling, TLI has not

been widely used, but the predictive power of this assay suggests that it is of value in centers experienced in its use, and in a general sense is supportive of the aggressive exploration of other technically simpler methods for measuring proliferation.

S-phase fraction
The most widely used measure of proliferative rate is S-phase fraction estimates derived by DNA flow cytometry. A consensus conference,[67,68] addressing the use of this technique, found that an overview of the literature supported the use of flow cytometric S phase, but noted that there was a lack of standardization of the processing of tissue for this technique and also a lack of standardization in the estimation of S phase from the resulting histograms. As a result of this limitation, it was recommended that each laboratory establish its own cut-offs for defining subsets with different expected prognoses. Some of the complexity of the clinical literature in this area is conveyed by Table 3.6. Studies evaluating S phase differ in terms of the type of tissue used (frozen vs paraffin embedded), the cut-offs used to distinguish high- and low-risk groups, and whether

Table 3.6 Studies of the prognostic value of S phase derived from DNA flow cytometry as a prognostic factor in NN breast cancer

Study	Subset	n	Follow-up (months)	Tissue	Cut-off point (%)	High (%)	Univariate		Multivariate (RR)	
							DFS	OS	DFS	OS
Winchester[69]	D	71	80	P	4	63	ND	+	ND	+(2?)
Winchester[69]	An	198	80	P	10.3	50	ND	NS	ND	NS
Merkel[70]	All	248	76	P	9	43	+	+	NS	+(2.3)
Dressler[71]	All	294	55	P	6.97	50	+	ND	+(?)	ND
Dresser[71]	D	150	55	P	6.97	18	+	ND	+(?)	ND
Dresser[71]	An	144	55	P	6.97	68	+	ND	+(?)	ND
Muss[72]	All	84	51	F	12.5	50	NS	+	NS	NS
Clark[73]	D	112	59	F	6.7	13	+	+	+(4.0)	+(3.9)
Clark[73]	An	233	59	F	6.7	Any	NS	NS	NS	NS
Sigurdsson[74]	All	367	48	?	<7.7– >11.9	45, 18, 37	+	+	+(1.5)	+(2.1)
Isola[75]	All	289	104	P	8	?	ND	+	ND	+(3.8)
Ewers[76]	All	217	120	F	7.3	48	ND	NS	ND	NS
Silvestrini[77]	All	291	48	F	?	–	NS	ND	NS	ND
Balslev[78]	All	421	81	F	9.0	75	ND	+	ND	+(2.0)

D, diploid; An, non-diploid; All, combined analysis; F, done on fresh or frozen tissue; P, done on paraffin-embedded tissue; ND, not done; NS, $p > 0.05$.

diploid and aneuploid histograms are interpreted the same way or using different cut-offs. In most studies, high S-phase fraction was associated with a poorer prognosis at least in univariate analysis, but the multiplicity of techniques and interpretations makes it impossible to state whether, for a given method, S-phase fraction adds independent prognostic information, and what RR is conferred.

Immunohistochemical methods of measuring proliferative rate

Many proteins play a role in the control of the cell cycle or are expressed at higher levels during specific phases of the cell cycle. Some of these have been studied in breast cancer specimens as markers of proliferative rate and as possible prognostic factors. The most widely used of these tests is for an antigen detected by the Ki67 monoclonal antibody.[79] This nuclear antigen is expressed in the S, G2 and M phase of the cell cycle. A limitation of the original monoclonal antibody used was that it would not stain fixed paraffin-embedded sections, but a newer monoclonal antibody, MIB1, appears suitable for staining both fresh and fixed preparations.[80] Table 3.7 shows an overview of seven studies in which Ki67 or MIB1 was used. Although in most of these studies there was evidence that Ki67 was a univariate predictor, the evidence that it is an independent predictor on multivariate analysis is still incomplete.

Table 3.7 Studies of the prognostic value of Ki67/MIB1 used in IHC as a prognostic factor in breast cancer

Study	Subset	n	Follow-up (months)	Tissue	Cut-off point (%)	High (%)	Univariate		Multivariate (RR)	
							DFS	OS	DFS	OS
Brown[81]	NN	674	72	IHCF	5	25	+	NS	+(1.8)	NS
Railo[82]	All	327	32	IHCF	?	?	+	NS	ND	ND
Veronese[83]	All	129	42	IHCF	20	25	+	+	ND	ND
Pinder[84]	All	177	>60	IHCP	<17	27, 31,	NS	+	NS	+(2.4)
				MIB1	>34	42?				
Gaglia[85]	All	385	<48	IHCF	9	50	+	ND	+(?)	ND
Gasparini[86]	All	168	60	IHCF	10	~50	+	+	ND	ND
Rudas[87]	All	184	73	IHCF	<3.5	31, 41,	NS	NS	NS	NS
					>10.5	28				

IHCF, done on fresh frozen tissue; IHCP, done on paraffin-embedded tissue; ND, not done; NS, $p > 0.05$.

There are other proteins that may find use in measuring proliferative rate such as PCNA,[88,89] the various cyclins[90,91] and mitosin,[92] but the studies to evaluate their use as prognostic makers are even more preliminary than for Ki67/MIB1. A particularly interesting proliferation marker is Ki-S1, which has recently been shown to be identical to topoisomerase II α.[93] This is of particular relevance because topoisomerase II is the target of a number of anti-cancer drugs such as the anthracyclines and podophyllotoxins. Two studies using Ki-S1 reached conflicting conclusions as to its prognostic value[94,95] so this marker is far from clinical usage, although one might hope that it will be shown to be a predictor of response to anthracyclines.

Proteases and the extracellular matrix

Proteases play important roles in control of the basement membrane, and in cell motility and invasion, and might thus indicate the invasive and metastatic potential of a tumor.

Cathepsin D
Of the proteases, cathepsin D is the most widely examined in prognostic studies. It was initially described as a lysosomal enzyme,[96] but has been suggested to play other roles such as a growth factor for some cell types. There are a number of methodologies for measuring cathepsin D expression in tissue which include immunoassays on cytosols, immunoblotting, direct measurement of cathepsin D activity and immunohistochemistry.

The most widely studied assays for cytosolic cathepsin D are based on the antibodies D7E3 and M1G8.[97] Table 3.8 shows the results from 10 studies using the two antibody assays on cytosols in an IRMA (immunoradiometric assay) format. In most studies, cathepsin D was a predictor of outcome at least in univariate analysis, with higher levels of cathepsin D correlating with early relapse, and also perhaps with shorter

Table 3.8 Studies of the prognostic value of cathepsin D as a prognostic factor in breast cancer using immunoassays done on cytosols

Study	Subset	n	Follow-up (months)	Tissue	Cut-off point (pmol/ml)	High (%)	Univariate		Multivariate (RR)	
							DFS	OS	DFS	OS
Sehadri[98]	All	858	31	IRMA	25	~50	+	ND	+(1.7)	ND
Sehadri[98]	NN	342	31	IRMA	25	~50	+	ND	+(1.2)	ND
Sehadri[98]	NP	239	31	IRMA	25	~50	+	ND	+(1.9)	ND
Foekens[99]	All	710	48	IRMA	70	25	+	+	+(1.9)	+(1.6)
Foekens[99]	NN	285	48	IRMA	70	25	+	NS	+(2.5)	ND
Foekens[99]	NP	420	48	IRMA	70	25	+	+	+(1.8)	ND
Namer[100]	All	413	68	IRMA	35	51	ND	+	ND	+(?)
Namer[100]	NN	246	68	IRMA	35	45	NS	NS	NS	NS
Namer[100]	NP	166	68	IRMA	35	45	+	+	+(?)	+
Ferno[101]	NN	217	37	IRMA	45	61	NS	ND	NS	ND
Ferno[101]	NP	404	37	IRMA	45	61	NS	ND	NS	ND
Gion[102]	All	267	39	IRMA	31	?	+	+	+(2.9)	+(2.2)
Janicke[103]	All	229	30	IRMA	50	48	NS	ND	NS	NS
Janicke[103]	NN	101	30	IRMA	50	34	NS	ND	NS	NS
Granata[104]	NN	199	87	IRMA	67	50	NS	NS	NS	NS
Kute[105]	NN	162	29	IRMA	63	33	+	+	+(>3)	+(>3)
Spyratos[106]	All	122	55	IRMA	70	23	+	ND	+(3.7)	ND
Romain[107]	All	85	58	IRMA	30	68	NS	+	NS	+(3.7)

survival. An examination of the four studies which included more than 500 patients reveals why this assay has not been widely endorsed for evaluation of prognosis. None of these studies used a prospectively defined cut-off for defining high- and low-risk subsets. All these studies used all or some of the patients to define the cut-off point in order to optimize the apparent statistical power of the test. In addition the cut-offs used were quite different, making it unclear as to how best to interpret assay results.

Immunoblotting as a technique used to measure cathepsin D levels no longer seems to be an area of active investigation, with a first study by Tandon et al[108] suggesting that it was a highly predictive assay, and a follow-up study failing to validate these results.[109] The relative complexity of immunoblotting and the need for using cytosols has limited the number of investigations. There is one study by Kute et al[105] in which the enzymatic activity of cathepsin D was directly measured in cytosols. In this study cathepsin D enzymatic activity was a highly predictive factor, but there have been no validation studies. There have been numerous studies of the potential prognostic value of cathepsin D measured by IHC. Although there have been studies suggesting that cathepsin D was a predictor,[110,111] most large studies failed to confirm[112–115] the predictive value of cathepsin D expression. Interpretation of these studies is complicated by differences in the primary antibodies used, the type of cells scored (tumor vs stromal vs macrophage) and the scoring method used.

The practical use of cathepsin D as a prognostic marker is a matter of some debate,[116,117] but of the assays available for measuring cathepsin D levels, the double antibody assay using the IRMA methodology appears promising. However, this assay has not been subjected to rigorous validation by a large study with a prospectively defined cut-off in the NN subset of patients, and therefore the cut-off to be used and the RR conferred by high levels are uncertain.

Urokinase plasminogen activator system
The urokinase plasminogen activator (uPA) plays an important role in the remodeling of the extracellular matrix. Thus, it potentially plays a role in the motility, invasiveness and metastatic potential of cancer cells.[118] A number of studies have addressed whether elevated uPA levels are predictive of elevated risk of metastasis and death resulting from breast cancer (Table 3.9).

Overall these studies suggest that elevated uPA levels are an independent predictor of early relapse and death with three out of the four large studies finding uPA a statistically significant predictor even in multivariate analysis. In the study by Bouchet[120] the predictive value in multivariate analysis was perhaps obscured by the inclusion of other non-routine prognostic variables.

A major caveat to the use of uPA in the prognostic assessment of breast cancer patients is the non-standardization of assay techniques which has resulted in a broad range of cut-off values. The differences in cut-off values are the result partly of methodologic differences and partly of the exploratory analysis used in some of these studies to find the best possible cut-off (a process that may make the apparent RRs appear somewhat larger than they actually are). None of these studies is a true validation of prior studies. In addition, no study addresses, in a convincing way, the value of uPA in the NN subset of patients,[121] the subset where it has potentially the greatest value. Thus, uPA may be of value but assay standardization and prospective validation studies are needed.

The uPA system is complex with receptors for uPA (uPAR) and also inhibitors for uPA (PAI-1 and PAI-2). Early studies of these factors suggest that high levels of uPAR are predictive of poor prognosis,[122] whereas high levels of PAI-1 may be protective.[123] Unexpectedly, high levels of the inhibitor, PAI-2, may actually predict poor prognosis. It is quite possible that the *ratios* of the major elements of the uPA system will be shown to be of particular value.

Table 3.9 Studies of the prognostic value of uPA as a prognostic factor in breast cancer

Study	Subset	n	Follow-up (months)	Tissue	Cut-off point (ng/ml)	High (%)	Univariate		Multivariate (RR)	
							DFS	OS	DFS	OS
Foekens[119]	All	671	48	ELSA	1.15	32	+	+	+(2.0)	+(1.7)
Bouchet[120]	All	314	84	ELSA	0.52	32	±	+	NS	NS
Janicke[103]	All	229	30	ELSA	2.97	39	+	+	+(3.0)	+(3.1)
Duffy[118]	All	166	35	ELSA	10.0	49	+	+	+(4.4)	+(11)

Peptide hormone receptors

Although much of the focus in breast cancer research has been on steroid hormone receptors, it is clear that peptide hormones can exert important roles in controlling breast cancer cell proliferation. Two peptide hormone receptors have been most thoroughly researched: c-erbB-2 and the epidermal growth factor receptor.

c-erbB-2

HER-2/neu, the protein product of the c-erbB-2 gene, is a transmembrane tyrosine kinase that is a receptor for a family of peptide ligands thought to stimulate cell growth. The first studies of the possible prognostic significance of this gene and its protein product focused on gene amplification, but more recently most studies have used IHC to measure the protein product. There seems to be a good agreement between these two measures.

The first study addressing the possible prognostic significance of c-erbB-2 gene amplification was published in 1987 by Slamon.[124] This study in 187 patients (both NP and NN) showed c-erbB-2 gene amplification to be strongly correlated in both univariate and multivariate analysis, with shortened disease-free survival and overall survival in the subset of 86 NP patients. Slamon then replicated the result, as reported in 1989 in a 526 patient series.[125] c-erbB-2 amplification was again found to be predictive of poorer disease-free survival and overall survival only in the NP subset (in both univariate and multivariate analyses), but not in the NN subset. However, further work by the same group in 210 NN patients suggested that, at least in univariate analysis, c-erbB-2 amplification did correlate with worsened disease-free survival.[126] Attempts to replicate these results by others have had mixed success, with some studies finding that c-erbB-2 gene amplification was an independent predictor in breast cancer patients,[127,128] and others failing to find any useful correlations.[129–133] Thus, overall, these studies correlating c-erbB-2 gene amplification with either disease-free survival or overall survival have produced no uncontested evidence for using this test in the evaluation of the prognosis of those breast cancer patients most in need of prognostic information – NN patients.

The results with IHC for c-erbB-2 are similar to those for gene amplification. The test has been a major disappointment as a prognostic factor in NN breast cancer patients with only one of 11 studies in NN patients finding that c-erbB-2 overexpression was an independent marker of poor prognosis (Table 3.10). Thus c-erbB-2 appears to have little practical value as a prognostic factor for predicting breast cancer outcome. However, the apparently greater value of c-erbB-2 in NP rather than NN has led to the suggestion that perhaps it is a marker of resistance to adjuvant therapy.

There is growing evidence that high levels of c-erbB-2 expression do correlate with resistance to adjuvant therapy. If c-erbB-2 overexpression were predictive of resistance to adjuvant therapy, then studies stratifying adjuvant therapy patients between no (or minimal) therapy and more intensive therapy would be expected to show predictive value of c-erbB-2 only or primarily in the groups getting more intensive therapy. This is borne out by some but not all studies. As positive examples (Table 3.11), in the study by Têtu and Brisson,[145] for the untreated NP patients c-erbB-2 was not a significant predictor of either disease-free survival or overall survival, whereas it was a powerful predictor of both for patients treated with either adjuvant chemotherapy or hormone therapy. Another study supporting this concept is the Ludwig study,[146] in which the NN population that received no adjuvant therapy showed no predictive value of c-erbB-2, whereas in the NN group that did receive adjuvant therapy (a single perioperative cycle) c-erbB-2 was a significant predictor of overall survival. Similar effects were seen in the NP population in that study, where patients were randomized between a less intensive therapy (one cycle of perioperative chemotherapy) and a more conventional multicycle, multidrug, adjuvant regimen. A greater predictive value of c-erbB-2 was noted in the more heavily treated group than in those receiving less intensive therapy. However, not all studies have agreed that c-erbB-2 is more

Table 3.10 Major studies of the prognostic value of *c-erbB*-2 measured by IHC as a prognostic factor in NN breast cancer

Reference	n	Follow-up (months)	Univariate		Multivariate	
			DFS	OS	DFS	OS
Thor[134]	141	102	NS	NS	ND	ND
Lovekin[135]	250	?~60	ND	NS	ND	ND
McCann[136]	113	48	ND	NS	ND	ND
Kallionemi[137]	174	118	ND	+	ND	+
Tanner[138]	105	36	NS	NS	ND	ND
Yuan[139]	101	>120	+	+	NS	NS
Alfred[140]	453	61	NS	NS	ND	ND
Noguchi[141]	151	?~60	NS	NS	NS	NS
Gusterson[142]	760	42	NS	+	NS	NS
Press[143]	210	108	+	ND	ND	ND
Bianchi[144]	230	>84	+	+	NS	NS

ND, not done; NS, $p > 0.05$.

Table 3.11 Relative risks for positive *c-erbB*-2 status in treated versus untreated (or less treated) patients

Reference	Site	No.	Patients	Treatment	Relative risks	
					DFS	OS
Têtu[145]	Montréal	232	NP	No adj	1.3	1.2
		656	NP	Adj	2.1*	2.4*
Gusterson[146]	Ludwig	260	NN	No adj	0.9	1.6
		500	NN	Peri adj	1.5	1.8*
		255 only	NP	Peri	1.3	1.8*
		491	NP	Adj	1.7*	2.4*

*Significant: $p < 0.05$. peri, perioperative ; adj, adjuvant.

predictive in the more heavily treated patients – a recent report by Muss et al[147] of a trial randomizing patients between different intensities of adjuvant chemotherapy can be interpreted as showing that c-erbB-2 overexpression was predictive of an increased sensitivity to chemotherapy. Whether this apparent discrepancy between different trials is the result of differences in the types of chemotherapy used, the relative doses, statistical aberrations or other factors is unclear at this time.

There is also more direct preclinical and clinical evidence that c-erbB-2 may be a predictor of treatment resistance. For example, Benz et al[148] have shown that, in animal models, transfection of breast tumor cells with c-erbB-2 results in treatment resistance to tamoxifen. Wright et al.[149] addressed this effect of c-erbB-2 overexpression on resistance to tamoxifen in 65 patients with recurrent metastatic breast cancer. Response rates were 7% in the c-erbB-2-positive patients and 37% in the c-erbB-2-negative patients ($p < 0.05$). Although the subsets were small, c-erbB-2 expression appeared predictive of treatment failure in estrogen receptor-positive patients, with response rates of 20% (1/5) in the ER-positive/c-erbB-2-positive patients and 48% (12/25) in ER-positive/c-erbB-2-negative patients. The work of Klijn et al[150] is consistent with these tamoxifen results, although the conclusion was not bolstered by a multivariate analysis. Paradoxically, Klijn et al also found that c-erbB-2 overexpression was actually a predictor of *good* response to cyclophosphamide, methotrexate and 5-fluorouracil (CMF) chemotherapy in patients with metastatic disease.

Overall c-erbB-2 does not appear to be useful in defining patient prognosis. There are several lines of evidence, however, that it may be a predictor of treatment response. These suggestive studies are largely based on retrospective analyses. Important validation studies are ongoing.

Epidermal growth factor receptor

The epidermal growth factor receptor (EGF-R) was one of the first peptide growth factor receptors described. It is overexpressed in a number of cancers. It is the receptor for transforming growth factor-α and has been implicated in autocrine regulation of breast cancer growth.[151] Its overexpression might therefore be expected to be associated with a more aggressive clinical course. This expectation seems to be borne out in women with breast cancer, with most studies showing a trend towards worsened prognosis in patients with high levels of EGF-R expression (Table 3.12). There are, however, a great many variations of ligand binding assays and IHC techniques. Reviewers of the prognostic significance of EGF-R expression often express frustration with the multiple assay techniques used, with the great variation in the cut-points used to define high- and low-risk subsets, and with the failure of EGF-R in most studies to be an independent predictor when multivariate analysis is done.

A more exciting prospect is that EGF-R might predict resistance to endocrine therapy. Data from some studies suggest that it does. For example, in the study by Wright et al[149] response rates to front-line endocrine therapy were 48% (11/23) if a patient was ER-positive and EGF-R-negative, 29% (2/7) if ER-positive and EGF-R-positive, 36% (4/11) if ER-negative and EGF-R-negative and 12% (3/24) if ER-negative and EGF-R-positive. Although the number of cases is small it appears that EGF-R positivity is a predictor of relative insensitivity to endocrine therapy. Studies that evaluate the value of EGF-R expression, predicting response to endocrine therapy (finding expression is predictive of low response rates),[159,160] are difficult to evaluate if they do not include ER in the analysis, because of the strong known correlation of EGF-R expression and ER negativity. Taken as a whole, the evidence that EGF-R predicts resistance to endocrine therapy is still tentative. Studies like that of Wright et al suggest that, when ER is taken into account, EGF-R may help refine estimates of hormone sensitivity, but that ER-positive, EGF-R-positive patients still have a high enough response rate that endocrine therapy should not be abandoned in a patient simply because they were EGF-R overexpressing.

Overall, until validation studies are done with a well-standardized technique, the use of EGF-R in defining prognosis and predicting

Table 3.12 Studies of the prognostic value of EGF-R as a prognostic factor in breast cancer

Study	Subset	n	Follow-up (months)	Assay	Cut-off point (fm/mg)	High (%)	Univariate		Multivariate (RR)	
							DFS	OS	DFS	OS
Studies dependent on non-IHC techniques										
Koenders[207]	All	376	24	Ligand	50	22	+	+	NS	NS
Fox[208]	All	370	18	Ligand	10	47	NS	NS	NS	NS
Seshadri[209]	All	345	57	Ligand	15	20	+	+	+(1.8)	+(2.3)
Seshadri[209]	NN	112	57	Ligand	10	20	?	?	NS	NS
Spyratos[152]	All	319	72	IE	6	31	+[a]	ND	+(2.4)	ND
Bolla[153]	All	229	34	Ligand	3	55	NS	NS	NS	NS
Harris[154]	All	221	24	Ligand	10	33	+	+	+(?)	+(?)
Klijn[155]	All	214	102	Ligand	2	33	NS	NS	NS	NS
Toi[156]	All	115	48	Ligand	1	35	+	ND	+(?)	ND
Studies dependent on IHC technique										
Gasparini[157]	All	165	60?	IHC	Any	56	+	NS	ND	NS
Toi[156]	All	126	48	IHC	++	16	+	ND	+(?)	ND
Newby[158]	All	88	39	IHC	>35%	22	+	+	NS	NS

[a]High levels of EGF-R were associated with low risk. IE, an assay using anti-EGF-R antibodies on cytosols; NS, $p > 0.05$; ND, not done.

response to therapy would appear to be investigational.

p53 and proteins regulating apoptosis

p53 is a nuclear protein that plays a role as a tumor suppressor and may play roles in the control of transcription, the cell cycle and apoptosis. It has been measured in tumor cells by a number of techniques aimed at defining mutations and levels of protein expression. Most mutations lead to forms of p53 that are abnormally stable, leading to increased expression.

p53 has been most widely studied by IHC. In studies of NN patients p53 overexpression has often[161–167] but not always[168–171] been shown to be an independent predictor of poor prognosis (Table 3.13). Some of the differences between studies may be explained by the different antibodies used to do the immunostaining for p53. In a study of five different antibodies to p53 used for staining 169 tumor samples, the Spearman correlation coefficients ranged from 0.63 to 0.83, and it appeared that some antibodies (1801) were better prognosticators for outcome than others, whereas some (CM1) were of little or no prognostic value.[179] Nevertheless, in clinical studies none of the antibodies is associated exclusively with prognostic or non-prognostic results.

Table 3.13 Studies of the prognostic value of p53 detected by IHC as a prognostic factor in NN breast cancer

Study	Subset	n	Follow-up (months)	Assay	Cut-off point (%)	High (%)	Univariate		Multivariate (RR)	
							DFS	OS	DFS	OS
Studies dependent on IHC technique										
Allred[172]	NN	700	54	1801, 240	Any	52	+	ND	+(2.5)	ND
Rosen[173]	NN	440	119	1801	10	22	NS	NS	NS	NS
MacGrogan[174]	NN	398	118	DO7	Any	32	+	+	NS	NS*
Haerslev[175]	NN	315	127	DO7	Any	32	NS	NS	NS	NS
Isola[176]	NN	289	104	CM1	20	14	ND	+	ND	+(2.7)
Silvestrini[177]	NN	256	72	1801	5	44	+	+	+(3.2)	+(2.6)
Gasparini[188]	NN	254	62	1801	Any	28	+	NS	+(3.1)	NS
Domagala[178]	NN	136	>60	CM1	10	35	ND	NS	ND	NS

NS, $p > 0.05$; ND, not done.

Other methodologies have been used to measure p53. For example, the study of Caleffi et al[180] examined exons 5–9 of p53. This study found 22% of 192 tumors had mutations in this region. In this relatively small study with a follow-up of 48 months, p53 mutations did not correlate with either disease-free survival or overall survival. The study by Elledge et al[181,182] also identified 14% of the patients as having mutations in one of the exons of p53 (5–9). In this study, p53 mutations did correlate with a more unfavorable outcome even in multivariate analysis.

Perhaps one of the more provocative and surprising aspects of p53 research is the suggestion that the presence in the serum of antibodies to p53 is associated with poor prognosis in breast cancer patients. In a 353 patient study Peyrat et al[183] found that the presence of antibodies to p53 (which occurred in 12% of their study population) was associated with a statistically significant independent increased relative risk of 1.4 and 1.9 for relapse and early death. This work, while provocative, awaits replication.

Taken together, the studies of p53 suggest that overexpression or abnormalities in p53 are associated with a poor outcome. The multiplicity of the assay types and interpretations used, the fact the some studies are definitively negative and the lack of prospective studies prevent a simple recommendation as to which assays are predictive, and which are not.

The Bcl-2 family
In hematologic malignancies *Bcl-2* has been associated with resistance to influences that trigger apoptosis.[184] If this role was played by *Bcl-2* in breast cancer, then one might expect high levels of *Bcl-2* to be associated with poor prognosis. This does not seem to be true. In the study by Silvestrini et al[185] high levels of *Bcl-2* correlated with favorable outcome in univariate analyses. However, the inclusion of p53 values in multivariate analyses caused *Bcl-2* not to be included. *Bcl-2*-positive tumors are reported to be more likely ER-positive, EGF-R-negative, *c-erbB-2*-negative and p53-negative.[186] This constellation of correlations with favorable features

may explain why *Bcl-2* expression correlates with favorable outcome in univariate analyses, but not in multivariate analyses.

A family of genes that share strong sequence homology with *Bcl-2* has been identified (*Bax*, *Bcl-X_l*,[187] *Bcl-X_s*,[188] *Mcl-1*,[189] etc.). Interactions between these proteins play important roles in the control of apoptosis.[190] *Bax* is a homologue of *Bcl-2* which promotes apoptosis in model systems. A study of patients with metastatic disease showed that, like *Bcl-2*, low levels of *Bax* expression were associated with a worsened overall prognosis, with a lower response rate to combination chemotherapy (6% versus 42% objective response rate), and a shortened time to treatment failure and shortened overall survival.[191] Direct measures of apoptosis also have been evaluated as prognostic factors. Lipponen et al have shown that high apoptotic rates are associated with high rates of relapse on univariate but not multivariate analyses.[192]

These results with *Bcl-2* and related genes suggest that an understanding of this family of apoptosis-related proteins will perhaps be worth while in determining the prognosis and predicting treatment response of breast cancer patients, but we are only at the start of this process.

ANGIOGENESIS

Angiogenesis is a process critical to the growth of any tissue, and neoplastic tissues are clearly capable of stimulating this process.[193] Intense interest has followed the publication of the initial small study suggesting that active angiogenesis, as measured by high microvessel density (MVD), correlates with poor clinical outcome for patients with early breast cancer.[194] This initial study has been expanded by its original authors and by others. The usual technique used is to stain the tissue immunohistochemically for an antigen expressed in microvessels, and then to count the number of vessels per unit area. There are six studies that have addressed the prognostic significance of MVD in node-negative patients (Table 3.14). Although three of these studies suggested that high MVD was a predictor of poor outcome, the

Table 3.14 Studies of the prognostic value of angiogenesis (as measured by IHC-detected microvessel counts) as a prognostic factor in NN breast cancer

Study	Subset	*n*	Follow-up (months)	Assay	Cut-off point (count/ mm²)	High (%)	Univariate		Multivariate (RR)	
							DFS	OS	DFS	OS
Studies dependent on IHC-based technique										
Gasparini[195]	NN	254	62	IHC	108	~50	+	+	+(5.8)	+(?)
Toi[196]	NN	130	56	IHC	tertiles	33	+	ND	+(?)	ND
Axelsson[197]	NN	110	138	IHC	~150	50	NS	NS	NS	NS
Fox[198]	NN	109	25	IHC	6[b]	~50	+	+	+(3.5)	+(6.6)
Von Hoef[199]	NN	93	155	IHC	C	–	NS	NS	NS	NS
Sittonen[200]	NN	77[a]	96	IHC	2.5[a]	50	ND	NS	ND	NS

[a]Microvessels as percentage of total tumor area.
[b]Vessels per ×250 magnification field. C, as a continuous variable per ×200 magnification field.

other three studies were unable to document this correlation. It should be noted that all these studies were relatively small, and none truly prospective. In addition, a wide variety of antibodies and scoring techniques was used. There may be specific issues in the scoring of MVD (average tumor areas or 'hot spots') and interobserver variation in scoring (in the carefully done study of Axelsson et al[197] this was noted to be very high). The use of angiogenesis in the prognostic assessment of breast cancer patients clearly is very promising, but in practical terms awaits large validation studies with well-standardized methodologies.

THE IMPORTANCE OF PROGNOSTIC MODELS

Given the large number of prognostic variables available, and in general the non-quantitative way in which much of this information is presented, it is perhaps not surprising that, when presented with simple clinical scenarios, clinicians often make quite different estimates of prognosis.[201] There is in fact no standardized method for integrating prognostic information. Nor is such a method likely to emerge in the near future given the non-standardization of measurement of prognostic factors.

How would such a prognostic model ideally perform? First, it would be based on the analysis of a large database in which the factors were measured by standardized techniques. Second, it would use much of the data as continuous variables (much information is lost or poorly presented by simple dichotomy). Third, it would produce estimates as continuous numbers (i.e. percentage risk of relapse at 5 years, rather than assigning patients to two or three prognostic categories). Fourth, it would need to be validated on an independent data set. There is no ideal model at this time, but even the non-ideal models have the potential to improve prognostic estimates.

The first prognostic index for breast cancer prognostic evaluation was the Nottingham index, which was derived from data on 387 patients, and used tumor size, lymph node staging and histologic grade to define three groups of patients.[202] The Nottingham index has been validated by the prospective inclusion of several times as many patients at the same center.[203] Confirmations of the Nottingham index are complicated by the unique lymph node staging system used in this index, and this makes direct comparisons with other data sets problematic. Perhaps the closest such comparison can be made in patients who are lymph node negative. In a study of NN patients in the Danish database, the Nottingham index discriminated high-, moderate- and low-risk patients, although the numerical estimates of outcome differed slightly from those in Nottingham.[204]

An example of a model that incorporates tumor size, number of involved nodes, S phase and ER is that proposed by Clark et al for predicting outcome of NP patients.[205] This model was successfully validated on a second data set.[206]

CHALLENGES AND OPPORTUNITIES FOR THE FUTURE

There are several important considerations which will affect and perhaps change the use of prognostic and predictive factors in the near future. First, the basic pathologic staging of breast cancer may change, with new sentinel node biopsy techniques perhaps changing the classic, more complete, axillary node staging that is now usually performed. Second, with the size of the average tumor decreasing, biochemical assays, such as the ligand binding assay for the estrogen receptor, will not be possible on an increasing number of patients and methodologies that can be performed on small sample sizes, and/or on paraffin-embedded material, will become particularly important. Third, with an increasing percentage of patients receiving adjuvant therapy, the use of tests that predict response to adjuvant therapy, and prognosis in patients treated with adjuvant therapy, will become increasingly important. Fourth, with increasing economic pressures and regulation, it will become increasingly important that prognostic factors be measured by standardized methodologies and demonstrably affect patient outcome. Over the next decade prognostic factor work will be more focused on clinical applicability, and should play an increasingly important role in decisions about adjuvant therapy and therapy for metastatic breast cancer.

REFERENCES

1. McGuire WL, Carbone PP, Sears ME, Eschert GC. Estrogen receptors in human breast cancer: an overview. In: *Estrogen Receptors in Human Breast Cancer* (McGuire WL, Carbone PP, Vollmer EP, eds). New York: Raven Press, 1975:1–7.

2. Anonymous. Early stage breast cancer: consensus statement. NIH consensus development conference, June 18–21, 1990. In: *Adjuvant Therapy of Breast Cancer* (Henderson IC, ed.). Norwell, MA: Kluwer Academic, 1992:383–93.

3. Goldhirsch A, Wood WC, Senn H-J. International consensus panel on the treatment of primary breast cancer. *Eur J Cancer* 1995; **31A:**1754–9.

4. Henson DE, Fielding LP, Grignon DJ, et al. College of American Pathologists Conference XXVI on clinical relevance of prognostic markers in solid tumors. *Arch Pathol Lab Med* 1995; **119:**1109–12.

5. Bast RC, Desch CE, Ravdin PM, Smith TJ. Clinical practice guidelines of the use of tumor markers in breast and colorectal cancer: Adopted on May 17, 1996 by the American Society of Clinical Oncology. *J Clin Oncol* 1996; **14:**2843–77.

6. Levine MN, Browman GP, Gent M, Roberts R, Goodyear M. When is a prognostic factor useful? A guide for the perplexed. *J Clin Oncol* 1991; **9:**348–56.

7. McGuire WL. Breast cancer prognostic factors: evaluation guidelines. *J Natl Cancer Inst* 1991; **83:**154–5.

8. Early Breast Cancer Trialists' Collaborative Group. Systemic treatment of early breast cancer by hormonal, cytotoxic, or immune therapy. *Lancet* 1992; **339:**1–15, 71–85.

9. Pereira H, Pinder SE, Sibbering DM, et al. Pathological prognostic factors in breast cancer. IV: Should you be a typer or a grader? A comparative study of two histological prognostic features in operable breast carcinoma. *Histopathology* 1995; **27:**219–26.

10. International Union Against Cancer, Committee on TNM Classification. *TNM Classification of Malignant Tumors*, 2nd edn. Geneva: International Union against Cancer, 1974.

11. Carter CL, Allen C, Henson DE. Relation of tumor size, lymph node status, and survival in 24,740 breast cancer cases. *Cancer* 1989; **63:**181–7.

12. Rosen PP, Groshen S, Saigo PE, et al. Pathological prognostic factors in stage I (T1N0M0) and stage II (T1N1M0) breast carcinoma: A study of 644 patients with median follow-up of 18 years. *J Clin Oncol* 1989; **7:**1239–51.

13. Moon TE, Jones SE, Bonnadona G, et al. Development and use of a natural history data base of breast cancer studies. *Am J Clin Oncol* 1987; **10:**396–403.

14. Quiet CA, Ferguson DJ, Weichselbaum RR, Hellman S. Natural history of node-negative breast cancer: A study of 826 patients with long-term follow-up. *J Clin Oncol* 1995; **13:**1144–51.

15. Moore MP, Ihde JK, Crowe JP, et al. Inflammatory breast cancer. *Arch Surg* 1991; **126:**304–6.

16. Wong JH, Kopald KH, Morton DL. The impact of microinvasion on axillary node metastases and survival in patients with intraductal breast cancer. *Arch Surg* 1990; **125:**1298–301.

17. Rosner D, Lane WW, Penetrante R. Ductal carcinoma in situ with microinvasion. A curable entity using surgery alone without need for adjuvant therapy. *Cancer* 1991; **67:**1498–503.

18. Solin LJ, Fowble BL, Yeh IT, et al. Microinvasive ductal carcinoma of the breast treated with breast-conserving surgery and definitive irradiation. *Int J Radiat Oncol Biol Phys* 1992; **23:**961–8.

19. Kinne DW, Petrek JA, Osborne MP, Fracchia AA, DePalo AA, Rosen PP. Breast carcinoma in situ. *Arch Surg* 1989; **124:**33–6.

20. de Mascarel I, Bonichon F, Coindre JM, Trojani M. Prognostic significance of breast cancer axillary lymph node micrometastases assessed by two special techniques: reevaluation with longer follow-up. *Br J Cancer* 1992; **66:**523–7.

21. Clayton F, Hopkins CL. Pathologic correlates of prognosis in lymph node-positive breast carcinomas. *Cancer* 1993; **71:**1780–90.

22. Elson CE, Kufe D, Johnston WW. Immunohistochemical detection and significance of axillary lymph node micrometastases in breast carcinoma. A study of 97 cases. *Analyt Quantit Cytol Histol* 1993; **15:**171–8.

23. Byrne J, Horgan PG, England S, et al. A preliminary report on the usefulness of monoclonal antibodies to CA 15-3 and MCA in the detection of micrometastases in axillary lymph nodes draining primary breast carcinoma. *Eur J Cancer* 1992; **28:**658–60.

24. Anonymous. Prognostic importance of occult axillary lymph node micrometastases from breast cancers. International (Ludwig) Breast Cancer Study Group. *Lancet* 1990; **335:**1565–8.

25. Noguchi S, Aihara T, Motomura K, et al. Detection of breast cancer micrometastases in axillary lymph nodes by means of reverse transcriptase-polymerase chain reaction. Comparison between MUC1 mRNA and keratin 19 mRNA amplification. *Am J Pathol* 1996; **148:**649–56.

26. Bloom HJ, Richardson WW. Histological grading and prognosis in breast cancer. *Br J Cancer* 1957; **11:**359–77.

27. Elston CW, Ellis IO. Pathological prognostic factors in breast cancer. I. The value of histological grade in breast cancer: Experience from a large study with long-term follow-up. *Histopathology* 1991; **19:**403–10.

28. Gilchrist KW, Kalish L, Gould VE, et al. Interobserver reproducibility of histopathological features in stage II breast cancer: An ECOG study. *Breast Cancer Res Treat* 1985; **5:**3–10.

29. Dalton LW, Page DL, Dupont WD. Histologic grading of breast carcinoma. A reproducibility study. *Cancer* 1994; **73:**2765–70.

30. Robbins P, Pinder S, de Klerk N, et al. Histological grading of breast carcinomas: a study of interobserver agreement. *Hum Pathol* 1995; **26:**873–9.

31. Henson DE, Ries L. Relationship among outcome, stage of disease and histologic grade in 22,616 cases of breast cancer. *Cancer* 1991; **68:** 2142–9.

32. Toikkanen S, Joensuu H, Klemi P. Nuclear DNA content as a prognostic factor in T1–2N0 breast cancer. *Am J Clin Pathol* 1990; **93:**471–9.

33. Quiet CA, Ferguson DJ, Weichselbaum RR, Hellman S. Natural history of node-negative breast cancer: A study of 826 patients with long-term follow-up. *J Clin Oncol* 1995; **13:** 1144–51.

34. Axelsson K, Ljung B-M, Moore DH, et al. Tumor angiogenesis as a prognostic assay for invasive ductal breast carcinoma. *J Natl Cancer Instit* 1995; **87:**997–1008.

35. Page DL, Ellis IO, Elston CW. Histologic grading of breast cancer. Let's do it. *Am J Clin Pathol* 1995; **103:**123–4.

36. Hillner BE, Smith TJ. Efficacy and cost effectiveness of adjuvant chemotherapy in women with node-negative breast cancer. *N Engl J Med* 1991; **324:**160–8.

37. Albain KS, Allred DC, Clark GM. Breast cancer outcome and predictors of outcome: Are there age differentials? *Monogr Natl Cancer Inst* 1994; **16:**35–42.

38. de la Rochefordiere A, Asselain B, Campana F, et al. Age as prognostic factor in premenopausal breast carcinoma. *Lancet* 1993; **341:**1039–43.

39. Bonnier P, Romain S, Charpin C, et al. Age as a prognostic factor in breast cancer: relationship to pathologic and biologic features. *Int J Cancer* 1995; **62:**138–44.

40. Nixon AJ, Neuberg D, Hayes DF, et al. Relationship of patient age to pathologic features of the tumor and prognosis for patients with Stage I or II breast cancer. *J Clin Oncol* 1994; **12:**888–94.

41. Lee CG, McCormick B, Mazumdar M, Vetto J, Borgen PL. Infiltrating breast carcinoma in patient age 30 years and younger: Long term outcome for life, relapse, and second primary tumors. *Int J Radiat Oncol Biol Phys* 1992; **23:**969–75.

42. Marcus JN, Watson P, Page DL, et al. Hereditary breast cancer: pathobiology, prognosis, and BRCA1 and BRCA2 gene linkage. *Cancer* 1996; **77:**697–709.

43. Fisher B, Redmond C, Fisher ER, et al. Relative worth of estrogen or progesterone receptor and pathologic characteristics of differentiation as indicators of prognosis in node negative breast cancer patients: Findings from National Surgical Adjuvant Breast and Bowel Project Protocol B-06. *J Clin Oncol* 1988; **6:**1076–87.

44. Silvestrini R, Daidone MG, Luisi A, et al. Biologic and clinicopathologic factors as indicators of specific relapse types in node-negative breast cancer. *J Clin Oncol* 1995; **13:**697–704.

45. Arriagada R, Rutqvist LE, Skoog L, et al. Prognostic factors and natural history in lymph node-negative breast cancer patients. *Breast Cancer Res Treat* 1992; **21:**101–9.

46. Berger U, Wilson P, Thethi S, et al. Comparison of an immunocytochemical assay for progesterone receptor with a biochemical method of measurement and immunocytochemical examination of the relationship between progesterone and estrogen receptors. *Cancer Res* 1989; **49:**5176–9.

47. Foekens JA, Portengen H, van Putten WLJ, et al. Prognostic value of estrogen and progesterone receptors measured by enzyme immunoassays in human breast tumor cytosols. *Cancer Res* 1989; **49:**5823–8.

48. Andersen J, Thorpe SM, King WJ, et al. The prognostic value of immunohistochemical estrogen receptor analysis in paraffin-embedded and frozen sections versus that of steroid-binding assays. *Eur J Cancer* 1990; **26:**442–9.

49. Hilsenbeck SG, Ravdin PM, de Moor CA, et al. Paradoxical decrease in prognostic utility as data sets mature: time-dependent lack of proportional hazards in prognostic factors in primary breast cancer. *Breast Cancer Res Treat* 1995; **37:**35.

50. Rutqvist LE. The significance of hormone receptors to predict the endocrine responsiveness of human breast cancer. *Acta Oncol* 1990; **29:**371–7.

51. Ravdin PM, Green S, Melink-Dorr T, et al. Prognostic significance of progesterone receptor levels in estrogen receptor-positive patients with metastatic breast cancer treated with tamoxifen: Results of a prospective Southwest Oncology Group Study. *J Clin Oncol* 1992; **10:**1284–91.

52. Thim L. A new family of growth factor-like peptides. 'Trefoil' disulphide loop structures as a common feature in breast cancer associated peptide (pS2), pancreatic spasmolytic polypeptide (PSP), and frog skin peptides (spasmolysins). *FEBS Lett* 1989; **250:**85–90.

53. Zaretsky JZ, Weiss M, Tsarfaty I, et al. Expression of genes coding for pS2, c-erbB2, estrogen receptor and the H23 breast tumor-associated antigen. *FEBS Lett* 1990; **265:**46–50.

54. Gion M, Mione R, Pappagallo GL, et al. PS2 in breast cancer – alternative or complementary tool to steroid receptor status? Evaluation of 446 cases. *Br J Cancer* 1993; **68:**374–9.

55. Predine J, Spyratos F, Prudhomme JF, et al. Enzyme-linked immunosorbent assay of pS2 in breast cancers, benign tumors, and normal breast tissues. *Cancer* 1992; **69:**2116–23.

56. Foekens JA, Rio MC, Sequin P, et al. Prediction of relapse and survival in breast cancer patients by pS2 protein status. *Cancer Res* 1990; **50:**3832–7.

57. Foekens JA, van Putten WLJ, Protengen H. Prognostic value of PS2 and Cathepsin D in 710 human primary breast tumors: multivariate analysis. *J Clin Oncol* 1993; **11:**899–908.

58. Soubeyran I, Coindre J-M, Wafflart J, et al. Immunohistochemical determination of pS2 in invasive breast carcinomas: A study on 942 cases. *Breast Cancer Res Treat* 1995; **34:**119–28.

59. Thor AD, Koerner FC, Edgerton SM, et al. pS2 expression in primary breast carcinomas: Relationship to clinical and histological features and survival. *Breast Cancer Res Treat* 1992; **21:**111–19.

60. Henry JA, Piggott NH, Mallick UK, et al. pNR-2/pS2 immunohistochemical staining in breast cancer: Correlation with prognostic factors and endocrine response. *Br J Cancer* 1991; **63:**615–22.

61. Cappelletti V, Coradini D, Scanziani E, et al. Prognostic relevance of pS2 status and proliferative activity in node-negative breast cancer. *Eur J Cancer* 1992; **28A:**1315–18.

62. Silvestrini R. Feasibility and reproducibility of the ^{3}H thymidine labelling index in breast cancer. *Cell Proliferation* 1991; **24:**437–45.

63. Silvestrini R, Daidone MG, Luisi A, et al. Biologic and clinicopathologic factors as indicators of specific relapse types in node-negative breast cancer. *J Clin Oncol* 1995; **13:**697–704.

64. Cooke TG, Stanton PD, Winstanley J, et al. Long-term prognostic significance of thymidine labelling index in primary breast cancer. *Eur J Cancer* 1992; **28:**424–6.

65. Courdi A, Hery M, Dahan E, et al. Factors affecting relapse in node-negative breast cancer. A multivariate analysis including the labeling index. *Eur J Cancer Clin Oncol* 1989; **25:**351–6.

66. Tubiana M, Pejovic MH, Koscielny S, et al. Growth rate, kinetics of tumor cell proliferation and long-term outcome in human breast cancer. *Int J Cancer* 1989; **44:**17–22.

67. Hedley DW. DNA flow cytometry and breast cancer. *Br Cancer Res Treat* 1993; **28:**51–3.

68. Hedley DW, Clark GM, Cornelisse CJ, et al. Consensus review of the clinical utility of DNA cytometry in carcinoma of the breast. *Br Cancer Res Treat* 1993; **28:**55–9.

69. Winchester DJ, Duda RB, August CZ, et al. The importance of DNA flow cytometry in node-negative breast cancer. *Arch Surg* 1990; **125:**886–9.

70. Merkel DE, Wichester DJ, Goldschmidt RA, et

al. DNA flow cytometry and pathologic grading as prognostic guides in axillary lymph node-negative breast cancer. *Cancer* 1993; **72:**1926–32.

71. Dressler LG, Eudry L, Gray R, et al. Prognostic significance of DNA flow cytometry measurements in node-negative breast cancer patients: Preliminary analysis of an intergroup study (INT 0076). *J Natl Cancer Inst Monog* 1992; **11:**167–72.

72. Muss HB, Kute TE, Case LD, et al. The relation of flow cytometry to clinical and biologic characteristics in women with node negative primary breast cancer. *Cancer* 1989; **64:**1894–900.

73. Clark GM, Dressler LG, Owens MA, et al. Prediction of relapse or survival in patients with node-negative breast cancer by DNA flow cytometry. *N Engl J Med* 1989; **320:**627–33.

74. Sigurdsson H, Baldetorp B, Borg A, et al. Indicators of prognosis in node-negative breast cancer. *N Engl J Med* 1990; **322:**1045–53.

75. Isola J, Visakorpi T, Holli K, Kallioniemi O-P. Association of overexpression of tumor suppressor protein p53 with rapid cell proliferation and poor prognosis in node-negative breast cancer patients. *J Natl Cancer Inst* 1992; **84:** 1114–19.

76. Ewers S-B, Attewell R, Baldetorp B, et al. Prognostic significance of flow cytometry DNA analysis and estrogen receptor content in breast carcinomas – a 10 year survival study. *Br Cancer Res* 1992; **24:**115–26.

77. Silvestrini R, Daidone MG, Del Bino G, et al. Prognostic significance of proliferative activity and ploidy in node-negative breast cancers. *Ann Oncol* 1993; **4:**213–19.

78. Balslev I, Christennsen BJ, Rasmussen BB, et al. Flow cytometry DNA ploidy defined patients with poor prognosis in node-negative breast cancer. *Int J Cancer* 1994; **56:**16–25.

79. Gerdes J, Schwab U, Lemke H, et al. Production of mouse–monoclonal antibody reactive with a human nuclear antigen associated with cell proliferation. *Int J Cancer* 1983; **31:**13–20.

80. Key G, Peterson JL, Becker MHG, et al. New antiserum against Ki-67 antigen suitable for double immunostaining of paraffin wax sections. *J Clin Pathol* 1993; **46:**1080–4.

81. Brown RW, Allred DC, Clark GM, et al. Prognostic value of Ki67 compared to S-phase fraction in axillary node-negative breast cancer. *Clin Cancer Res* 1996; **2:**585–92.

82. Railo M, Nordling S, von Boguslawsky K, et al. Prognostic value of Ki-67 immunolabelling in primary operable breast cancer. *Br J Cancer* 1993; **68:**579–83.

83. Veronese SM, Gambacorta M, Gottardi O, et al. Proliferation index as a prognostic marker in breast cancer. *Cancer* 1993; **71:**3926–32.

84. Pinder SE, Wencyk P, Sibbering DM, et al. Assessment of the new proliferation marker MIB1 in breast carcinoma using image analysis: associations with other prognostic factors and survival. *Br J Cancer* 1995; **71:**146–9.

85. Gaglia P, Bernardi A, Venesio T, et al. Cell proliferation of breast cancer evaluated by anti-Brd-U and anti-Ki67 antibodies: its prognostic value on short term recurrences. *Eur J Cancer* 1994; **29A:**1509–13.

86. Gasparini G, Boracchi P, Verderio P, Bevilacqua P. Cell kinetics in human breast cancer: comparison between the prognostic value of cytofluorimetric S-phase fraction and that of the antibodies to Ki67 and PCNA antigens. *Int J Cancer* 1994; **57:**822–9.

87. Rudas M, Gnant MFX, Mittlbock M, et al. Thymidine labeling index and Ki67 growth fraction in breast cancer: comparison and correlation with prognosis. *Breast Cancer Res Treat* 1994; **32:**165–75.

88. Siitonen SM, Kallioniemi O-P, Isola NJ. Proliferating cell nuclear antigen immunohistochemistry using monoclonal antibody 19A2 and a new antigen retrieval technique has prognostic impact in archival paraffin-embedded node-negative breast cancer. *Am J Pathol* 1993; **142:**1081–9.

89. Aaltomaa S, Lipponen P, Papinaho S, Syrjanen K. Proliferating-cell nuclear antigen (PC10) immunolabelling and other proliferation indices as prognostic factors in breast cancer. *J Cancer Res Clin Oncol* 1991; **119:**228–94.

90. Sutherland RL, Hamilton JA, Sweeney KJ, et al. Expression and regulation of cyclin genes in breast cancer. *Acta Oncol* 1995; **34:**651–6.

91. Dutta A, Chandra R, Leiter LM, Lester S. Cyclins as markers of tumor proliferation: immunocytochemical studies in breast cancer. *Proc Natl Acad Sci USA* 1995; **92:**5386–90.

92. Zhu X, Mancini MA, Chang KH, et al. Characterization of a novel 350-kilodalton nuclear phosphoprotein that is specifically involved in mitotic-phase progression. *Mol Cell Biol* 1995; **15:**5017–29.

93. Boege F, Andersen A, Jensen S, et al. Proliferation associated nuclear antigen Ki-S1 is identical with topoisomerase II-alpha. *Am J Pathol* 1995; **146:**1302–8.

94. Sampson SA, Kreipe H, Gillet CE, et al. Ki-S1 – a novel monoclonal antibody which recognizes proliferating cells: evaluation of its relationship to prognosis in mammary carcinoma. *J Pathol* 1992; **168**:179–85.

95. Morris ES, Elston CW, Bell JA. An evaluation of the cell cycle associated monoclonal antibody KiS1 as a prognostic factor in primary invasive adenocarcinoma of the breast. *J Pathol* 1995; **176**:55–62.

96. Morisset M, Capony F, Rochefort H. The 52 kDa estrogen-induced protein secreted by MCF7 cells is a lysosomal acidic protease. *Biochem Biophys Res Commun* 1986; **138**:102–9.

97. Rogier H, Freiss G, Basse M-G, et al. Two site immunoenyzmatic assay for the 52 kDa cathepsin D in cytosols of breast cancer tissues. *Clin Chem* 1989; **35**:81–5.

98. Sehadri R, Horsfall DJ, Firgaira F, et al. The relative prognostic significance of total cathepsin D and HER-2/neu oncogene amplification in breast cancer. *Int J Cancer* 1994; **56**:61–5.

99. Foekens JA, van Putten WLJ, Protengen H. Prognostic value of PS2 and Cathepsin D in 710 human primary breast tumors: multivariate analysis. *J Clin Oncol* 1993; **11**:899–908.

100. Namer M, Ramaioli A, Fontana X, et al. Prognostic value of total cathepsin D in breast tumors. *Br Cancer Res Treat* 1991; **19**:85–93.

101. Ferno M, Baldetorp B, Borg A, et al. Cathepsin D, both a prognostic and a predictive factor for the effect of adjuvant tamoxifen in breast cancer. *Eur J Cancer* 1994; **30A**:2042–8.

102. Gion M, Mione R, Pappagallo GL, et al. Biochemical parameters for prognostic evaluation in patients with breast cancer. *Anticancer Res* 1994; **14**:693–8.

103. Janicke F, Schmitt M, Pache L, et al. Urokinase (uPA) and its inhibitor PAI-1 are strong and independent prognostic factors in node-negative breast cancer. *Breast Cancer Res Treat* 1993; **24**:195–208.

104. Granata G, Coradini D, Cappelletti, Di Fronzo G. Prognostic relevance of cathepsin D versus oestrogen receptors in node-negative breast cancers. *Eur J Cancer* 1991; **27**:970–2.

105. Kute TE, Shao L-M, Sugg NK, et al. Cathepsin D as a prognostic indicator for node-negative breast cancer patients using both immunoassays and enzymatic assays. *Cancer Res* 1992; **52**:1–6.

106. Spyratos F, Brouillet J-P, Defrenne A. Cathepsin D: An independent prognostic factor for metastasis of breast cancer. *Lancet* 1989; **327**:115–18.

107. Romain S, Muracciole X, Varette I, et al. La cathepsin-D: un facteur pronostique indepen-dent dans le cancer du sein. *Bull Cancer* 1990; **77**:439–47.

108. Tandon AK, Clark GM, Chamness GC, et al. Cathepsin D and prognosis in breast cancer. *N Engl J Med* 1990; **322**:297–302.

109. Ravdin PM, Tandon AK, Allred DC, et al. Cathepsin D by western blotting and immuno-histochemistry: Failure to confirm correlations with prognosis in node-negative breast cancer. *J Clin Oncol* 1994; **12**:467–474.

110. Isola J, Weitz S, Visakorpi T, et al. Cathepsin D expression detected by immunohistochemistry has independent prognostic value in axillary node-negative breast cancer. *J Clin Oncol* 1993; **11**:36–43.

111. Tetu B, Brisson J, Cote C, et al. Prognostic significance of cathepsin D expression in node-positive breast carcinoma: an immunohisto-chemical study. *Int J Cancer* 1993; **55**:429–35.

112. Kandalft PL, Chang KL, Ahn CW. Prognostic significance of immunohistochemical analysis of cathepsin D in low-stage breast cancer. *Cancer* 1993; **71**:2756–63.

113. Joensuu H, Toikkanen S, Isola J. Stromal cell cathepsin D expression and long-term survival in breast cancer. *Br J Cancer* 1995; **71**:155–9.

114. Hurlimann J, Gebhard S, Gomez F. Oestrogen receptor, progesterone receptor, PS2 ERD5, HSP27, and D in invasive ductal breast carcino-mas. *Histopathology* 1993; **23**:239–48.

115. Eng Tan P, Benz CC, Dollbaum C, et al. Prognostic value of cathepsin D expression in breast cancer: immunohistochemical assess-ment and correlation with radiometric assay. *Ann Oncol* 1994; **5**:329–36.

116. Rochefort H, Cathepsin D in breast cancer: a tissue marker associated with metastasis. *Eur J Cancer* 1992; **28A**:1780–3.

117. Ravdin PM. Evaluation of cathepsin D as a prognostic factor in breast cancer. *Br Cancer Res Treat* 1993; **24**:219–26.

118. Duffy, MJ. Urokinase plasminogen activator and malignancy. *Fibrinolysis* 1993; **7**:295–302.

119. Foekens JA, Schmitt M, van Putten WLJ, et al. Prognostic value of urokinase-type plasmino-gen activator in 671 primary breast cancer patients. *Cancer Res* 1992; **52**:6101–5.

120. Bouchet C, Spyratos F, Martin PM, et al. Prognostic value of urokinase-type plasmino-gen activator (uPA) and plasminogen activator inhibitors PAI-1 and PAI-2 in breast cancers. *Br*

J Cancer 1994; **69**:398–405.

121. Duffy MJ, Reilly D, McDermott E, et al. Urokinase plasminogen activator as a prognostic marker in different subgroups of patients with breast cancer. *Cancer* 1994; **74**:2276–80.

122. Grondahl-Hansen J, Peters HA, van Putten WLJ. Prognostic significance of the receptor for urokinase plasminogen activator in breast cancer. *Clin Cancer Res* 1995; **1**:1079–87.

123. Grondahl-Hansen J, Christensen IJ, Rosenquist C, et al. High levels of urokinase-type plasminogen activator and its inhibitor PAI-1 in cytosolic extracts of breast carcinomas are associated with prognosis. *Cancer Res* 1993; **53**:2513–21.

124. Slamon DJ, Clark GM, Wong SG, Levin WJ, Ullrich A, McGuire WL. Human breast cancer: Correlation of relapse and survival with amplification of the Her-2/neu oncogene. *Science* 1987; **235**:177–82.

125. Slamon DJ, Godolphin W, Jones LA, et al. Studies of the HER-2/neu proto-oncogene in human breast and ovariancancer. *Science* 1989; **244**:707–12.

126. Press MF, Pike MC, Chazin VR, et al. Her-2/neu expression in node-negative breast cancer: direct tissue quantitation by computerized image analysis and association of overexpression with increased risk of recurrent disease. *Cancer Res* 1993; **53**:4960–70.

127. Winstanley J, Cooke T, Murray GD, et al. The long term prognostic significance of c-erbB-2 in primary breast cancer. *Br J Cancer* 1991; **63**:447–50.

128. Paterson MC, Dietrich KD, Danyluk J, et al. Correlation between c-erbB-2 amplification and risk of recurrent disease in node-negative breast cancer. *Cancer Res* 1991; **51**:556–7.

129. Berns EM, Klijn JG, van Putten WL, van Staveren IL, Portengen H, Foekens JA. c-myc amplification is a better prognostic factor than HER2/neu amplification in primary breast cancer. *Cancer Res* 1992; **52**:1107–13.

130. Ali IU, Campbell G, Lidereau R, Callahan R. Lack of evidence for the prognostic significance of c-erbB-2 amplification. *Oncogene Res* 1988; **3**:139–46.

131. Clark GM, McGuire WL. Follow-up study of HER-2/neu amplification in primary breast cancer. *Cancer Res* 1991; **51**:944–8.

132. Tsuda H, Hirohashi S, Shimosato Y, et al. Immunohistochemical study on overexpression of c-erbB-2 protein in human breast cancer: its correlation with gene amplification and long-term survival of patients. *Jpn J Cancer Res* 1990; **81**:327–32.

133. Borg Å, Tandon AK, Sigurdsson H, et al. HER-2/neu amplification predicts poor survival in node-positive breast cancer. *Cancer Res* 1990; **50**:4332–7.

134. Thor AD, Schwartz LH, Koerner FC, et al. Analysis of c-erbB-2 expression in breast carcinomas with clinical follow-up. *Cancer Res* 1989; **49**:7147–52.

135. Lovekin C, Ellis IO, Locker A, et al. c-erbB-2 oncoprotein expression in primary and advanced breast cancer. *Br J Cancer* 1991; **63**:439–43.

136. McCann AH, Dervan PA, O'Regan M, et al. Prognostic significance of c-erbB-2 and estrogen receptor status in human breast cancer. *Cancer Res* 1991; **51**:3296-303.

137. Kallioniemi O-P, Holli K, Visakorpi T, Koivula T, Helin HH, Isola JJ. Association of c-erbB-2 protein over-expression with high rate of cell proliferation, increased risk of visceral metastasis and poor long-term survival in breast cancer. *Int J Cancer* 1991; **49**:650–5.

138. Tanner B, Friedberg T, Mitze M, Beck T, Oesch F, Knapstein PG. c-erbB-2 oncogene expression in breast carcinoma: analysis by S1 nuclease protection assay and immunohistochemistry in relation to clinical parameters. *Gynecol Oncol* 1992; **47**:228–33.

139. Yuan J, Hennessy C, Givan AL, et al. Predicting outcome for patients with node negative breast cancer: a comparative study of the value of flow cytometry and cell image analysis for determination of DNA ploidy. *Br J Cancer* 1992; **65**:461–5.

140. Allred DC, Clark GM, Tandon AK, et al. HER-2/neu in node-negative breast cancer: prognostic significance of overexpression influenced by the presence of in situ carcinoma. *J Clon Oncol* 1992; **10**:599–605.

141. Noguchi M, Koyasaki N, Ohta N, et al. c-erbB-2 oncoprotein expression versus internal mammary lymph node metastases as additional prognostic factors in patients with axillary lymph node-positive breast cancer. *Cancer* 1992; **69**:2953–60.

142. Gusterson BA, Gelber RD, Goldhirsch A, et al. Prognostic importance of c-erbB-2 expression in breast cancer. International (Ludwig) Breast Cancer Study Group. *J Clin Oncol* 1992; **10**:1049–56.

143. Press MF, Pike MC, Chazin VR, et al. Her-

2/neu expression in node-negative breast cancer: direct tissue quantitation by computerized image analysis and association of overexpression with increased risk of recurrent disease. *Cancer Res* 1993; **53**:4960–70.

144. Bianchi S, Paglierani M, Zampi G, et al. Prognostic significance of c-erbB-2 expression in node negative breast cancer. *Br J Cancer* 1993; **67**:625–9.

145. Têtu B, Brisson J. Prognostic significance of HER-2/neu oncoprotein expression in node-positive breast cancer. The influence of the pattern of immunostaining and adjuvant therapy. *Cancer* 1994; **73**:2359–65.

146. Gusterson BA, Gelber RD, Goldhirsch A, et al. Prognostic importance of c-erbB-2 expression in breast cancer. International (Ludwig) Breast Cancer Study Group. *J Clin Oncol* 1992; **10**: 1049–56.

147. Muss HB, Thor AD, Berry DA, et al. c-erbB-2 expression and response to adjuvant therapy in women with node-positive breast cancer. *N Engl J Med* 1994; **330**:1260–6.

148. Benz CC, Scott GK, Sarup JC, et al. Estrogen-dependent, tamoxifen-resistant tumorigenic growth of MCF-7 cells transfected with HER2/neu. *Breast Cancer Res Treat* 1993; **24**:85–95.

149. Wright C, Nicholson S, Angus B, et al. Relationship between c-erbB-2 protein product expression and response to endocrine therapy in advanced breast cancer. *Br J Cancer* 1992; **65**:118–21.

150. Klijn JG, Berns EM, Bontenbal M, Foekens J. Cell biological factors associated with the response of breast cancer to systemic treatment. *Cancer Treat Rev* 1993; **19** (suppl B):45–63.

151. Valverius EM, Bates SE, Stampfer MR, et al. Transforming growth factor alpha production and epidermal growth factor receptor expression in normal and oncogene transformed human mammary epithelial cells. *Mol Endocrinol* 1989; **3**:203–14.

152. Spyratos F, Martin PM, Hacene K, et al. Prognostic value of a solubilized fraction of EGF receptors in primary breast cancer using an immunoenzymatic assay – a retrospective study. *Br Cancer Res Treat* 1994; **29**:85–95.

153. Bolla M, Chedin M, Coonna M, et al. Lack of prognostic value of epidermal growth factor receptor in a series of 229 N0T1/T1 breast cancers with well defined prognostic parameters *Breast Cancer Res Treat* 1994; **29**:265–70.

154. Harris AL, Nicholson S, Sainsbury RC, et al. Epidermal growth factor receptors in breast cancer: Association with early relapse and death, poor response to hormones and interactions with neu. *J Steroid Biochem* 1989; **34**:123–31.

155. Klijn JGM, Look MP, Portengen H, et al. The prognostic value of epidermal growth factor receptor (EGF-R) in primary breast cancer: Results of a 10 year follow-up study. *Br Cancer Res Treat* 1994; **29**:73–83.

156. Toi M, Tominaga T, Osaki A, Tetsuya T. Role of epidermal growth factor receptor expression in primary breast cancer: results of a biochemical study and an immunocytochemical study. *Breast Cancer Res Treat* 1994; **29**:51–8.

157. Gasparini F, Boracchi P, Bevilacqua P, et al. A multiparametric study on the prognostic value of epidermal growth factor receptor in operable breast cancer. *Breast Cancer Res Treat* 1994; **29**:59–71.

158. Newby JC, A'Hern RP, Leek RD, et al. Immunohistochemical assay to epidermal growth factor receptor on paraffin-embedded sections: validation against ligand-binding assay and clinical relevance in breast cancer. *Br J Cancer* 1995; **71**: 1237–42.

159. Archer SG, Eliopoulos A, Spandidos D, et al. Expression of ras p21, p53, and c-erbB-2 in advanced breast cancer and response to first line hormonal therapy. *Br J Cancer* 1995; **72**:1259–66.

160. Nicholson RI, McClelland RA, Finlay P. Relationship between EGF-R, c-erbB-2 protein expression and Ki67 immunostaining in breast cancer and hormone sensitivity. *Eur J Cancer* 1993; **29A**:1018–23.

161. Borg Å, Lennerstrand J, Stenmark-Askmalm M, et al. Prognostic significance of p53 overexpression in primary breast cancer; a novel luminometric immunoassay applicable on steroid receptor cytosols. *Br J Cancer* 1995; **71**:1013–17.

162. Beck T, Weller EE, Weikel W, et al. Usefulness of immunohistochemical staining for p53 in the prognosis of breast carcinomas: Correlation with established prognosis parameters and with the proliferation marker MIB-1. *Gynecol Oncol* 1995; **57**:96–104.

163. Stenmark-Askmalm M, Stal O, Sullivan S, et al. Cellular accumulation of p53 protein: an independent prognostic factor in stage II breast cancer. *Eur J Cancer* 1994; **30A**:175–80.

164. Marks JR, Humphrey PA, Wu K, et al. Overexpression of p53 and HER-3/neu proteins

as prognostic markers in early stage breast cancer. *Ann Surg* 1994; **219**:332–41.

165. MacGrogan C, Bonichon F, de Mascarel I, et al. Prognostic value of p53 in breast invasive ductal carcinoma: an immunohistochemical study of 943 cases. *Breast Cancer Res Treat* 1995; **27**: 95–102.

166. Thor AD, Moore DH, Edgerton SM, et al. Accumulation of p53 tumor suppressor gene protein: an independent marker of prognosis in breast cancers. *J Natl Cancer Inst* 1992; **84**: 845–55.

167. Barnes DM, Dublin EA, Fisher CJ. Immunohistochemical detection of p53 protein in mammary carcinoma. *Hum Pathol* 1993; **24**:469–76.

168. Haerslev T, Jacobsen GK. An immunohistochemical study of p53 with correlations to histopathological parameters, c-erbB-2, proliferating cell nuclear antigen, and prognosis. *Hum Pathol* 1995; **26**:295–301.

169. Domagala W, Striker G, Szadowska A, et al. p53 protein and vimentin in invasive ductal NOS breast carcinoma-relationship with survival and sites of metastases. *Eur J Cancer* 1994; **30A**: 1527–34.

170. Schimmelpenning H, Eriksson ET, Zetterberg A, Auer GU, Association of immunohistochemical p53 tumor suppressor gene protein overexpression with prognosis in highly proliferative human mammary adenocarcinomas. *World J Surg* 1994; **18**:827–33.

171. Lipponen P, Aaltomaa HJI, Syrjanen S, Syrjanen K. p53 protein expression in breast cancer as related to histopathological characteristics and prognosis. *Int J Cancer* 1993; **55**:51–6.

172. Allred DC, Clark GM, Elledge R, et al. Association of p53 protein expression with tumor cell proliferation rate and clinical outcome in node-negative breast cancer. *J Natl Cancer Inst* 1993; **85**:200–6.

173. Rosen PP, Lesser ML, Arroyo CD, et al. p53 in node-negative breast carcinoma: an immunohistochemical study of epidemiologic risk factors, histologic features, and prognosis. *J Clin Oncol* 1995; **13**:821–30.

174. MacGrogan C, Bonichon F, de Mascarel I, et al. Prognostic value of p53 in breast invasive ductal carcinoma: an immunohistochemical study of 943 cases. *Breast Cancer Res Treat* 1995; **36**:71–81.

175. Haerslev T, Jacobsen GK. An immunohistochemical study of p53 with correlations to histopathological parameters, c-erbB-2, prolifer-

ating cell nuclear antigen, and prognosis. *Hum Pathol* 1995; **26**:295–301.

176. Isola J, Visakorpi T, Holli K, Kallioniemi O-P. Association of overexpression of tumor suppressor protein p53 with rapid cell proliferation and poor prognosis in node-negative breast cancer patients. *J Natl Cancer Inst* 1992; **84**: 1114–19.

177. Silvestrini R, Benini E, Daidone G, et al. p53 as an independent prognostic marker in lymph node-negative breast cancer patients. *J Natl Cancer Inst* 1993; **85**:965–70.

178. Domagala W, Striker G, Szadowska A, et al. p53 protein and vimentin in invasive ductal NOS breast carcinoma – relationship with survival and sites of metastases. *Eur J Cancer* 1994; **30A**: 1527–34.

179. Elledge RM, Clark GM, Fuqua SAW, Yu YY, Allred DC. p53 protein accumulation detected by five difference antibodies: Relationship to prognosis and heat shock protein 70 in breast cancer. *Cancer Res* 1994; **54**:3752–7.

180. Caleffi M, Teague MW, Jensen RA. p53 gene mutation and steroid receptor status in breast cancer. *Cancer* 1994; **73**:2147–56.

181. Elledge RM, Fuqua SAW, Clark GM, et al. The role and prognostic significance of p53 gene alterations in breast cancer. *Breast Cancer Res Treat* 1993; **27**:95–102.

182. Elledge RM, Fuqua SAW, Clark GM, et al. Prognostic significance of p53 gene alterations in node-negative breast cancer. *Breast Cancer Res Treat* 1993; **26**:225–35.

183. Peyrat J-P, Bonneterre J, Lubin R, et al. Prognostic significance of circulating antibodies in patients undergoing surgery for locoregional breast cancer. *Lancet* 1995; **345**:621–2.

184. Hockenberry D, Nunez G, Milliman C, et al. Bcl-2 is an inner mitochondrial membrane protein that blocks programmed cell death. *Nature* 1990; **348**:334-6.

185. Silvestrini R, Veneroni S, Daidone MG, et al. The Bcl-2 protein: a prognostic indicator strongly related to p53 protein in lymph node-negative breast cancer patients. *J Natl Cancer Inst* 1994; **86**: 499–504.

186. Leek RD, Kaklaminis L, Pezzella F, et al. bcl-2 in normal human breast and carcinoma, association with oestrogen receptor-positive, epidermal growth factor receptor-negative tumors and in situ cancer *Br J Cancer* 1994; **69**: 135–9.

187. Boise LH, Gonzalez-Garci M, Posterna CE, et al.

bcl-x, a bcl-2-related gene that functions as a dominant regulator of apoptotic cell death. *Cell* 1993; **74**:597–608.

188. Ealovega MW, McGinnis PK, Sumantran VN, et al. bcl-xs gene therapy induces apoptosis of human mammary tumor in nude mice. *Cancer Res* 1996; **56**:1965–9.

189. Bodrug SE, Aime-Sempe C, Sato T, et al. Biochemical and functional comparisons of Mcl-1 and Bcl-2 proteins: evidence for a novel mechanism of regulating Bcl-2 family protein function. *Cell Growth Differ* 1995; **2**:173–82.

190. Oltvai Z, Milliman C, Korsmeyer SJ, Bcl-2 homodimerizes in vivo with a conserved homolog, Bax, that accelerates programmed cell death. *Cell* 1993; **74**:609–19.

191. Krajewski S, Blomqvist C, Fransilla K, et al. Reduced expression of the proapoptotic gene BAX is associated with poor response to combination chemotherapy and shorter survival in women with metastatic breast adenocarcinoma. *Cancer Res* 1995; **55**:4471–8.

192. Lipponen P, Aaltomaa S, Kosma VK, Syrjannen K. Apoptosis in breast cancer as related to histopathologic characteristics and prognosis. *Eur J Cancer* 1994; **30A**:2068–73.

193. Folkman J. Angiogenesis and breast cancer. *J Clin Oncol* 1994; **12**:441–3.

194. Weidner N, Semple JP, Welch WR, et al. Tumor angiogenesis and metastasis-correlation in invasive breast cancer. *N Engl J Med* 1991; **324**:1–8.

195. Gasparini G, Weidner N, Bevilacqua P, et al. Tumor microvessel density, p53 expression, tumor size, and peritumoral lymphatic vessel invasion are relevant prognostic markers in node-negative breast cancer. *J Clin Oncol* 1994; **12**:454–66.

196. Toi M, Inada K, Suzuki H, Tominaga T. Tumor angiogenesis in breast cancer: Its importance as a prognostic indicator and the association with vascular endothelial growth factor expression. *Breast Cancer Res Treat* 1995; **36**:193–204.

197. Axelsson K, Ljung B-M, Moore DH, et al. Tumor angiogenesis as a prognostic assay for invasive ductal breast carcinoma. *J Natl Cancer Inst* 1995; **87**:997–1008.

198. Fox SB, Leek RD, Smith K, et al. Tumor angiogenesis in node-negative breast carcinomas – relationship with epidermal growth factor receptor, estrogen receptor and survival. *Br Cancer Res Treat* 1994; **29**:109–16.

199. Van Hoef MEHM, Knox WF, Dhesi SS, Howell A, Schor AM. Assessment of tumor vascularity as a prognostic factor in lymph node negative invasive breast cancer. *Eur J Cancer* 1993; **29A**: 1141–5.

200. Sittonen SM, Haapasalo HK, Rantala IS, et al. Comparison of different immunohistochemical methods in the assessment of angiogenesis: Lack of prognostic value in a group of 77 selected node-negative breast carcinomas. *Modern Pathol* 1995; **8**:745–52.

201. Loprinzi CL, Ravdin PM, de Laurentiis M, Novotny P. Do American oncologists know how to use prognostic variables for patients with newly diagnosed primary breast cancer? *J Clin Oncol* 1994; **12**:1422–6.

202. Haybrittle JL, Blamey RW, Elston CW, et al. A prognostic index in primary breast cancer. *Br J Cancer* 1982; **45**:361–6.

203. Galea MH, Blamey RW, Elston CE, Ellis IO. The Nottingham prognostic index in primary breast cancer. *Breast Cancer Res Treat* 1992; **22**:207–19.

204. Balslev I, Axelsson CK, Zedeler K, et al. The Nottingham index applied to 9,149 patients from studies of the Danish Breast Cancer Cooperative Group. *Breast Cancer Res Treat* 1994; **32**:281–90.

205. Clark GM, Hilsenbeck SG, Ravdin PM, et al. Prognostic factors: rationale and methods of analysis and integration. *Breast Cancer Res Treat* 1994; **32**:105–12.

206. Clark GM, Hilsenbeck SG, Ravdin PM, et al. Validation of a model that identifies high risk breast cancer patients for clinical trials of intensive therapy. *Proc Annu Meet Am Soc Clin Oncol* 1995; **14**:A69.

207. Koenders P, Beex L, Kienhuis C, et al. Epidermal growth factor in human breast cancer: a prospective study. *Breast Cancer Res Treat* 1993; **25**:21–7.

208. Fox SB, Smith K, Hollyer J, et al. The epidermal growth factor receptor as a prognostic marker: Results of 370 patients and review of 3009 patients. *Breast Cancer Res Treat* 1994; **29**:41–9.

209. Seshadri R, McLeay WRB, Horsfall DJ, et al. Prospective study of the prognostic significance of epidermal growth factor receptor in primary breast cancer. *Int J Cancer* 1996; **69**:23–7.

4

The management of inherited breast cancer risk

James Mackay, Bruce AJ Ponder

CONTENTS • **Background** • **Risk estimation from family history** • **Mammographic screening** • **Genetic testing** • **Options available to mutation carriers** • **Psychological issues** • **Financial and social issues**

There has been public and professional interest in the fact that a proportion of breast cancer has a strong genetic component. This interest has been fanned by the identification and sequencing of strongly predisposing breast cancer susceptibility genes. The result is that there has been a great increase in anxiety coupled with a lack of accurate knowledge. There is a clear need for accurate and effective information to be given to relatives of women with breast cancer. This chapter concentrates on delineating the important concepts the physician needs to get over to relatives of breast cancer patients.

BACKGROUND

In a general practice list of 2000 patients, 50 will have a relative with breast, ovarian or colorectal cancer.[1] Of these 50 individuals, 10 will have a relative who developed breast, ovarian or colorectal cancer under the age of 50. Yet only a small percentage of women who have a relative with these cancers are at significantly increased risk of developing cancer themselves. This is represented diagrammatically in Figure 4.1. All the relatives of breast cancer patients are at slightly increased risk of developing breast

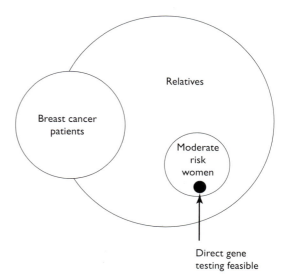

Figure 4.1 Diagrammatic representation of risk for relatives of women with breast cancer. Breast cancer patients are represented by the circle on the left, with their relatives represented by the larger circle. The smaller circle indicates those who are at significantly increased risk of developing breast cancer themselves.

cancer themselves. Among those who are at significantly increased risk of developing breast cancer are a few for whom the recent discovery of two highly penetrant breast cancer susceptibility genes[2,3] may allow genetic testing in the foreseeable future. It is important that a clinician faced with a woman who has a family history of breast cancer has a clear idea of how these circles are defined, in order to place the women seeking advice into the appropriate group. In this chapter we attempt to provide a conceptual framework by which to clarify a woman's risk status. We also suggest appropriate management strategies, although we accept that much of this field has yet to be evaluated.

RISK ESTIMATION FROM FAMILY HISTORY

Several models have now been developed which allow clinicians to predict a woman's risk of developing inherited breast cancer, based on: the number of women in the family with breast cancer;[4–6] the age at which the breast cancer was diagnosed;[7–10] whether the breast cancer is bilateral;[4–11] and several hormonal factors.[12–14] It is possible to refine these models further to give a more precise risk figure. However, several studies have now shown that the accuracy of this risk figure is not reflected in the patient's own perception of her risk.[15–18] In this case, putting a great deal of time and effort into providing a more accurate risk figure may be misplaced.

Defining a set of easily understood criteria to define those at significantly increased risk would probably be more productive. The criteria outlined in Table 4.1 define women who are at approximately three or more times the population risk of developing breast cancer by the age of 50. These correspond to the 'moderate-risk women' in Figure 4.1. The choice of a cut-off at three times the general population risk is of course completely arbitrary and criteria could be established to set the significant risk level at any level. The value of the clinical criteria set out in Table 4.1 is that they allow clinicians to make a relatively accurate estimation of whether a woman is at significantly increased risk, quickly, in the clinic.

Table 4.1   Moderate risk criteria
A woman who has:
1. One first-degree female relative with breast cancer diagnosed under the age of 40 or one first-degree male relative with breast cancer at any age
2. Two first- or second-degree relatives with breast cancer diagnosed under the age of 60 or with ovarian cancer at any age on the same side of the family
3. Three first- or second-degree relatives with breast or ovarian cancer on the same side of the family
4. A first-degree relative with bilateral breast cancer

A first-degree female relative is mother, sister or daughter. A second-degree female relative is grandmother, granddaughter, aunt or niece.

MAMMOGRAPHIC SCREENING

The mortality reduction obtained by offering mammographic screening to the general female population aged over 50 years is between 10% and 30%.[19–24] This has been discussed elsewhere (Chapter 1). Re-analysis of the Swedish Two Counties Study has suggested that a mortality reduction similar to that obtained by the British National Breast Screening Programme (BNBSP) may also be obtained by offering annual mammography to women between the ages of 40 and 50.[25–29] No randomized control trials of mammographic screening have been performed in female populations known to be at a significantly increased risk of developing inherited breast cancer. There has been much debate about the ethics and practicalities of randomized studies in these high-risk populations, with a control group randomized to no mammographic screening. A more practical and acceptable approach may be an observational study in which all those considered at significantly increased risk are offered a research-based, age-related, mammographic screening programme and in which all mammographic, surgical and pathological data are carefully collected. Such a study could be set up in a cohort of women at threefold increased risk by the criteria defined in Table 4.1. These women are seen in the breast clinic, a family history is taken and their risk estimated; those with a significant risk are offered mammographic screening.

Within this cohort there are a small number of women with very strong family histories who are at a much higher risk of developing inherited breast cancer. These individuals come from families in which a strong breast cancer susceptibility gene is likely to be present. We need to identify these families and offer them intervention based on recent molecular genetic advances. Our current arbitrary definition of this group is families with four or more relatives affected with breast and/or ovarian cancer in two to three generations, in which one affected relative is alive and willing to give blood for DNA extraction. These families are seen in the cancer genetics clinic.

GENETIC TESTING

Two strong breast cancer susceptibility genes have now been identified. *BRCA*1 (*br*east *ca*ncer 1), located on chromosome 17q12-21, was identified in 1994.[2,30,31] It is a large gene, with a coding sequence of 5592 base-pairs, encoding a protein of 1863 amino acids. Women with a *BRCA*1 mutation have an 85% risk of developing breast cancer, and an estimated risk between 26% and 65% of ovarian cancer, by the age of 80.[32–34] The second gene, *BRCA*2, is located on chromosome 13q12-13. It is even larger than *BRCA*1, with a coding sequence of 10 254 base-pairs, encoding 3418 amino acids.[3,35,36] *BRCA*1 and *BRCA*2 are between them responsible for most families with four or more women affected with either breast cancer before 60 years of age or ovarian cancer (S Gayther, personal communication; DF Easton, personal communication). The proportion of smaller families, with only two or three affected

members, which are due to *BRCA*1 or *BRCA*2 mutations is still unclear but may be considerably lower.

In the Cancer Genetics Clinic, it is now possible to offer to institute a search for a faulty copy of *BRCA*1 or *BRCA*2 in a family. It is, however, important to realize that such a search is technically demanding and may not produce a useful result. *BRCA*1 and *BRCA*2 are large genes. The mutations tend to differ from family to family, and occur at any point along the length of the gene. Extensive analysis may therefore be needed before a mutation is found; even then, a negative result is no guarantee that no mutation is present. Perhaps 20% of mutations in *BRCA*1 and *BRCA*2 are missed with current techniques.[37] In some families, predisposition is not the result of *BRCA*1 or -2 but of other as yet unidentified genes, which cannot therefore be analysed. Genetic prediction is therefore possible only in the case when a predisposing mutation has been clearly identified in the family, and other family members can be tested to determine whether or not they have inherited it. Failure to find a mutation in the family may mean that no mutation is present and the family history is not caused by inherited predisposition, but this is not a safe conclusion because it may also be that a mutation is present but has not been found. If no mutation is found in the family, genetic prediction is not possible.

For these reasons, genetic testing is currently being offered mostly to families in which there is a high chance of finding a mutation in *BRCA*1 or *BRCA*2. As indicated above, in the authors' clinic testing has currently been restricted to families with four or more relatives affected with breast and/or ovarian cancer in two to three generations and one living affected relative who is willing to give blood. Plans for extending testing to families with less strong family histories of cancer will be made in the light of this experience. Once a faulty copy of *BRCA*1 or -2 has been found in a family, it is possible to offer direct gene testing to unaffected members in that particular family.

Technically, the performance of a direct gene test once the mutation has been found is simple,

Table 4.2 Protocol for *BRCA*1 gene testing	
Step	**Action/Information received**
First interview with cancer geneticist	Risks of developing breast or ovarian cancer
	How a gene test is done
	Implications of a positive result
	Implications of a negative result
	Timing of the test
	Contact name and number
One month later: interview with cancer genetic nurse/associate to discuss	Understanding of implications of testing
	Reasoning behind decision-making
	Knowledge of breast/ovarian cancer
	Understanding of preventive options
	Offer of session with surgeon
Two weeks later: clinic appointment	Blood sample taken
	Appointment for result in 2 weeks
Exactly 2 weeks later: appointment for result	Result given at clinic appointment
	Follow-up plan made to suit
Follow-up plan if a mutation is not present	Discussion about stopping further screening
	Letter sent giving result and offer of appointment for further discussion
Follow-up plan if a mutation is present	Discussion regarding further action and exploration of all options
	Letter sent giving result and explanations about discussion

but the emotional and psychological issues may be quite complex.[38,39] Genetic testing in Huntington's disease has been available for some years.[40] The Huntington's Disease International Consortium has laid down clear and strict guidelines for offering direct gene testing to unaffected individuals.[41] Building on these guidelines[42] we have adopted a modified protocol for breast and ovarian cancer families, which is shown in Table 4.2.

The important points of this protocol are as follows. An initial consultation with a cancer geneticist is made to discuss the possibility of gene testing, the options available to gene carriers, the options available to those shown to be non-carriers, the advantages and disadvantages of entering a testing programme, and the fact that entry into a genetic testing programme remains that individual's absolute choice. This session attempts to provide accurate up-to-date information and to ensure that each individual is aware that there is no compulsion whatsoever to go forward with gene testing. This is important because pressure may often be exerted by relatives. Some time later, the individual is seen by a genetic nurse/associate and, at this consultation, understanding of the information given in the first consultation is checked. The various options are again discussed, and the motivation for going forward with testing explored. This includes understanding and expectations of possible results, the action that the particular individual can take if it is shown that she either does or does not have the mutation, and implications for other family members, e.g. children. It is also important to be clear who should and who should not have access to the test result, for example, the GP or other family members. Once these points are clear, and the individual wishes to proceed, a blood sample is taken with informed consent for a gene test to be performed. A definite appointment is made to give the result in a further face-to-face consultation. Alternatively, if the individual is undecided, further thinking time can be suggested.

OPTIONS AVAILABLE TO MUTATION CARRIERS

As the best management is unclear, it is recommended that, wherever possible, those shown to carry a mutation in one of the highly penetrant breast cancer susceptibility genes should enter a research study. The options include the following:

- Entry into research-based screening programmes, for example, mammography with clinical examination, or other modalities such as magnetic resonance imaging (MRI).
- Entry into trials of experimental drug intervention, for example, the current tamoxifen trial.[43]
- Entry into studies of prophylactic surgery. Research-based mammographic screening programmes have been discussed previously.

A randomized control trial of tamoxifen versus placebo in those at significantly increased risk of developing breast cancer is currently under way and the results are awaited.[43,44]

A cohort of currently unaffected gene carriers is being collected by the International Breast Cancer Consortium for similar prevention studies in the future. Contacts for patient entry to these studies are given at the end of this chapter. The two prophylactic surgery options available are prophylactic bilateral mastectomy and prophylactic oophorectomy. The operation of prophylactic bilateral subcutaneous mastectomy removes a large percentage of the breast tissue, however (depending on the precise nature of the operation), leaving some tissue in the chest wall and some around the nipple.[45–48] There is a risk that breast cancer may develop in the tissue that has been left.[49–51] If a prosthesis has been inserted, it becomes very difficult to offer effective mammographic screening. The actual magnitude of the risk of breast cancer after different types of prophylactic mastectomy is not known and studies to address this question are needed.

Prophylactic oophorectomy is the removal of normal ovaries in order to reduce the risk of ovarian cancer. Some surgeons recommend that total hysterectomy and salpingectomy be done at the same time.[52] An argument for this is that, in younger women, it makes it possible to give hormone replacement therapy with oestrogen alone without risk of endometrial cancer. There have been several well-documented cases of women developing ovarian cancer at considerable time intervals after removal of normal ovaries.[53–55] It is therefore clear that prophylactic oophorectomy does not completely remove the risk of developing inherited ovarian cancer, although it probably reduces it. Accurate figures for reduction of that risk are not yet available and there are several ongoing studies that address this question.

PSYCHOLOGICAL ISSUES

The use of family history information and genetic testing in breast cancer management has the potential for harm from individual anxiety, family disruption, and social effects such as insurance and employability. As a result, psychological evaluation is part of most genetic testing programmes, which initially involve mostly large families in which there are a high number of women affected with breast or ovarian cancer. These families are often very sophisticated with regard to knowledge of genetic research, in which they will often have taken part, of the management of breast cancer and of the shortcomings of mammographic screening. Many of the women in these families have been aware for some time of their familial risk and of the possibility of gene testing, and will have already made up their minds as to which course of action they wish to follow. It is therefore likely that the institution of direct - gene-testing programmes in these families will be possible without great psychological morbidity.[56,57] It is important to remember that the women in these families are very atypical in their knowledge. The application of genetic testing to women without a strong family history and with no previous awareness may well result in considerably greater psychological distress.

The pathway taken by a patient is outlined in Figure 4.2: first consulting the GP, then a familial breast clinic referral and a cancer genetic clinic referral, eventually to being offered a search for a gene 'faulty copy' or mutation in the family, and then a direct gene test.

The first important patient decision is made before going to see the GP. Then the patient goes through the strategy outlined, with some minor decision points along the route, until a mutation search is offered in the cancer genetics clinic. Only if a mutation is found in a consenting affected relative in the family can a direct gene test be offered which involves a further major decision point. In many ways the first part of this journey is similar to the experiences of patients presenting with a history of one of the common medical symptoms, such as breathlessness or haematuria, who end up going down a relatively well-defined investigative and treatment pathway from primary to tertiary care. The second part of this journey is much more unusual because of the major implications for other family members stemming from the mutation search decision point.

Consider the pedigree in Figure 4.3. The arrowed woman comes to the cancer genetics clinic with a significant family history. Her sister, mother and grandmother all developed premenopausal breast cancer. Her maternal aunt developed ovarian cancer. Her sister with breast cancer is willing to give a blood sample for analysis. In the cancer genetics clinic we offer institution of a mutation search. The arrowed individual, the key individual, decides to accept this offer. She may or may not have discussed this with her unaffected sister and her unaffected brother. Her affected sister will be aware of some of the implications of instituting a mutation search, but may not have considered them all. The sister's consent is obtained and there is a delay after the decision has been made, while the laboratory staff search for a mutation in a blood sample from the affected sister, as represented in Figure 4.4. Once a mutation has been identified, suddenly a large number of family members will be faced

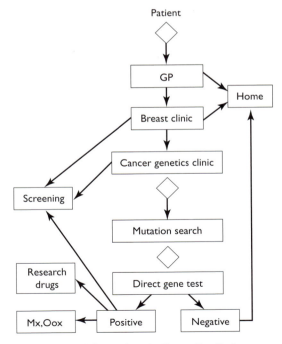

Figure 4.2 Decision points in the patient's journey. ◇, a decision point: Mx, prophylactic mastectomy; Oox, prophylactic oophorectomy.

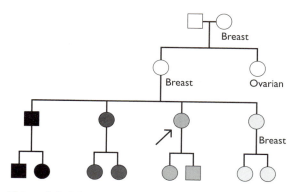

Figure 4.3 A breast/ovarian family pedigree. Key individual arrowed; ■/●, unaffected brother and his offspring, unaffected sister and her offspring; ○, affected individuals.

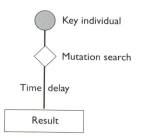

Figure 4.4 The key individual makes a decision to institute a mutation search. ◇, a decision point.

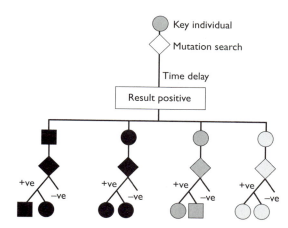

Figure 4.5 A cascade of decision making once the mutation has been found. ◇, decision point; ■/● , unaffected brother and his offspring, unaffected sister and her offspring; ○, affected individuals.

with an important personal decision point, as represented in Figure 4.5.

The key woman has to decide if she wants a direct gene test. If she does have a gene test and she has the mutated copy of the gene, her adult children have to decide if they want a test. Her unaffected sister and brother have to make a decision and, again, if found to have a mutated gene, their children have to make a decision. This cascade effect should be stressed in the consultation before the institution of a mutation search. Another important factor to stress is the length of the time delay. Many of our present laboratory techniques only pick up between 60% and 80% of *BRCA1* mutations and therefore, as mentioned, failure to find a mutation does not allow a clear conclusion. To avoid false reassurance, the current practice in most cancer genetics clinics is to inform family members only once a mutation has been identified. This open-ended time frame may cause considerable anxiety and distress, which could potentially be avoided.[58,59] Research urgently needs to be focused on some of these issues.

FINANCIAL AND SOCIAL ISSUES

In addition to the complicated psychological issues involved in identifying a cohort of individuals at high risk of developing breast cancer, there are a host of financial and social issues to consider. In the USA, two companies are offering *BRCA1* mutation testing to individuals willing and capable of paying for it. These tests are only available through a licensed physician and both companies stress that testing should only be carried out as part of a package including accurate information giving and supportive counselling.[60,61] Any registered physician, without necessarily having had training in cancer or genetics, can access testing. There is concern that the understandable financial incentive to maximize test marketing will result in individuals being tested without the support and information widely regarded to be essential. In the UK, the question of 'over-the-counter' genetic testing is being considered by the Advisory Committee on Genetic Testing. A preliminary report from this Committee,[62] in agreement with recommendations from a working group on cancer and genetic services,[63] has suggested that testing for adult-onset cancer susceptibility genes should not be made available outside the National Health Service (NHS) Specialists' Clinical Genetic Clinics. It is likely that, over the next few years in the UK, *BRCA*1 genetic testing within the NHS will be confined to carefully evaluated research programmes. The private sector may well contribute to the laboratory provision of such tests. The report on cancer and genetics services[63] recommends that testing be provided within a counselling framework. This, however, is encouragement, not legislation. Other countries are actively considering these issues and we are likely to see a variety of legislative and advisory recommendations over the next few years.[64,65]

Testing for disease genes in asymptomatic individuals may well affect the ease with which that individual can obtain life insurance or medical insurance.[39] These issues have already surfaced in several other adult-onset genetic diseases such as Huntington's disease.[66] The present situation in the UK for life insurance to underwrite, for example, a mortgage is that premiums may be increased in those individuals with a family history of cancer. The British Association of Insurers have accepted a moratorium on the use of testing for cancer susceptibility genes in determining life insurance premiums until the situation becomes clearer.[67,68] The Committee on Genetic Testing will also consider this issue in the near future. Any woman thinking of proceeding with genetic testing for *BRCA*1 mutations should be advised before blood has been taken that the result of the test may affect the ease with which she can obtain life or medical insurance in the future. As the pace of identifying genes responsible for many of the other common diseases that reduce life expectancy (such as diabetes, hypertension and ischaemic heart disease) increases, so more and more individuals will be shown to carry genes detrimental to their health. The insurance business will have to reach an equitable solution to a problem encompassing more than the narrow area of

*BRCA*1 testing, but it is likely that considerable time will be needed before such a solution is reached.

Similar broad considerations apply when determining an individual's suitability for certain types of employment for which particular genotypes may be at increased risk. Recent progress in the identification of many genes involved in the pathogenesis of the common diseases will force society to examine these difficult issues.

Even a superficial consideration of the complex issues involved underlines how important it is for there to be vigorous and critical evaluation of programmes that attempt to identify those with strong cancer susceptibility genes. Above all, genetic testing should not be offered to families or individuals without careful attention to the need for them to understand the potential limitations as well as benefits and the range of complex issues involved.

Below are addresses of contact points for the studies being carried out:

- International Breast Cancer Intervention Study (Tamoxifen Study): Claire O'Neil, IBIS Coordinating Centre, PO Box 123, Lincolns Inn Fields, London WC2A 3PX.
- International Breast Cancer Consortium Study:
  UK Contact: Dr Doug Easton, Director CRC Genetic Epidemiology Unit, Institute of Public Health, University Forvie Site, Robinson Way, Cambridge.
  International Contact: Dr David Goldgar, Chief, Unit of Genetic Epidemiology, International Agency for Research into Cancer, 150 cours Albert-Thomas, 69372 Lyon cedex 08, France.

REFERENCES

1. Department of Health. Advances in the genetics of common diseases: implications for the NHS. *Report of a workshop held at Royal Society of Arts in May 1995.* London: Department of Health, 1995.
2. Miki Y, Swevson J, Shattuck-Eidens D, et al. A strong candidate for the breast and ovarian cancer susceptibility gene BRCA1. *Science* 1994; **266:**66–71.

3. Wooster R, Bignell G, Swift S, et al. Identification of the BRCA2 gene. *Nature* 1995; **378:**789–92.

4. Anderson DE. Genetic predisposition to breast cancer: Identification of a high risk group. *Cancer* 1974; **34:**1090–7.

5. Sattin RW, Rubin GL, Webster LA, et al. Family history and the risk of breast cancer. *JAMA* 1985; **253:**1908–13.

6. Mettlin C, Croghan I, Natarajan N, Lane W. The association of age and familial risk in a case-control study of breast cancer. *Am J Epidemiol* 1990; **131:**961–72.

7. Schildkraut JM, Risch N, Thompson WD. Evaluating genetic association among ovarian, breast and endometrial cancer: evidence for a breast/ovarian cancer relationship. *Am J Hum Genet* 1989; **45:**521–9.

8. Houlston RS, McCarter E, Parbhoo S, et al. Family history and risk of breast cancer. *J Med Genet* 1992; **29:**154–7.

9. Goldgar DE, Easton DF, Cannon-Albright LA, Skolnick MH. Systematic population-based assessment of cancer risk in first degree relatives of cancer probands. *J Natl Cancer Inst* 1994; **86:**1600–7.

10. Claus EB, Risch N, Thompson WD. Age of onset as an indicator of familial risk of breast cancer. *Am J Epidemiol* 1990; **131:**961–72.

11. Ottman R, Pike MC, King M-C, Casagrande JT, Henderson BE. Familial breast cancer in population based series. *Am J Epidemiol* 1986; **123:**15–21.

12. Claus EB, Risch N, Thompson WD. Genetics analysis of breast cancer in cancer and steroid hormone (CASH) study. *Am J Hum Genet* 1991; **48:**232–42.

13. Claus EB, Risch N, Thompson WD. Autosomal dominant inheritance of early-onset breast cancer. *Cancer* 1994; **73:**643–51.

14. Gail MH, Brinton LA, Byar DP, et al. Projecting individualised probabilities of developing breast cancer for white females who are being examined annually. *J Natl Cancer Inst* 1989; **81:**1879–86.

15. Evans DGR, Burnell LD, Hopwood P, Howell A. A perception of risk in women with a family history of breast cancer. *Br J Cancer* 1993; **67:**612–14.

16. Evans DGR, Blair V, Greenhalgh R, Hopwood P, Howell A. The impact of genetic counselling on risk perception in women with a family history of breast cancer. *Br J Cancer* 1994; **70:**934–8.

17. Kash KM, Holland JC, Hapler MS, Miller DG. Psychological distress and surveillance behav-iours of women with a family history of breast cancer. *J Natl Cancer Inst* 1992; **84:**24–30.

18. Audrian J, Lerman C, Rimer B, Cella D, Steffens R, Gomez-Caminero A. Awareness of heightened breast cancer risk among first-degree relatives of recently diagnosed breast cancer patients. *Cancer Epidemiology, Biomarkers and Prevention* 1995; **4:**561–5.

19. Shapiro S, Venet W, Strax P, Venet L. Current results of the breast cancer screening randomised trial: The Health Insurance Plan (HIP) of Greater New York Study. In: *Screening for Breast Cancer* (Miller A, Day N, eds). Toronto: Hans Huber, 1988.

20. Tabar L, Fagerberg G, Duffy SW, Day NE, Gad A, Grontoft O. Update of the Swedish two-county programme of mammographic screening for breast cancer. *Radiol Clin North Am* 1992; **30:**187–210.

21. Anderson I, Aspegren K, Janzon L, et al. Mammographic screening and mortality from breast cancer: the Malmo screening trial. *BMJ* 1988; **297:**943–8.

22. Frisell J, Eklund G, Hellstrom L, Lidbrink E, Rutqvist L-E, Somell A. Randomised study of mammography – preliminary report on mortality in the Stockholm trial. *Breast Cancer Res Treat* 1991; **18:**49–56.

23. Alexander FE, Anderson TJ, Muir BB, et al. The Edinburgh randomised trial of breast cancer screening: results after 10 years of follow up. *Br J Cancer* 1994; **70:**542–8.

24. Nystrom N, Rutqvist L-E, Wall S, et al. Breast cancer screening with mammography: overview of Swedish randomised trials. *Lancet* 1993; **341:**973–8.

25. Chen HH, Duffy SW, Tabar L. A Markov chain method to estimate the tumour progression rate from preclinical to clinical phase, sensitivity and positive predictive value for mammography in breast cancer screening. *The Statistician* 1996; **45:**307–17.

26. Duffy SW, Chen HH, Tabar L, Day NE. Estimation of mean sojourn time in breast cancer screening using a Markov chain model of both entry to and exit from the preclinical detectable phase. *Stat Med* 1995; **14:**1531–43.

27. Tabar L, Fagerberg G, Chen HH, et al. Efficacy of breast cancer screening by age: new results from the Swedish two county trial. *Cancer* 1995; **75:**2507–17.

28. Tabar L, Fagerberg G, Chen HH, et al. Tumour development, histology and grade of breast can-

cers: prognosis and progression. *Int J Cancer* 1996; **66:**413–19.

29. Duffy SW, Chen HH, Tabar L, et al. Sojourn time, sensitivity, and positive predictive value of mammography screening for breast cancer in women aged 40–49. *Int J Epidemiol* 1997; in press.

30. Futreal PA, Liu Q, Schattuck-Eidens D, et al. BRCA1 mutations in primary breast and ovarian carcinomas. *Science* 1994; **266:**120–2.

31. Shattuck-Eidens D, McClure M, Simard J, et al. A collaborative survey of 80 mutations in the BRCA1 breast and ovarian cancer susceptibility gene. *JAMA* 1995; **273:**535–41.

32. Easton DF, Bishop DT, Ford D, et al. Genetic linkage analysis in familial breast and ovarian cancer: results from 214 families. *Am J Hum Genet* 1993; **52:**678–701.

33. Easton DF, Ford D, Bishop DT, and the Breast Cancer Linkage Consortium. Breast and ovarian cancer incidence in BRCA1 mutation carriers. *Am Hum Genet* 1993; **56:**265–71.

34. Ford D, Easton DF, Bishop DT, et al. Risks of cancer in BRCA1 mutation carriers. *Lancet* 1994; **343:**692–5.

35. Wooster R, Neuhausen SL, Mangion J, et al. Localisation of a Breast Cancer susceptibility gene, BRCA2 to Chromosome 13q12-13. *Science* 1994; **265:**2088–90.

36. Phelan CM, Lancaster JM, Tonin P, et al. Mutation analysis of the BRCA2 gene in 49 site-specific breast cancer families. *Nature Genetics* 1996; **13:**120–2.

37. Gayther SA, Harrington P, Russell P, et al. Rapid detection of regionally clustered germ-line BRCA1 mutations by multiplex heteroduplex analysis. *Am J Hum Genet* 1996; **58:**451–6.

38. Mackay J, Crosbie AE, Steel CM, Smart GE, Smyth JF. Clinical and ethical dilemmas in familial ovarian cancer. In: *Ovarian Cancer* vol. 4 (Sharp F, Blackett T, Leake R, Berek J, eds). London: Chapman & Hall, 1996:81–90.

39. Collins F. BRCA1 – lots of mutations, lots of dilemmas. *N J Engl Med* 1996; **334:**186–8.

40. Lazarou LP, Meredith AL, Myring JM, et al. Huntington's disease: predictive testing and the molecular genetics laboratory. *Clin Genet* 1993; **43:**150–6.

41. Craufurd D, Tyler A, the UK Huntington's Prediction Consortium. Predictive testing for Huntington's disease: protocol of the UK Huntington's Prediction Consortium. *J Med Genet* 1992; **29:**915–18.

42. Harper P. Ethical issues in genetic testing for Huntington's disease: lessons for the study of familial cancers. *Disease Markers* 1992; **10:**189–93.

43. Powles TJ, Hardy JR, Ashley SE, et al. A pilot trial to evaluate the acute toxicity and feasibility of tamoxifen for prevention of breast cancer. *Br J Cancer* 1989; **60:**126–31.

44. Powles TJ, Jones AL, Ashley SE, et al. The Royal Marsden Hospital pilot tamoxifen chemoprevention trial. *Breast Cancer Res Treat* 1994; **31:**73–82.

45. Wapnir IL, Rabinowitz B, Greco RS. A reappraisal of prophylactic mastectomy. *Surg Gynecol Obstet* 1990; **171:**171–84.

46. Horton CE, Dascombe WH. Total mastectomy: indications and techniques. *Clin Plast Surg* 1988; **15:**677–87.

47. Fisher J, Maxwell GP, Woods J. Surgical alternatives in subcutaneous mastectomy reconstruction. *Clin Plast Surg* 1988; **15:**667–76.

48. Temple W, Lindsay R, Magi E, Urbanski S. Technical considerations for prophylactic mastectomy in patients at high risk for breast cancer. *Am J Surg* 1991; **161:**413–15.

49. Goodnight JE Jr, Quagliana JM, Morton DL. Failure of subcutaneous mastectomy to prevent the development of breast cancer. *J Surg Oncol* 1984; **26:**198–201.

50. Eldar S, Meguid M, Beatty JD. Cancer of the breast after prophylactic subcutaneous mastectomy. *Am J Surg* 1984; **148:**692–3.

51. Ziegler L, Kroll S. Primary breast cancer after prophylactic mastectomy. *Am J Clin Oncol* 1994; **14:**451–4.

52. NIH Consensus Development Panel on Ovarian Cancer. Ovarian Cancer: Screening, treatment and follow-up. *JAMA* 1995; **273:**491–7.

53. Tabacman JK, Tucker MA, Kase R, et al. Intra-abdominal carcinomatosis after prophylactic oophorectomy in ovarian cancer-prone families. *Lancet* 1992; **ii:**795–7.

54. Kemp GM, Hsiu JG, Andrews MC. Papillary peritoneal carcinomatosis after prophylactic oophorectomy. *Gynecol Oncol* 1993; **47:**395–7.

55. Piver MS, Jishi MF, Tsukada Y, Nava G. Primary peritoneal carcinoma after prophylactic oophorectomy in women with a family history of ovarian cancer. A report of the Gilda Radner Familial Ovarian Cancer Registry. *Cancer* 1993; **71:**2751–5.

56. Watson M, Murday V, Lloyd S, et al. Genetic testing in breast/ovarian cancer (BRCA1) families. *Lancet* 1995; **346:**583.

57. Watson M, Lloyds SM, Eeles R, et al. Psychosocial impact of testing (by linkage) for

the BRCA1 breast cancer gene: An investigation of two families in the research setting. *Psycho-oncology* 1996; **5**:233–40.

58. Wiggins S, Whyte P, Huggins M, et al. The psychological consequences of predictive testing for Huntington's disease. *N Engl J Med* 1992; **327**:1401–5.

59. Michie S, McDonald V, Marteau T. Understand responses to predictive genetic testing: a grounded theory approach. *Psychology and Health* 1996; **11**:455–70.

60. Genetic Analysis for Risk of Breast and Ovarian Cancer. *Is it right for you?* Salt Lake City, Utah: Myriad Genetic Laboratories, Inc., 1996.

61. *Hereditary Breast Cancer: Questions and Answers for Physicians.* Gaithersburg, MA: Oncormed, Inc., 1996.

62. Advisory Committee on Genetic Testing. *Draft Consultation Document On 'Over the Counter' Genetic Testing*, 1996.

63. Genetics and Cancer Services. *Report of a Working Group for the Chief Medical Office*, Department of Health. December 1996.

64. Statement of the American Society of Human Genetics on genetic testing for breast and ovarian cancer predisposition. *Am J Hum Gen* 1994; **55**:i–iv.

65. Presymptomatic genetic testing for heritable breast cancer risk. Press release of the National Breast Cancer Coalition. Washington DC, September 28, 1995.

66. Harper PS. Insurance and genetic testing. *Lancet* 1993; **341**:224–7.

67. Nuffield Council on Bioethics. *Genetic Screening Ethical Issues.* London: Nuffield Council on Bioethics, 1993:73.

68. Bowley R. The insurance implications of the new genetics. In: *Report of a Conference on Cancer Genetics.* London: The King's Fund, 1994.

5

Current role of the surgeon in collaborating with medical oncologists

John F Forbes

Although breast cancer has been primarily diagnosed and treated in the past by surgeons, increasingly these steps must involve early collaboration with medical oncologists to ensure optimal outcomes. As distinct from almost every other specialty, breast disease has lacked a medical equivalent to the surgical specialty – as exists, for example, for colon, kidney and lung cancers. This has restricted research to clinical research including clinical trials until recently, because few surgeons were equipped to undertake laboratory studies in breast cancer biology. It has also meant that many patients had their therapy confined to local treatment of the breast alone, with no or late involvement of medical oncologists in patient care.

It is not now acceptable for surgeons to treat breast cancer without consultation with medical oncologists, as this may lead to omission of potentially life-saving adjuvant chemotherapy. This includes many patients once thought to be obtaining an optimal outcome from local breast treatment alone, e.g. patients classified as 'axillary lymph node negative', who until recently did not often have any adjuvant systemic therapy, and postmenopausal patients with 'positive nodes and positive oestrogen receptors (ER)' who have previously been treated with tamoxifen alone as their only adjuvant therapy.

Optimal collaboration between surgical and medical oncologists should be based on an understanding by both of important principles. These include the following:

1. Patients must receive consistent advice from both the surgical and medical oncologist. This dictates that both be closely aware of both surgical and medical oncology treatment programmes, their aims, as well as their limitations, potential benefits and the details of their components, timing and sequencing (Tables 5.1–5.3).
2. As it is impossible for the medical oncologist to attend every consultation with new breast patients, it is essential that effective communication processes be in place. This usually requires full-time, on-site surgeons and medical oncologists.
3. As patients with breast cancer require access to a large number of specialist staff, patients are best treated at a multi-discipline centre. This does not mean that patients must be seen in multi-discipline clinics; these have a role for uncommon problems when there are no clinical trials or treatment protocols, but are not usually beneficial for patients.

Table 5.1 Clinical care policies requiring agreement for effective collaboration: joint policies

Diagnostic investigations to be done:
  On all new patients suspected of having breast cancer
  After breast cancer is confirmed

Pathology reporting:
  Terminology
  Content
  Format of report

Criteria for defining patient risk

Timing of interdisciplinary consultations:
  Preoperative
  After diagnosis
  After definitive surgery

Clinical trial protocols:
  Definition of the patient population
  Eligibility criteria
  Process for queries and consultation
  Responsibility for randomization

Follow-up:
  Who is responsible?
  Investigations and schedule

Table 5.2 Policies requiring multi-discipline understanding for effective collaboration: medical oncology policies

Chemotherapy treatment outside of clinical trials
1. Patient population definition for no routine chemotherapy
2. Definition of group for chemotherapy to be added to tamoxifen
3. Patients requiring special consideration before chemotherapy
4. Details of chemotherapy regimen and schedule to be used
5. Patient definition for high-dose chemotherapy
6. Patient definition for primary chemotherapy
7. Policy and scheduling for tamoxifen and chemotherapy to be used together
8. Policy and schedules for radiotherapy and chemotherapy to be given to the same patient

4. The surgical and medical oncologist musthave complete agreement on criteria for diagnostic assessment, investigations after diagnosis is confirmed, criteria for assessing risk and pathology reporting expectations (Table 5.4). In most cases, treatment plans will initially be addressed by the surgeon – often in response to questions from the patient (see Table 5.3).

Policies may be developed by the surgeons, the medical oncologists or both, but in each case, it is essential that there is understanding by both of all of these policies, which should include:

(a) *Clinical trial protocols* (see Table 5.1): including a clear understanding of eligibility criteria for each current protocol and a readily available and effective query process for checking these. It must also be understood who is responsible for obtaining consent and completing randomization, at which stage of assessment this is permissible, and the policy for follow-up in addition to the postoperative care planned.

(b) *The indications for adjuvant chemotherapy outside of clinical trial protocols* (see Table 5.2):
  (i) patient groups who will not require routine adjuvant chemotherapy, e.g. patients with pure tubular, grade 1, ER-positive tumours, <5 mm in size;

Table 5.3 Policies requiring multi-discipline understanding for effective collaboration: surgical oncology policies

Cytology:

Process for obtaining specimens (methods, personnel)

Indications and agreed limitations, e.g. axillary dissection not done if cytology is the only tissue specimen

Core biopsy:

Indications and agreed limitations

Methods for obtaining specimen (e.g. clinical, ultrasonography, stereotaxis)

Specimen handling and tests to be undertaken on the specimen

Pathology report content

Acceptable core biopsy methods, e.g. Mammotome, ABBI

Protocol if breast cancer is 'removed'

Protocol if core biopsy is negative

Open biopsy:

Indications

Specimen handling, definition of CLE

Definition of clear margins

Policy if status of margins is uncertain

Mastectomy:

Indications for in early disease

Timing of and indications for in advanced disease

Radiotherapy after complete local excision:

Indications for

Timing of delivery if chemotherapy is given

Axillary dissection:

Definition of patient population for not doing axillary dissection, e.g. pure duct carcinoma in situ (DCIS), or very small, grade 1, pure tubular tumours

Extent of axillary dissection

Number of nodes to be examined

Method of processing lymph nodes

Frozen section:

Indications

Agreed limitations and extent of reporting permitted

ABBI, advanced breast biopsy instrument: CLE, complete local excision.

(ii) postmenopausal groups who will be offered adjuvant chemotherapy in addition to or instead of tamoxifen, e.g. 'patients with large (>20 mm), grade 3 or ER-negative tumours';

(iii) patients who require special consideration before chemotherapy,

Table 5.4 Pathology reporting: content

Macroscopic description

Type of specimen and state of delivery, e.g. fresh, ice, formalin

Apparent side and position in the breast

Presence of orientation markers and their type, e.g. clips, sutures

Presence or not of lesions and dimensions

Special features

Microscopic description

Invasive breast cancer

Present or not

Extent and size in two largest dimensions

Type of invasive cancer

Grade of tumour

Relationship of invasive cancer to margins

Presence of vascular (blood vessel and lymphatic) invasion

Duct carcinoma in situ (DCIS)

Present or not

Extent and size in largest dimension, whether within or beyond invasive cancer

Nuclear grade: 1–3

Type of architecture pattern

Whether or not necrosis is present

Calcification: present or absent and type (secretory or necrotic)

Relationship of DCIS to margins

Axillary lymph nodes

Number identified

Number positive

Presence of any special features, e.g. extracapsular spread

Status of margins

Closest distance between cancer and margins

Whether margins are judged to be involved or not

Oestrogen and progesterone receptors

Whether tissue has been taken or not

Result (positive or negative), quantitative result, type of assay

Special assays

Type of assay and result

e.g. pregnant women, patients with compromised hepatic and renal function, and patients with other illnesses or advanced age, e.g. over 80 years;

(iv) the chemotherapy regimen to be given for each important patient subgroup: this may vary from three cycles of oral CMF (cyclophosphamide, methotrexate and 5-fluorouracil), to combinations of doxorubicin and cyclophosphamide or sequential therapy with differing regimens. These have implications for follow-up and the timing of radiotherapy;

(v) the patient population for whom high-dose chemotherapy will be considered and the type of support therapy (peripheral stem cell support or marrow transplant) to be used, e.g. patients with 10 or more positive lymph nodes or at least five positive lymph nodes and a grade 3 or ER-negative tumour;

(vi) the patient group for whom primary chemotherapy will be used and the type of regimen, e.g. patients with advanced local disease; the policy for reviewing response and considering subsequent surgery and radiotherapy must be clear;

(vii) the policy for combining tamoxifen and similar agents with chemotherapy, e.g. sequential or concurrent therapies;

(viii) the policy for delivering both chemotherapy and radiotherapy to the same patient, e.g. chemotherapy first followed by radiotherapy, or 'CMF' given concurrently with radiotherapy. Variations in policy for radiotherapy timing, as a result of the regimen of chemotherapy to be used, also need to be understood by the surgeon.

5. The medical oncologist must have a clear understanding of surgical policies and the basis for and limitations of different treatments (see Table 5.3). These include:

(a) the biological basis of surgery for early breast cancer including the aims, limitations and benefits;

(b) the alternative strategies for obtaining a pathological diagnosis and the components of a complete diagnosis as a basis for treatment planning – including further surgery, radiotherapy and chemotherapy (see Table 5.4);

(c) the alternative steps in treatment and their implications and limitations;

(d) the impact of preoperative and perioperative chemotherapy on surgery and wound healing, in particular the impact of high-dose chemotherapy on surgery;

(e) the questions commonly asked of surgeons by patients and the agreed responses to be given; it is particularly important that questions about prognosis are answered in a comparable manner by both surgeon and medical oncologist;

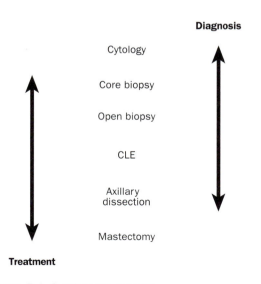

Diagnosis

Cytology

Core biopsy

Open biopsy

CLE

Axillary dissection

Mastectomy

Treatment

Figure 5.1 Surgical procedures.

(f) the changing role of core biopsy and newer surgical procedures and their limitations including, for example, the Mammotome and ABBI core biopsy procedures (Figure 5.1).

Collaboration enhances the effectiveness of both surgical and medical oncologists and the likelihood of patients receiving optimal care. Medical oncologists need to be aware of the role of surgery in diagnosis and treatment of breast cancer to enable collaboration to occur.

THE PRINCIPLES OF LOCAL TREATMENT

Modern surgery for early breast cancer aims to ensure certainty and completeness of diagnosis, complete removal of all local disease, optimal cosmesis and effective multi-disciplinary care. Assessment of axillary lymph nodes remains important for assessment of the risk of systemic disease and the need for systemic therapy. Hence, axillary dissection is important for most women with early breast cancer.

Systemic adjuvant chemotherapy has an established role in improving survival of patients with early breast cancer.[1,2] Local treatments can only treat local disease and are very unlikely to have important effects on survival, because even if local recurrences occur, a lump in the breast on its own is not a fatal illness. The exception would be if a local recurrence was the only disease present and became the source of systemic life-threatening metastasis. Several prospective clinical trials have shown that variations in local treatment – mastectomy, or breast preservation with or without radiotherapy – do not impact on survival. These include trials that have compared different local treatments for invasive breast cancer, mastectomy or breast preservation for ductal carcinoma in situ (DCIS), and the international overviews of trials evaluating radiotherapy as part of the local treatment.[3-11]

The underlying principle is that, after the establishment of a complete diagnosis and completion of breast and axillary surgery, the provision of chemotherapy or other systemic therapy that can control potentially life-threatening distant metastases is a higher priority than local radiotherapy for patient survival.

SURGERY AND THE DIAGNOSIS OF BREAST CANCER

Diagnostic steps may include cytology, core biopsy and open biopsy. Core biopsy is being used increasingly to obtain a preoperative diagnosis of invasive disease. The aim of open biopsy should be to obtain a 'complete local excision' (Table 5.5) as a single surgical step for breast preservation together with axillary dissection in almost all patients. This demands that a diagnosis of invasive breast cancer be obtained preoperatively where possible.

The role of surgery as both a diagnostic and a treatment procedure is undergoing substantial change, and it is important that medical oncologists and patients are aware of the basis of the changes and the limitations of new approaches. This is particularly important when use of pre-operative chemotherapy is considered. New core biopsy approaches, including the Mammotome suction device for rapid, multiple-core biopsies and the advanced breast biopsy instrument (ABBI), using a large-core device, may change core biopsy from a purely diagnostic procedure to, at least partly, a therapeutic procedure. Before widely implementing such new approaches, it is essential that their limitations and advantages are carefully evaluated and understood.[12]

It is essential that a complete pathology diagnosis is available to allow assessment of the probability of metastatic disease being present, assessment of lymph node status and margins and details of the type of tumour, including invasive and in situ components. Oestrogen receptor and progesterone receptor status are important in deciding potential value of chemotherapy and endocrine therapy. This is important for planning whether to give adjuvant chemotherapy, the type of chemotherapy and whether to give postoperative radiotherapy.

A number of special assays may have value

Table 5.5 Steps to ensure a complete local excision (CLE) and complete pathology assessment

Preoperative steps

1. Complete mammography
2. Localization for subclinical lesions
3. Discussion between surgeon and radiologist
4. Discussion with the pathologist if prior core biopsy or excision has been done

Operative steps

1. Review of all relevant radiographs in the operating room
2. Assessment of position, length and direction of the localization device
3. Placement of incision to allow optimal excision, including 1 cm of normal surrounding breast tissue
4. Avoidance of diathermy damage to margins
5. Orientation of the excised tissue by an agreed method
6. Avoid incising the lesion during and after the excision
7. Specify clearly the side of the lesion and the position of the abnormality in the breast
8. Transfer of the specimen for specimen radiographs

Specimen radiograph

1. Complete as a routine on all specimens
2. Avoid specimen compression during the procedure
3. The specimen radiological report is conveyed to the surgeon
4. The specimen and specimen radiographs with the report are transferred to the pathologist

Pathology specimen handling and reporting

1. Margins are marked for identification for microscopic assessment
2. The lesion is identified on the specimen radiographs
3. Specimen slices are cut and labelled
4. Radiographs are taken of the slices
5. Appropriate blocks are taken for pathology reporting
6. Microscopic assessment is completed and reported
7. Particular attention is given to reporting of margins

---

for selecting treatment or for assessing the risk of systemic metastasis. These might include assessment of tumour angiogenesis, breast cancer cells in bone marrow and *c-erbB*-2 expression. If particular specimen-handling requirements are required for a successful assay, it is essential that the surgeon is aware of this. The markers to be used in chemotherapy treatment decisions must be known by the surgeon.

Cytology: advantages and limitations

Medical oncologists will most often use cytology for assessment of possible recurrence of breast cancer. The use of cytology for primary diagnosis and its limitations must also be understood.

Obtaining a cytology sample is usually quick, cheap, well tolerated by patients and, with experienced cytologists, is reliable for detecting the presence of malignant cells. False positives, usually as a result of sampling error, are uncommon. Sensitivity as high as 98% and specificity of 100% have been reported,[13] but false negatives – either for the presence of any malignancy or for the presence of invasion when only 'malignant' cells are identified – are more common. An experienced cytologist may be able to diagnose 'invasion' on a cytology specimen, but this is not a sufficient basis for undertaking an axillary dissection. If a patient has only DCIS, then an axillary dissection is not required because it should be negative except for the small number of patients (1–2%) in whom positive lymph nodes are present – presumably because an invasive focus of disease has been missed. Thus, if cytology is the only preoperative tissue assessment procedure available, it will be difficult for a large number of patients to have a single, definitive operative procedure, because too many will have presurgical doubt as to the presence of invasion and hence whether axillary dissection is required.

Cytology cannot be used for confident diagnosis of a benign lesion, because false-negative results for breast cancer are likely. The exception is a young woman (e.g. in her teens and early 20s) who has a typical fibroadenoma clinically and ultrasonography confirms this. Cytology will detect characteristic bipolar cells and breast cancer can be excluded. Such patients may still require an excisional biopsy, but this will be for patient preference and not for medical reasons.

Cytology can be readily completed for palpable lumps and can be used for impalpable lumps with the aid of stereotactic localization or ultrasonography.

Core biopsy: advantages and limitations

Core biopsy produces a large tissue sample with architectural structure preserved, and can be used to diagnose subclinical lesions.[12] Hence, it can be used for definitive distinction between invasive and in situ disease, and it is an important surgical tool in both a screening programme and clinical practice to reduce the number of open biopsies done for benign disease. False-negative core biopsies can occur through sampling error, and false-negative results will still occur, including sampling errors where no malignant cells are found at all, and also patients in whom only DCIS is diagnosed but who in fact have invasive disease. For small, stellate lesions detected on mammography, for example, a diagnosis of invasive disease on core biopsy allows a single step, including axillary dissection, to be planned with a better informed patient and savings in operating room and hospital bed costs.[12]

Stereotactic large-core biopsy is being developed in the 1990s and includes the use of dedicated, prone biopsy tables, 14-gauge biopsy needles and automatic biopsy guns. Miss rates as low as 2%, with no false-positive results, have been documented in large series using open biopsy as the reference.[14–16] Needle tract seeding of tumour cells is theoretically possible but has rarely been documented.[17] Nevertheless, when cancer is diagnosed, the needle tract should be excised whenever possible during subsequent open biopsy.

Core biopsy can be undertaken by the surgeon for palpable lesions; for lesions more than 2 cm in diameter most can have invasive breast cancer confirmed preoperatively.[18] Increasingly, however, core biopsies are taken by the radiologist using ultrasonography to guide the needle, or by localization using a stereotactic device, digital radiography and a prone table. Many benign lesions can be confidently diagnosed on core biopsy, provided it is clear that the sample has come from the suspicious area of breast. Benign calcification can be diagnosed only if the calcification is seen in the core specimen.[19] If there is doubt about the adequacy of sampling, the patient must be managed as if the core result was not available, and she must subsequently have an open biopsy or an early repeat of mammograms, as appropriate.

Usually five or more core samples are taken when a prone table and stereotactic localization are used, because this reduces the number of false-negative results.[20] More recently, techniques to allow multiple and larger core samples to be taken have been introduced. These also have treatment implications and are discussed below.

Open biopsy and complete local excision

Open breast biopsy may be required for: (1) diagnosis, if this is not completed preoperatively; (2) local treatment of the breast; or (3), depending on the size and type of lesion, both. The aim should usually be complete local excision (CLE), which is a functional procedure, involving critical preoperative and postoperative steps, as well as the surgical procedure on the breast. Although several terms have been used to describe breast tumour excision – lumpectomy, wide excision, quadrantectomy, segmentectomy – all refer to anatomically based surgical procedures which do not encompass the purpose of the procedure or the additional essential steps that are necessary to ensure that the aims are reached. A complete local excision implies that all detectable tumour has been removed from the breast. The most effective and 'complete' local excision is a total mastectomy.

The careful assessment required to determine the completeness of excision involves preoperative, operative and postoperative steps (see Table 5.5). The aim is to assess whether excision margins are likely to be free of tumour and hence whether further surgery is required. When there is doubt as to the completeness of excision, further surgery should be undertaken.

There are few data from prospective, randomized, clinical trials to determine the relevance of involved excision margins and the role of radiotherapy in treating them. Veronesi et al[9,21] reported a clinical trial, from the Milan Cancer Institute, of different extents of local surgery in patients undergoing breast preservation with radiotherapy. A lower local recurrence rate was seen when the breast surgery was a quadrantectomy (5.3%) than when it was a lumpectomy (13.3%). The same group have reported that local recurrence rates are higher when margins are involved (17.4%) than when

they are not (8.6%).[9] Others have reported an increase of local recurrence when margins are involved.[22,23] The treatment of 'involved' margins is not, however, clear cut. Radiotherapy should not be used as an alternative to adequate surgery if there is doubt about the completeness of the excision, because it generates costs and morbidity and is of uncertain value. Surgery removes tumour but compromises the cosmetic result. Further clinical trials are required to evaluate the role of both surgery and radiotherapy in patients with positive margins. Such trials will be of particular importance in defining optimal local treatment for patients who commence their treatment with an 'excisional core biopsy', and this group is likely to increase in size.

Problems with frozen section

Frozen section examination of breast biopsies should not be used often. When mastectomy was the predominant treatment for breast cancer, frozen section was used to confirm a diagnosis before breast removal under the same anaesthetic. This was relatively simple for the pathologist to complete reliably as the specimen was usually large. There were substantial disadvantages of this sequence, however, for the patient, as women did not know preoperatively whether they would wake up with their breast intact or not.

For small lesions detected on mammography, frozen section may compromise the definitive pathology assessment and may be inaccurate in distinguishing between DCIS and invasive breast cancer or between malignancy and some benign lesions. Most patients prefer to know before surgery whether or not mastectomy will occur and will not accept the uncertainty of a single surgical step with 'frozen section and proceed'. The exception might be a lesion that clinically and/or radiologically is overtly malignant and where, in addition, malignant cells are obtained by cytology but a definitive diagnosis of invasion has not been made. The patient can be told that she has breast cancer and that axillary dissection can be completed concurrent with the breast surgery if the frozen section confirms that the breast cancer is invasive during the operation. This allows the surgery to be completed with a single anaesthetic, without any misdiagnosis, and preoperative uncertainty about axillary dissection is not as alarming as uncertainty about mastectomy. If the frozen section is not possible nothing is lost. A second procedure may still be required as would be the case if the frozen section were not done.

SURGERY ISSUES IN THE TREATMENT OF BREAST CANCER

Surgery is important for removal of breast cancer in the breast and for removal of axillary lymph nodes, as part of the assessment of early disease before systemic treatment. It is also essential for diagnostic procedures during follow-up. All such procedures require close collaboration with the medical oncologist.

Local treatment of the breast

Local treatment of the breast can involve surgery with or without radiotherapy. Radiotherapy should not be used as a substitute for adequate surgery because it does not destroy all cancer cells and adds to morbidity and costs. The two procedures that can be used for local treatment of the breast are total mastectomy and CLE. Both procedures aim to remove all of the cancer in the breast and axillary dissection is usually completed with both, i.e. total mastectomy + axillary dissection and CLE + axillary dissection.

Mastectomy
The type of mastectomy that should be completed for early breast cancer is a total mastectomy, i.e. with the intent to remove all breast tissue. Old and ambiguous terms such as radical mastectomy, Halsted mastectomy, Patey mastectomy and 'subtotal' mastectomy should be discarded. Radiotherapy should not be used as a routine for all patients after mastectomy,

because if the surgery is complete there will be no breast cancer cells remaining to be irradiated. No worthwhile survival advantage has been demonstrated and few patients gain advantage in terms of local recurrence. There is evidence that patients having radiotherapy may have a real but small increase in mortality, although this may be confined to node-negative patients.[10,11] There is no established value for routine irradiation of supraclavicular nodes or internal mammary nodes. Radiotherapy can be used for treatment of residual local disease if, for example, a tumour was found to be attached to the pectoral muscle and a subsequent pathology report noted muscular invasion.

Breast preservation
The breast surgery for preservation should aim to be a CLE as discussed previously. This will usually be supplemented by radiotherapy to the residual breast tissue as part of the preservation procedure, i.e. CLE + radiotherapy + CLE, if this is thought to be in the patients' interest, taking into account all relevant factors (see below).

Radiotherapy should not, however, delay the early commencement of chemotherapy which can prolong survival and for which timing is important. The radiotherapy has no impact on survival, and delay in commencement of the radiotherapy, at least for some months after surgery to allow chemotherapy to be completed, does not appear to cause disadvantage in terms of survival or local control.

Recently published results from randomized trials have addressed this issue. The Joint Center for Radiation Therapy in Boston randomized patients with early breast cancer who had a 'substantial risk of systemic metastases', and who were having breast preservation with radiotherapy after their breast surgery, to receive either their cytotoxic chemotherapy followed by radiotherapy or the reverse sequence. The patients who had chemotherapy first had lower rates for recurrence (5-year actuarial rates: 31% vs 38%) and systemic recurrence rates (20% vs 32%, $p = 0.07$), and a higher overall survival rate (81% vs 73%). Hence, if the delay in starting the radiotherapy was important, it was more than compensated for by the early commencement of the chemotherapy.[24]

The second trials addressed timing of radiotherapy in a different way. Two trials of the International Breast Cancer Study Group (IBCSG), studies 6 and 7, included patients who had breast preservation with or without radiotherapy. In study 6, node-positive premenopausal patients were randomized to have 3 or 6 months of chemotherapy and radiotherapy was withheld until chemotherapy was completed (433 patients having breast preservation with radiotherapy). Patients were also randomized to receive an additional late course of three cycles of the same chemotherapy, but all radiotherapy was completed by this time. In study 7, node-positive postmenopausal patients were randomized to receive either tamoxifen alone and no immediate postoperative chemotherapy, or tamoxifen and an initial three postoperative cycles of chemotherapy (285 patients having breast preservation and radiotherapy). Patients having radiotherapy were scheduled to receive it either early postoperatively if no chemotherapy was being given, or after the three cycles of chemotherapy were completed. After 4-years of median follow-up, there was no evidence of any deleterious effect on actuarial total failure rates, systemic recurrence rates or overall survival if the radiotherapy was delayed for 3 or 6 months (study 6), or given early postoperatively or delayed 3 months (study 7).[25]

Hence, if chemotherapy is to be given it should be given before the radiotherapy. If chemotherapy is not going to be given and radiotherapy is planned after surgery for breast preservation, then the radiotherapy should be given soon after surgery because there is no evidence from randomized trials that delay of the radiotherapy is not disadvantageous in the absence of chemotherapy.

There is no established value from randomized trials for a radiotherapy boost of any type, and some of the best results from radiotherapy for breast preservation have been obtained without the use of a boost.[26]

The role of axillary dissection

Both the surgeon and medical oncologist must have the same understanding as to the indications and purpose of axillary dissection. This includes the way in which the status of axillary nodes will be used to determine clinical trial eligibility, how many axillary nodes are ideally to be removed, what the impact of extracapsular spread will be for assessment and possible radiotherapy to the axilla, what the indications will be for axillary dissection for patients who apparently have only DCIS, and whether 'micro-invasion' will be interpreted differently from invasion of nodes. The medical oncologist must also be aware what the surgeon tells the patient in each of these circumstances.

The pathological status of axillary lymph nodes remains the most reliable predictor of prognosis and systemic metastases.[27-30] There is no available test to determine the status of these nodes without removing them for pathological examination. Clinical assessment is unreliable.[18] If nodes are involved, the probability of systemic metastases is sufficiently high for the benefits of chemotherapy to outweigh the side effects of most regimens. If lymph nodes are not involved, it is likely that chemotherapy will not be used unless there is some additional marker of probable systemic metastases, such as a large, grade 3 tumour that is ER-negative.[31] Hence, it is important to know with confidence whether or not nodes are pathologically involved.

It is not possible to have a false-positive result from lymph node assessment. Hence, any involvement, even one positive node, is important for therapeutic decisions. The more nodes involved the poorer the prognosis and, by implication, the greater the risk of systemic metastases. A negative result is, however, partly ambiguous and particularly so if only a small number of nodes are dissected and examined. It has been demonstrated that about eight to ten lymph nodes must be examined before a negative result can be considered very likely to be a true negative result.[32] Careful examination of nodes by serial sections to detect micrometastases, in apparently negative nodes after less stringent examination, can identify patients with a worse prognosis than those who are still node negative after such examination.[33–35]

Removal of the axillary nodes is likely to be responsible for removal of the last residue of regional tumour cells in only a very small number of patients. The procedure should be looked on essentially as a staging and risk assessment procedure.

Axillary dissection causes morbidity in some patients,[36] but this is less if the dissection does not involve a complete removal of all nodes. As 10 or more nodes are sufficient for assessment of involvement, a more complete dissection should not be done unless there is overt macroscopic involvement. Axillary dissection prolongs hospital stay, particularly in patients who are having a CLE rather than mastectomy, because CLE can often be completed as an outpatient procedure. Arm oedema can be troublesome in a small minority of patients, but is detectable in a larger group if routine measurements of the arm are taken. It is probably less common if the axillary vein sheath is not closely dissected. It is substantially more common and troublesome if the axilla is irradiated after surgery of the axilla and this should be avoided except where it might be needed for local control for advanced axillary disease. Paraesthesia persists for some months if the intercostobrachial nerve is divided, and division of the nerve can usually be avoided. Lymph collection may be troublesome for a short period and may require aspiration. It invariably resolves.

Do all patients require an axillary dissection? The procedure is not required if there is no, or a very low (<2–3%), risk of node involvement, or if planned treatment is not dependent on the pathological lymph node status. Patients with pure DCIS should not have a routine axillary dissection. Some patients have extensive high-grade DCIS with associated tumour necrosis and a poor prognosis. Some of these patients may already have foci of invasion and axillary dissection should be considered, because these patients will usually require a mastectomy for treatment of their breast if the disease is extensive. Some patients, for example, those with very small (<5 mm) grade 1, pure tubular carcinoma, have a very low rate of positive glands and may not need routine axillary dissection, but for all tumours of 5 mm or less, axillary node positivity rates as high as 20% have been reported.[37] Patients with invasive tumours that are up to 10 mm or grade 2 or 3 have a node positive rate of 8–20% and should still have routine axillary dissection. The exception might be an elderly patient with a known ER-positive tumour, who might be treated with tamoxifen alone in the first instance after breast surgery, regardless of the status of the axillary nodes. Sentinel node biopsy has not replaced more extensive axillary dissection, but may prove to be valuable for patients who otherwise might not have axillary dissection completed unless there was some evidence of positive nodes, e.g. patients with a small grade 1 tumour.

Breast preservation versus mastectomy: what choice does the patient have?

Whether or not a woman has breast preservation depends on medical, cosmetic, personal and economic issues. In a minority of women, the risk of local recurrence is sufficiently high for mastectomy to be recommended as the best method of local control. A very large tumour in a relatively small breast, multifocal or multiple cancers, and extensive high-grade DCIS involving more than a quarter of the breast are examples where mastectomy is surgically indicated. Invasive lobular cancer has also been a relative indication for mastectomy, although there is some recent evidence that these patients are not compromised by breast preservation. There are few absolutes and some women may still prefer to keep their breast, even knowing that the risk of local recurrence and hence probably subsequent mastectomy to treat the recurrence might be as high as 50%.

If mastectomy is not indicated for surgical reasons (about 20% of patients), a woman can be more involved in the decision to choose either breast preservation or mastectomy. A patient should be made aware of the advantages and disadvantages of each procedure and choose the one that she is most comfortable with. For many women, the decision is not based only on loss of the breast or an increased risk of local recurrence, and provided women are informed and can relate the implications of each procedure to their personal needs then they can have more options. If the relevant issues are clearly discussed, most women will select what they are most comfortable with and understand the implications. They can be supported in their preference by the oncologist.

Women who have a total mastectomy and axillary dissection (AD) as their local treatment (TM + AD) do not gain any survival advantage and they lose their breast. They can usually have a reconstruction, early or later, but they will not have a normal breast. This may be the most important issue for them. They will have a very low rate of local recurrence, but they may have a longer stay in hospital. They will usually not require radiotherapy and hence will avoid the cost and morbidity associated with this.

Women who have breast preservation and axillary dissection with breast radiotherapy (RT) added (CLE + AD + RT) will retain their breast and usually get a good cosmetic result. They will also have a low rate of local recurrence and, hence, a low rate of subsequent surgery and mastectomy. If recurrence occurs, it will be somewhat more difficult to detect both clinically and on a mammogram than if radiotherapy was not given. Core biopsy has improved assessment of possible recurrence over needle cytology, because core biopsy has a high utility in providing a diagnosis for suspicious lesions. The radiotherapy will cause mild morbidity, skin redness, minor arm swelling, tiredness and breast discomfort for some months in a substantial number of patients; substantial morbidity occurs in a much smaller number – radiation pneumonitis (1%), rib fractures (1.8%), sarcoma (rarely), acute inflammation with blistering and ulcers, brachial plexopathy, induced lung and breast cancers (rarely) and cardiac damage.[38,39] The cost of the radiotherapy can be substantial. In one randomized trial it amounted to more than $US100 000 per recurrence prevented and a negative quality-adjusted life years (QUALY)

score in women over 60, who did not have invasive lobular cancer or calcification in their tumour (L Holmberg, 1996, personal communication). Mastectomy is more often required to treat recurrence that occurs in the breast after radiotherapy has been used.

Women who have breast preservation without radiotherapy (CLE + AD) usually obtain a very good cosmetic result, retain their breast and do not have to have radiotherapy. Overall, such patients have a higher rate of local breast recurrence and for many women this may be the most important consideration. However, there is no demonstrable survival disadvantage from avoiding the radiotherapy. If recurrence occurs, it can usually be detected more readily and can often be treated by a further excision without a mastectomy.

Several trials comparing outcome for patients having breast preservation with and without radiotherapy have failed to identify a group of patients uniformly for whom the recurrence rate was not clearly lower with radiotherapy.[4,7,8] In contrast Veronesi et al[9] found no advantage in a randomized trial for radiotherapy in breast preservation, for women over 55 years, in whom the 3-year local relapse rate was 3.8%. Reduction in local relapse rates is not, however, the critical or the only important question for the patient. Medical oncologists have long understood that proportional risk reductions are similar, regardless of risk, and that some patients have a risk of relapse so low that the morbidity and cost of chemotherapy given to reduce it further cannot be justified. Patients also understand this. The question for patients having breast preservation and considering radiotherapy is 'What is their absolute risk of relapse without radiotherapy', noting that whether or not they have radiotherapy will have little or no impact on their cure and survival. Many patients with relapse rates of less than 15–20% may choose not to have radiotherapy. Younger patients in particular should, however, have radiotherapy recommended because of their higher relapse rate, and all patients choosing not to have it should be told of the higher risk of local recurrence in the breast. They should also be reminded that this in itself has not been shown to impact on survival.

Taken together, the two Milan trials, which show an advantage for quadrantectomy over lumpectomy when radiotherapy is given, and the failure to find any advantage for radiotherapy for breast preservation for women over 55, suggest that radiotherapy can be withheld in women aged over 55 if adequate surgery is completed.

Patients must, however, be informed of the relevant issues. The analysis of trade-offs for mastectomy, breast-conserving surgery and breast-conserving surgery plus radiotherapy for women with DCIS illustrates this. Modelling predicts 10-year survival rates of 91.7%, 91.0% and 86.9%, and 20-year survival rates with both breasts preserved of 0.0%, 56.0% and 64.2%, respectively. If survival advantage were the only issue, there would be a small advantage for mastectomy, but quality-adjusted survival favoured mastectomy only if the annual reduction in quality of life were less than 1%. Breast preservation with or without radiotherapy compared with mastectomy traded a very small survival difference for the value of breast preservation.[40] A similar analysis can and should be done for invasive breast cancer. Surgeons and medical oncologists must inform patients of these issues and convey all of the differences between treatment approaches, noting that the costs of treatments will also be an issue.[40]

In the future, some patient selection may be important to avoid cardiac damage from radiotherapy, because even with modern techniques the left anterior coronary artery is still irradiated[38,41] and cardiac damage may be more common if doxorubicin and radiotherapy are used in the same patients.[42] For example, patients who have existing ischaemic heart disease or who need to have doxorubicin, and particularly if younger with a good prognosis and a long survival expectancy, might be better to have a total mastectomy or CLE without radiotherapy. There may, however, also be long-term cardiac damage from doxorubicin.

THE SEQUENCE OF SURGICAL PROCEDURES

An understanding of the steps that may be involved in completing diagnosis and local treatment is important for the medical oncologist. This is particularly so while these procedures and their purpose are changing and because patients may present primarily to the medical oncologist.

If preoperative diagnosis is incomplete

This includes patients who have a diagnosis of cancer but without any distinction between invasive disease and DCIS. For patients for whom a diagnosis has not been completed before surgery, one or two surgical steps may be required. Two steps would involve an initial open biopsy and then definitive local treatment, e.g. open biopsy followed by CLE + AD or M + AD depending on the pathology. The initial biopsy should aim to be a CLE by following the steps in Table 5.5. For some patients who have not been able to complete a preoperative diagnosis but who are very likely, based on their clinical and radiological findings, to have invasive breast cancer, immediate pathology examination may allow the invasive breast cancer to be confirmed, thus avoiding a second surgical procedure. Frozen section examination should rarely be used, however.

If preoperative diagnosis is completed for invasive breast cancer

When the complete diagnosis is known, patients can usually have a single step procedure, e.g. CLE + AD or M + AD. Two steps may still be required in some patients if, for example, margins are thought to be involved, and hence CLE has not been achieved after the first step. A breast re-excision may be required to complete the CLE or, alternatively, this local breast procedure may be converted to a total mastectomy. On occasions, a patient may be so concerned to avoid a mastectomy that a second re-excision, i.e. a third attempt to obtain a CLE, may be done, although this will compromise the cosmetic result.

NEW APPROACHES TO DIAGNOSIS AND TREATMENT

Core biopsy was described in the 1970s for pre-operative diagnosis of palpable breast lumps.[18] More recently, automated firing devices, ultra-sonic guidance, and particularly prone tables with stereotactic localization devices and digital radiography, have all enhanced the use of core biopsy. The large majority of patients can now expect to have a preoperative diagnosis and better planning of their surgery.[12]

During 1996, two additional procedures have been introduced following advances in technology – the Mammotome multiple suction core biopsy (Biopsy Medical, Irvine, CA) and the ABBI device. Both promise to change substantially the way benign and malignant breast pathology are diagnosed and treated. Both also require careful evaluation to find their optimal and safe use.

The Mammotome was developed to obtain multiple core tissue samples with a single insertion of the outer sheath. This device enhances the taking of core biopsies by using a rotating blade to slice rather than chop the specimen off, a suction attachment to ensure that a more complete specimen is removed and a fixed outer sheath to facilitate rapid removal of multiple specimens. As the specimens are removed under radiological control, theoretically, at least, a small lesion could be completely excised. This device is clearly an effective diagnostic instrument. Substantial evaluation is required, with particular and careful assessment of margins on subsequent surgical excision of lesions previously 'excised' by multiple core biopsies. Following proper evaluation, the Mammotome is likely to have a role in diagnosis and removal of small breast cancers, and medical oncologists must remain aware of its status.

The ABBI device removes a large core, at present up to 20 mm. The biopsy requires a dedicated procedure room and a skin incision and closure, and can be carried out by a surgeon who would also be responsible for haemostasis. At present, this device is likely to be of greatest value in diagnosis and plausibly treatment of benign disease. If used to sample or 'remove' a breast cancer, there are likely to be problems with margins and, like the Mammotome, the ABBI device requires very careful and extensive prospective evaluation. Particular attention must be given to assessment of margins after surgical excision of the core biopsy cavity, and assessment of local recurrence rates with longer-term follow-up.

Both of these devices are experimental for tumour removal at present. It is well established that margins are an important determinant of recurrence and radiotherapy should not be used as a substitute for poor surgery when margins are involved. The most important biological message learned from the screening trials is that earlier diagnosis is better and, by implication, there is a time during which breast cancer is totally confined to the breast and is curable by local treatment alone.[43,44] The disease is more curable at this early stage than later. It would be unfortunate if the gains of screening and early diagnosis were eroded by inadequate treatment of early breast cancer by using new, as yet unestablished, core biopsy instruments for treatment. It would be equally unfortunate if potentially valuable new approaches were not properly evaluated to find their best place in diagnosis and perhaps treatment in the future.

If breast cancer can be completely removed as an outpatient procedure and with minimally invasive procedures, then very early systemic therapy can be given without the delays or compromises of surgery. It would also be possible to instil an appropriate chemotherapy agent into the biopsy cavity if this was considered to be potentially advantageous. Laser therapy could also be targeted directly to the tumour site. There are ample new questions to address by appropriate clinical trials.

TIMING OF CHEMOTHERAPY

Primary chemotherapy has become well established for treatment of locally advanced disease and is increasingly being used for smaller and earlier tumours. The theoretical advantages are potential reduction in occult systemic metastases and improved survival, increased breast preservation rates, and use of clinical and pathological response rates as predictors of outcome and for planning of subsequent therapy without knowledge of the nodal status. There are uncertainties about the extent of local control obtained with primary chemotherapy and whether breast preservation can be obtained more often.[45] This will require long follow-up in clinical trials. Uncontrolled data have demonstrated a high rate of breast preservation (90%), even in patients with tumours more than 3 cm in diameter at diagnosis. Careful surgical technique and attention to margins are also important.[46]

Most chemotherapy regimens used for treatment of early breast cancer have been postoperative regimens. This is largely a consequence of the fact that most patients still present first to a surgeon, and diagnosis has been a surgical procedure linked to surgical treatment. This is now changing. A large National Surgical Breast and Bowel Project (NSABP) clinical trial, B-18, randomized patients with early breast cancer to preoperative or postoperative adjuvant chemotherapy. Patients with preoperative chemotherapy had a lower node-positive rate at operation, a higher breast preservation rate and a high tumour response rate of 80%.[47,48] Whether these data will eventually be translated into a better outcome in terms of disease-free survival and overall survival remains to be seen.

It is plausible that a small number of patients will have systemic disease treated more effectively by neoadjuvant chemotherapy, but, for most, the earlier timing of the chemotherapy is probably not very important in the scale of total duration of survival. It is plausible that the surgery has a deleterious effect on the kinetics of tumour growth and that this can be obviated in part by preoperative chemotherapy. This requires longer follow-up to be properly addressed. It is also plausible that, after a good response to primary chemotherapy, breast preservation might safely be completed by radiotherapy alone. This also requires prospective clinical trials for evaluation. Recently, an evaluation of mammography to assess the response to primary chemotherapy was reported. Prediction of pathological response was not possible and five of eight patients with apparent complete clinical response had residual disease; there was no response at all for calcification on mammography.[49]

What is more likely, however, to lead to new evaluations of primary chemotherapy is the use of a core biopsy procedure such as the Mammotome to excise tumours. Chemotherapy could then truly be given from the time of diagnosis with potential for optimal efficacy.

The present treatment of breast cancer is soundly based on clinical trial data – pioneered particularly by Bonadonna, Veronesi, Fisher and Baum – three of these being surgeons. This more than anything else highlights the potential for progress from collaboration between surgical and medical oncologists. Continued commitment world wide to quality clinical trials research will ensure the progress continues.

REFERENCES

1. Bonadonna G, Valagussa P, Moliterni A, Zambetti M, Brambilla C. Adjuvant cyclophosphamide, methotrexate, and fluorouracil in node-positive breast cancer: The results of 20 years follow up. *N Engl J Med* 1995; **332**:901–6.
2. Early Breast Cancer Trialists Collaborative Group. Systemic treatment of early breast cancer by hormonal, cytotoxic, or immune therapy: 133 randomised trials involving 31,000 recurrences and 24,000 deaths among 75,000 women. *Lancet* 1992; **339**:1–15, 71–85.
3. Lichter AS, Lippman ME, Danford DN Jr, et al. Mastectomy versus breast conserving therapy in the treatment of stage I and II carcinoma of the breast: A randomised trial at the National Cancer Institute. *J Clin Oncol* 1992; **10**:901–6.
4. Fisher B, Redmond C. Lumpectomy for breast cancer: an update of the NSABP experience. *J Nat Cancer Inst Mon* 1992; **11**:7–13.
5. Blichert-Toft M, Rose C, Andersen JA, et al. Danish randomised trial comparing breast conservation therapy with mastectomy: six years of lifetable analysis. *J Natl Cancer Inst Mon* 1992; **11**:19–25.
6. van Dongen JA, Bartelink H, Fentiman IS, et al.

Randomised clinical trial to assess the value of breast conserving therapy in stage I and II breast cancer: EORTC 10801 trial. *J Natl Cancer Mon* 1992; **11**:15–18.

7. Liljegren G, Holmberg L, Adami H-O, et al. Sector resection with and without postoperative radiotherapy for stage I breast cancer: five-year results of a randomised trial. *J Natl Cancer Inst* 1994; **869**:717–22.

8. Clark R, McCulloch P, Levine M, Lipa M, Wilkinson R. Randomised clinical trial to assess the effectiveness of breast irradiation following lumpectomy and axillary dissection for node-negative breast cancer. *J Natl Cancer Inst* 1992; **328**:1587.

9. Veronesi U, Luini A, Del Vecchio M, et al. Radiotherapy after breast-preserving surgery in women with localised cancer of the breast. *N Engl J Med* 1993; **328**:1587–91.

10. Cuzick J, Stewart H, Peto R, et al. Overview of randomised trials of postoperative adjuvant radiotherapy in breast cancer. *Cancer Treat Rep* 1987; **71**:15–29.

11. Cuzick J, Stewart H, Rutqvist L, et al. Cause specific mortality in long-term survivors of breast cancer who participated in trials of radiotherapy. *J Clin Oncol* 1994; **12**:447–53.

12. Parker SH, Burbank F. A practical approach to minimally invasive breast biopsy. *Radiology* 1996; **200**:11–20.

13. Hermans J. The value of aspiration cytology examination of the breast: a statistical review of the medical literature. *Cancer* 1992; **69**:2104.

14. Parker SH, Lovin JD, Jobe WE, et al. Stereotactic breast biopsy with a biopsy gun. *Radiology* 1990; **176**:741–7.

15. Parker SH, Burbank F, Jackman RJ, et al. Percutaneous large-core breast biopsy: a multi-institutional study. *Radiology* 1994; **193**:359–64.

16. Liberman L, Dershaw DD, Rosen PP, Cohen MA, Hann LE, Abramson AF. Stereotactic core biopsy of impalpable spiculated breast masses. *AJR* 1995; **165**:551–4.

17. Harter LP, Curtis JS, Ponto G, Craig PH. Malignant seeding of the needle track during stereotaxic core needle breast biopsy. *Radiology*, 1992; **185**:713–14.

18 Hughes LE, Forbes JF. Early breast cancer. Part I: Surgical pathology and pre-operative assessment. *Br J Surg* 1978; **65**:753–63.

19. Liberman L, Evans WP III, Dershaw DD, et al. Radiography of microcalcifications in stereotaxic mammary core biopsy specimens. *Radiology* 1994; **190**:223–4.

20. Liberman L, Dershaw DD, Rosen PP, Abramson AF, Deutch BM, Hann LE. Stereotaxic 14-gauge breast biopsy: how many core biopsy specimens are needed? *Radiology* 1994; **192**:793–5.

21. Veronesi U, Volterrani F, Luini A, et al. Quadrantectomy versus lumpectomy for small size breast cancer. *Eur J Cancer* 1990; **26**:671–3.

22. Solin L, Fowble B, Schultz D, et al. The significance of the pathology margins of the tumour excision on the outcome of patients treated with definitive irradiation for early stage breast cancer. *Int J Radiat Oncol Biol Phys* 1991; **21**:279–87.

23. Schnitt SJ, Abner A, Gelman R, et al. The relationship between microscopic margins of resection and the risk of local recurrence in breast cancer patients treated with conservative surgery and radiotherapy. *Cancer* 1994; **74**:1746–51.

24. Recht A, Steven SC, Henderson CI, et al. The sequencing of chemotherapy and radiation therapy after conservative surgery for early-stage breast cancer. *N Engl J Med* 1996; **334**:1356–61.

25. Wallgren A, Bernier J, Gelber R, et al. Timing of radiotherapy and chemotherapy following breast-conserving surgery for patients with node-positive breast cancer. *Int J Radiat Oncol Biol Phys* 1996; **35**:649–59.

26. Fisher B, Anderson S, Redmond CK, Wolmark N, Wickerman DL, Cronin WM. Re-analysis and results after 12 years of follow-up in a randomised clinical trial comparing total mastectomy with lumpectomy with or without irradiation in the treatment of breast cancer. *N J Engl Med* 1995; **333**:1456–61.

27. Valagussa P, Bonadonna G, Veronesi U. Patterns of relapse and survival following radical mastectomy. *Cancer* 1978; **41**:1170–8.

28. Fisher B, Slack N, Katrych D, et al. Ten-year follow up results of patients with carcinoma of the breast in a cooperative clinical trial evaluating surgical adjuvant chemotherapy. *Surg Gynecol Obstet* 1975; **140**:528–34.

29. Fisher B, Anderson S, Fisher ER, et al. Significance of ipsilateral breast tumour recurrence after lumpectomy. *Lancet* 1991; **338**:327–31.

30. Ferguson D, Meier P, Karrison T, et al. Staging of breast cancer and survival rates: an assessment based on 50 years of experience with radical mastectomy. *JAMA* 1982; **248**:1337–41.

31. Neville AM, Bettleheim R, Gelber RD, et al., for the International Breast Cancer Study Group. Factors predicting treatment responsiveness and

prognosis in node-negative breast cancer. *J Clin Oncol* 1992; **10**:696–705.

32. Axelsson CK, Mouridsen HT, Zedeler K. Axillary dissection of level I and II lymph nodes is important in breast cancer classification. The Danish Breast Cancer Cooperative Group. *Eur J Cancer* 1992; **28A**:1415–18.

33. International Breast Cancer Study Group. Prognostic importance of occult axillary lymph node micrometastases from breast cancer. *Lancet* 1990; **335**:1565–8.

34. Neville AM, Bettelheim R, Gelber RD, Goldhirsch A. Occult axillary lymph-node micrometastases in breast cancer. *Lancet* 1990; **336**: 759.

35. Neville AM, Price K, Gelber RD, Goldhirsch A, for the International Breast Cancer Study Group. Axillary node micrometastases and breast cancer. *Lancet* 1991; **337**:1110.

36. Ivens D, Hoe AL, Podd TJ, et al. Assessment of morbidity from complete axillary dissection. *Br J Cancer* 1992; **66**:136–8.

37. Carter C, Allen C, Henson D. Relation of tumour size, lymph node status, and survival in 24,740 breast cancer cases. *Cancer* 1989; **63**:181.

38. Fuller SA, Haybittle JL, Smith REA, Dobbs HJ. Cardiac doses in post-operative breast irradiation. *Radiother Oncol* 1992; **25**:19–24.

39. Rutqvist LE, Johansson H. Mortality by laterality of the primary tumour among 55,000 breast cancer patients from the Swedish Cancer Registry. *Br J Cancer* 1990; **61**:866–8.

40. Hillner BE, Desch CE, Carlson RW, Smith TJ, Esserman L, Bear HD. Trade-offs between survival and breast preservation for three initial treatments of ductal carcinoma-in-situ of the breast. *J Clin Oncol* 1996; **14**:70–7.

41. Mallik R, Fowler A, Hunt P. Measuring irradiated lung and heart area in breast tangential fields using a simulator-based computerized tomography device. *Int J Radiat Oncol Biol Phys* 1995; **31**:411–17.

42. Valagussa P, Zambetti M, Biasi S, et al. Cardiac effects following adjuvant chemotherapy and breast irradiation in operable breast cancer. *Ann Oncol* 1994; **5**:209–16.

43. Taber L, Fagerberg CJG, Gad A, et al. Reduction in mortality from breast cancer after mass screening with mammography: randomised trial from the Breast Cancer Screening Working Group of the Swedish National Board of Health and Welfare. *Lancet* 1985; **i**:829–32.

44. Taber L, Fagerberg CJG, Gad A, et al. Update of the Swedish two-county program of mammographic screening for breast cancer. *Radiol Clin North Am* 1992; **30**:187–210.

45. Powles TJ, Hickish TF, Makris A, et al. Randomised trial of chemoendocrine therapy started before or after surgery for treatment of primary breast cancer. *J Clin Oncol* 1995; **13**: 547–52.

46. Bonadonna G, Veronesi U, Brambilla C, et al. Primary chemotherapy to avoid mastectomy in tumours with diameters of three centimetres or more. *J Natl Cancer Inst* 1990; **82**:1539–45.

47. Fisher B, Rockette H, Robidoux A, et al. Effect of preoperative therapy for breast cancer (BC) on loco-regional disease: First report of NSABP B-22. *ASCO* 1994; **13**:57.

48. Hyams DM, Mamounas EP, Petrelli N, et al. A clinical trial to evaluate the worth of preoperative multimodality therapy in patients with operable carcinoma of the rectum: a progress report of National Surgical Adjuvant Breast and Bowel Project Protocol R-03. *Dis Colon Rectum* 1997; **40**:131–9.

49. Vinnicombe SJ, MacVicar AD, Guy RZ, et al. Primary breast cancer: mammographic changes after neoadjuvant chemotherapy with pathological correlation. *Radiology* 1996; **182**:333–40.

6

Primary chemotherapy

Ian E Smith, Paul N Mainwaring

Primary chemotherapy for early breast cancer (sometimes referred to as neoadjuvant or preoperative chemotherapy) is a major new development with important implications for the future management of this disease. With this approach, the traditional roles of treatment are reversed and chemotherapy is given as first-line therapy *before* rather than after surgery. Concepts in the management of breast cancer have undergone a fundamental change over the last two or three decades, and primary chemotherapy represents the next logical step in this continuing process.

Surgery as the principal treatment for breast cancer has entirely dominated our approach to management for 100 years, influenced very much by the work and writings of William Steward Halsted, Professor of Surgery at Johns Hopkins University in the last decade of the nineteenth century.[1] Against such deep-rooted tradition, it is difficult to introduce new concepts in treatment. It is of historical interest to note, however, that some of Halsted's predecessors had a healthy scepticism for the limitations of their skill. In a survey of his colleagues' results in 1844, Jean-Jacques Leroy found that 18 of 1192 patients who had not had surgery lived for more than 30 years, whereas only 4 of 804 treated by surgery were alive after a similar interval; his conclusion was that operative treatment was more harmful than beneficial.[2] In 1852 James Paget came to a similar conclusion with the observation that women treated with surgery for scirrhous cancers died on average 13 months earlier than those not given an operation.[3] These cautionary views were submerged in the general enthusiasm for Halsted's advocacy of radical mastectomy. His hypothesis was that cancer spreads centrifugally from the breast into the regional nodes which serve as an initial barrier to the bloodstream. Treatment strategy was consequently surgical removal of the breast *en bloc* with regional nodes and the adjacent pectoralis muscle to prevent cancer spread and achieve cure. Subsequent generations of surgeons interpreted failure of this strategy and the appearance of metastases as a flaw not in the concept itself but in surgical technique.

Grudging acceptance that the hypothesis itself was wrong has come slowly and only within the past 20 years or so. Randomized trials have shown consistently, and without significant exception, that survival and the risk of metastatic recurrence in breast cancer are unrelated to the nature and intensity of local treatment.[4] Long-term follow-up has demonstrated that most patients with so-called early breast cancer eventually develop metastatic disease, irrespective of local treatment. The only reasonable explanation for these clinical observations is that blood-borne micrometastases must have been present at the time of initial clinical diagnosis, albeit undetectable. Modern immunohistochemical staining techniques have indeed now demonstrated microscopic metastases in the bone marrow of many patients with so-called early breast cancer. In other words, for most patients, breast cancer is a systemic disease at the outset and potentially curable only with effective medical therapies in addition to local treatment.

Acceptance of these views has led to two major changes in management. The first is conservative surgery rather than mastectomy for patients with small cancers. The second is the use of adjuvant medical therapy using chemotherapy, endocrine therapy or both, given immediately after surgery, to try to control clinically undetectable micrometastases in patients presenting with early, clinically localized cancer. The established survival benefit of adjuvant medical therapy is discussed in Chapters 7 and 8. An important limitation of this approach is, however, that such treatment is given 'blind', based on a statistical probability of activity but with no certainty that the individual patients' micrometastases are sensitive to the drugs selected.

Primary chemotherapy represents the next step in the management of breast cancer as a systemic disease. Its origins lie in the experience with locally advanced *inoperable* breast cancer, where medical treatment has been increasingly used for many years before local therapy to try to improve local control and prolong survival (see Chapter 9). Interest in primary chemotherapy developed from this starting point and focused, in particular, on the most appropriate management of patients with large but operable cancers, where mastectomy rather than conservative surgery was the only conventional option because of tumour size or central position. The prognosis for such patients is usually poor irrespective of local

treatment[5] and in those circumstances mastectomy is an unattractive option for many women. Such women would generally be offered adjuvant medical treatment anyway on prognostic grounds, and it therefore seemed a logical development to assess the role of medical treatment first; this provides the opportunity for the primary tumour to be used as an in vivo measure of sensitivity to treatment, and also offers the hope that downstaging of the primary might allow mastectomy to be avoided.

CLINICAL RESULTS IN NON-RANDOMIZED STUDIES

Primary chemotherapy in patients with large but operable breast primaries has shown considerable success in terms of response rates, downstaging and avoidance of mastectomy.

Forrest et al[6] and his group in Edinburgh were among the first to report on the use of primary endocrine therapy and/or chemotherapy, emphasizing the potential of the tumour itself as an in vivo measure of response, and their results were updated by Anderson et al.[7] Forty-seven patients received CHOP (cyclophosphamide, hydroxydaunorubicin, vincristine [Oncovin] and prednisone) chemotherapy, either as first-line treatment or following endocrine therapy failure, and of these 34 (72%) achieved 'a significant reduction in tumour volume', including 13 (28%) achieving complete clinical regression and 8 (17%) with no histological evidence of invasive carcinoma in their subsequent mastectomy or wide local excision specimens. No patient showed evidence of tumour progression during treatment with chemotherapy. Initially, at least, this study was not designed to try to avoid mastectomy.

The author's own initial experience with conventional chemotherapy at the Royal Marsden was very similar. Sixty-four patients were treated whose tumours were of sufficient size to require initial mastectomy (median diameter 6 cm) with either CMF (cyclophosphamide, methotrexate and 5-fluorouracil) or MMM (mitomycin C, methotrexate and mitozantrone) chemotherapy and, of these, 44 (69%) achieved an overall objective response of over 50%, including 11 (17%) who achieved complete clinical remissions. Only one patient (2%) had progressive disease on chemotherapy. In the initial part of this study, surgery was left to the discretion of the surgeon; in the second part, surgery was to be avoided where clinically possible; radical breast radiotherapy was used following chemotherapy and only 4 of 49 patients (8%) required a mastectomy.[8]

A major contributor to primary chemotherapy trials has been the Milan Cancer Institute which started a programme in 1988 for patients who would otherwise require radical mastectomy. Their cumulative results have recently been updated.[9] In their first prospective non-randomized study, sequential groups totalling 227 women with breast cancers of diameter over 3 cm (median 4.5 cm) were treated with five chemotherapy regimens based on CMF, anthracycline or mitozantrone-containing combinations, or doxorubicin alone, for three to four cycles. Of the patients 78% achieved an objective response, including 21% who achieved a complete clinical remission. There was no significant correlation between response and drug schedule used or duration of treatment.

In the second study at Milan, started in 1990, 210 patients with tumours over 2.5 cm in diameter (median 4 cm) were treated with doxorubicin alone for three cycles every 3 weeks. Overall response rate was 74% and complete remission rate 12%. In both studies only 3% of patients had tumour progression during treatment.

In these trials subsequent surgery involved conservative quadrantectomy and axillary resection for tumours less than 3 cm at their widest diameter, and modified radical mastectomy for larger or bifocal tumours. In the two studies, 91% and 83%, respectively, of patients were treated with conservative surgery, but only 3% of the resected specimens showed complete pathological remissions (absence of infiltrating or in situ carcinoma). The likelihood of conservative surgery was inversely related to the size of the original tumour; in the two studies the patients whose presenting tumours were less than 4 cm had a 97% and 92% chance of conservative surgery, respectively, compared with 73% and 57% for tumours over 5 cm initially. All patients with a breast-conserving procedure subsequently had radical breast radiotherapy.

French groups were also very active in early studies of primary chemotherapy. Jacquillat et al[10] initiated one of the earliest studies in 1980 with a mixed population of 250 potentially operable and inoperable patients. Primary chemotherapy consisted of vinblastine, thiotepa, methotrexate, 5-fluorouracil and prednisolone; in patients with tumours over 7 cm or locally advanced disease, doxorubicin was also used. There was a variation in treatment details between different patient groups; however, the overall response rate was 75% with 30% achieving complete clinical remission. After primary chemotherapy, radical radiotherapy was given to breast and regional nodes. Salvage mastectomy was required in only 11 patients (4.4%).

Chollet and colleagues have updated their findings of neoadjuvant chemotherapy consisting of doxorubicin (Adriamycin), vincristine, cyclophosphamide, 5-fluorouracil and methotrexate (AVCF ± M) for six cycles in 148 patients with non-inflammatory operable breast cancers of diameter 3 cm or more. The objective response rate was significantly higher after six cycles than after three ($p < 0.001$).[11]

Other groups have reported similar results and these are summarized in Table 6.1. The following are of particular note. Lara and colleagues[12] have reported, in abstract form, 26 patients with stage II–III breast cancer treated with first-line, platinum-based, combination chemotherapy consisting of cisplatin 100 mg/m^2, doxorubicin 50 mg/m^2 and cyclophosphamide 500 mg/m^2 on day 1 every 3 weeks for four cycles. All patients responded and 46% of patients were reported to demonstrate either microscopic or complete pathological remission. Di Blasio and colleagues[13] investigated the role of anthracyclines in a prospective randomized trial comparing CMF chemotherapy with the addition of epirubicin and vincristine (CMFEV). Two hundred and eleven patients with operable breast cancer (stages I and II, and

Table 6.1 Trials of primary chemotherapy
A. Non-randomized trials of primary chemotherapy

Trial	No. of patients	Inclusion criteria	Chemotherapy	Overall response (%)	Complete clinical response (%)	Complete pathological response (%)
Anderson[7]	27 chemo 20 Ctx + endo	≥ 4 cm Operable	CHOP	72	28	17
Jacquillat[10]	250	UICC I–IIIB	VTMFP ± ADX	75 > 75	30	radiotherapy
Choliet[11]	148	≥ 3 cm Operable	AVCMF	97	30	1
Smith[8]	64	≥ 4 cm Operable	CMF/M_1M_2M	67	11	NS
Calais[33]	158	> 3 cm	MVCF/EVCF	61	30	NS
Lara[12]	26	≥ 3 cm	PAC	100	46	15
Smith[15]	50	≥ 3 cm Operable	EC_iF_i	98	33	27
Bonadonna[9]	227	> 3 cm	CMF/FAC/FEC FNC/A	78	21	4
DiBlasio[13]	211	> 2.5 cm	CMF CMFEV	66 74	13 20	1 6

B. Randomized trials of primary chemotherapy

Trial	No. of patients	Inclusion criteria	Chemotherapy	Arm	Overall response (%)	Complete clinical response (%)	Disease-free survival	Overall survival
Mauriac[27]	138	> 3 cm operable	EVM/MTV	Adj	NS	NE	NS	p = 0.04
	134			Neoadj		33		
Scholl[28]	190	3–7 cm	CAF	Adj	65%	NE	NS	p = 0.04
	200			Neoadj		29		
Semiglazov[29]	134	UICC IIb–IIIa	TMF	RTX	57%	6	p = 0.04	NS
	137			CTX/RTX	69%	12		
NSABP	549	Operable	AC	Adj	80%	NE	NS	NS
				Neo-adj		37		
Danforth[30]	16	UICC II	FLAC	Adj	NS	NS	NS	NS

Adj; adjuvant; Neoadj, neoadjuvant; NE, NS, not stated; CTX, chemotherapy; RTX, radiotherapy.

tumours over 2.5 cm, or any tumour with axillary involvement proven on fine-needle aspiration cytology) received four cycles of neoadjuvant chemotherapy. In the CMFEV arm, each of the four drugs was omitted, in rotation, in the subsequent four cycles. In the CMF-only arm, 13% of patients achieved complete clinical remission with an overall response rate of 66%. In the anthracycline-containing arm, 20% of patients achieved complete clinical remission and the overall response rate was 74%. There were no significant differences between the two arms.

NOVEL THERAPIES

Infusional chemotherapy

After the results at the Royal Marsden with conventional chemotherapy, the authors carried out a pilot study using an infusion-based chemotherapy regimen consisting of epirubicin 50 mg/m^2 i.v. and cisplatin 60 mg/m^2 i.v. every 3 weeks, along with infusional 5-fluorouracil 200 mg/m^2 per day via a Hickman line and ambulatory pump, for six cycles. This programme was based on high activity in metastatic/locally advanced breast cancer.[14] Fifty patients with large operable breast cancer with a median tumour diameter of 6 cm (range 3–12 cm), who would normally require a mastectomy, were treated; 49 achieved an overall objective response (98%), including 33 complete clinical remissions (66%). Only three patients (6%) subsequently required mastectomy. As the trial proceeded the need for surgical excision in patients who had achieved complete remission was questioned, and 15 (30%) received no surgery. At the completion of treatment 34 patients had surgical excision of residual tumour or tumour bed and a further seven had a needle biopsy of the tumour bed. Eleven (27%) had a pathologically complete remission. It is possible that the overall complete pathological remission rate could have been higher, given that the best clinical remitters frequently did not have surgery.

In both the conventional and the infusional studies, a repeat needle biopsy of the tumour was carried out 3 weeks after the initial course of chemotherapy where possible, and residual tumour cellularity was scored 'blind'. Tumour cellularity was markedly reduced or absent in 21 of 26 repeat needle biopsies following one course of ECF (epirubicin, cisplatin and infusional 5-fluorouracil) compared with only 9 of 24 biopsies after conventional CMF or MMM (81% versus 36%, $p < 0.002$). A striking feature of the study was not merely the high response rate, but the very high complete clinical remission rate (66%) compared with other published studies[15]. The real success stories in cancer medicine, for example, in lymphomas, testicular cancers and paediatric malignancies, have evolved from novel chemotherapies that result in a high complete remission rate, which is an essential prerequisite for a significant increase in cures. Primary chemotherapy for large breast cancer offers an appropriate clinical model to test this hypothesis in a common epithelial cancer. Currently the authors are carrying out a multicentre randomized trial comparing infusional ECF with a conventional doxorubicin/cyclophosphamide regimen as used in the National Surgical Adjuvant Breast and Bowel Project (NSABP-18) trial (see below). The aims of this trial are to determine whether infusional ECF achieves higher complete remissions than a very active conventional chemotherapy schedule and whether this translates into prolonged survival.

Accelerated chemotherapy with G-CSF

Several groups have explored accelerated chemotherapy with cytokine support. Bernardo et al[16] have reported, in abstract form, on 36 patients treated with accelerated combination chemotherapy consisting of cyclophosphamide 600 mg/m^2 (day 1), epirubicin 65 mg/m^2 (day 1) and 5-fluorouracil 600 mg/m^2 (day 1) at 14-day intervals with granulocyte colony-stimulating factor (G-CSF) support (4–5 µg/kg s.c. on days 7–12). All patients achieved objective clinical response. Conservative surgery could be carried out on 29 patients (80.5%) and radical mastectomy was performed after two additional cycles in seven patients (19.5%). No pathological complete remission of the primary tumour was found. In a pilot study Charrier and colleagues[17] treated 40 women with at least two of the following poor prognostic features:

- tumour >3 cm
- inflammatory signs
- lymph node involvement
- SBR (Steel–Bloom–Richardson) grade III
- aneuploidy
- negative hormone receptors

with a semi-intensive neoadjuvant chemotherapy regimen consisting of THP–doxorubicin 20 mg/m^2 on days 1–3, vinorelbine 25 mg/m^2 on days 1 and 4, and cyclophosphamide 300 mg/m^2 and 5-fluorouracil 400 mg/m^2 on days 1–4 with 29 patients receiving G-CSF or GM-CSF (granulocyte–macrophage CSF) support. Nineteen patients had complete clinical responses (49%) with an overall response rate of 92%. Nine patients (23%) had complete pathological responses and two (5%) others had only in situ carcinoma in the breast.

It is the belief of the authors that primary chemotherapy offers an important test bed for other novel therapies, including new drugs, e.g. the taxoids, or high-dose chemotherapy in patients with high-risk tumours.

SCIENTIFIC RATIONALE FOR A SURVIVAL BENEFIT WITH PRIMARY CHEMOTHERAPY

So far, we have been considering primary chemotherapy principally in larger cancers where the immediate clinical aim is to downstage the tumour and avoid the need for mastectomy. There may also be a potential survival benefit with this approach, at least in theory, because the tumour can be used as an in vivo measurement of sensitivity to treatment with the option of switching to alternative treatment if early clinical response is deemed inadequate. This concept will be discussed in more detail below.

In addition there are, however, other theoretical reasons why preoperative rather than postoperative chemotherapy might improve

survival, irrespective of the initial size of the tumour.

Surgery and subsequent wound healing physiologically stimulate a variety of growth factors which could also promote residual tumour growth. In experimental tumour systems, it has been demonstrated that surgical removal of the primary neoplasm may result in an enhanced rate of growth for the residual metastatic disease. Simpson-Herren and colleagues[18] reported an increase in the thymidine index and growth rate with minimal changes in cell cycle parameters of lung metastases after non-curative resection of a primary, subcutaneous, Lewis lung tumour. Sham surgery also resulted in a reduction in median lifespan and an increase in the thymidine index of the undisturbed primary tumour. Fisher et al[19] showed, in six different tumour host systems, that there was an increase in labelling index of the metastasis 24 hours after removal of the primary tumour; this increase persisted for a variable period of days and resulted in a decrease in tumour doubling time and a measurable increase in tumour size. Further investigation of the underlying mechanism indicated that stimulation of metastatic cell growth after primary tumour removal resulted from a transmissible serum growth factor. When serum obtained from mice after tumour removal was injected intravenously into recipients bearing similar tumours to the donor, kinetic changes occurred which were identical to those observed when a primary tumour was removed. The intriguing feature of these studies was that cyclophosphamide chemotherapy (or tamoxifen or radiotherapy) given before surgery prevented these kinetic alterations, suppressed tumour growth and prolonged survival.[20] Likewise serum from mice treated preoperatively failed to stimulate tumour growth in isologous recipients.

It is well established that a significant minority of women with newly diagnosed breast cancer have immunohistochemically detectable micro-metastases in the bone marrow.[21,22] More recently immunohistochemical methods have demonstrated that around 10% of patients with early breast cancer have circulating micro-metastases within the peripheral blood.[23] The influence of surgery on the incidence of such circulating tumour cells and their long-term clinical significance have not yet been fully assessed. Their identification, however, gives reasonable grounds for concern, and indicates another potential mechanism whereby primary chemotherapy before surgery might be of survival benefit.

A theoretical benefit for primary chemotherapy has been argued based on the Goldie–Coldman hypothesis. This contends that, as a tumour cell population increases, there is an ever-expanding number of drug-resistant phenotypic variants which arise as a result of spontaneous somatic mutations which become increasingly difficult to eradicate.[24] In addition, it has been argued that not only the absolute numbers but also the percentage of resistant cells increase in the total population as the tumour grows; this is because resistant phenotypes multiply not only as a result of their own intrinsic growth rate but also as a consequence of the addition of new mutations from the pool of initially non-resistant cells. With enhanced proliferation of cells after tumour removal it can therefore be argued that the number of resistant phenotypes in the metastatic population will increase. Primary chemotherapy should therefore not only destroy cells made more sensitive by their kinetic alteration but also prevent cell proliferation and a consequent increase in resistant cells.

These arguments are of course hypothetical; the real measure of survival benefit, if any, with primary chemotherapy can only be determined by randomized trials.

PRIMARY CHEMOTHERAPY: RANDOMIZED CLINICAL TRIALS

The largest trial of preoperative chemotherapy in the treatment of early breast cancer was instituted in October 1988 by the NSABP Protocol B-18. In this trial 1523 patients with operable breast cancer of any size (T1–T3) in whom the diagnosis had been established by fine-needle aspiration cytology were stratified by age, clinical tumour size and clinical nodal status, either to surgery as appropriate followed by four courses of AC (doxorubicin/Adriamycin 60 mg/m^2, cyclophosphamide 600 mg/m^2) chemotherapy every 21 days or to the same chemotherapy given preoperatively followed by surgery as appropriate. Strikingly, over 70% of patients in this trial had tumours that were 2 cm or over in diameter. No survival data are available so far but preliminary results have shown that preoperative AC chemotherapy achieved an objective response in 80% of patients, with 37% achieving a complete clinical remission.[25] Complete remissions were more common in small tumours of 2 cm or more (50%) than in larger tumours of 2.1–4 cm (38%), and in tumours over 4 cm (18%). Limited surgery was carried out in 57% of patients receiving postoperative chemotherapy compared with 81% of patients receiving primary chemotherapy who achieved a complete remission, 61% of those who achieved a partial response and 50% of patients with stable or progressive disease. There was some downstaging of axillary nodal status with 41% of patients with involved axillary nodes after preoperative chemotherapy compared with 58% of those in the adjuvant group.

In a Royal Marsden trial, 212 patients were randomized to receive either adjuvant or primary combined chemotherapy and endocrine therapy (mitozantrone and methotrexate with tamoxifen) given for 3 months before and 3 months after surgery (primary arm) or after surgery (conventional adjuvant arm). It is of note that more than 50% of patients entered had initial tumours less than 3 cm in diameter. The overall objective response rate to primary chemoendocrine therapy was 85%, with 19% achieving a complete clinical remission and 30% only minimal residual nodularity after treatment. Complete pathological response rate was 10%. This trial confirmed, on a randomized basis, that the requirement for mastectomy was significantly reduced and was used in 13% of patients receiving primary chemotherapy compared with 28% in those receiving adjuvant therapy ($p < 0.005$). With a median follow-up of 28 months, only four patients have so far relapsed locally and 20 have developed metastatic disease.[26]

Three randomized trials of preoperative chemotherapy have so far published survival data. The first was started by Mauriac et al[27] in 1985; 272 evaluable patients were randomized either to mastectomy with axillary dissection followed by adjuvant chemotherapy or to primary chemotherapy using three cycles of epirubicin, vincristine and methotrexate, followed by a further three cycles of mitomycin C, thiotepa and vindesine in patients with breast cancers over 3 cm in diameter. Patients in the surgical arm with histologically involved axillary nodes or with negative oestrogen receptors were treated with adjuvant chemotherapy using the same drug schedule. Locoregional treatment in the patients receiving primary chemotherapy involved radiotherapy alone in patients achieving complete remission (33%), conservative surgery followed by radiotherapy in patients with residual tumours smaller than 2 cm (30%), and radical mastectomy in the remaining patients (37%). With 34 months of median follow-up (range 8–58 months) there was a trend for recurrence-free survival in favour of the primary chemotherapy arm ($p = 0.05$) and a survival benefit for patients receiving primary chemotherapy just reached statistical significance ($p = 0.04$). A larger proportion of patients received optimal chemotherapy; in terms of timing and dosage in the primary chemotherapy arm. Clinical tumour reduction was demonstrated to be superior in oestrogen receptor (ER)-negative tumours than ER-positive tumours ($p = 0.01$); however, patients who recurred after conservative therapy more often had ER-negative tumours.

In another French trial, Scholl et al[28] reported on 414 premenopausal patients with T2–T3 operable breast cancer randomized to receive either four courses of primary chemotherapy (cyclophosphamide, doxorubicin and 5-fluorouracil), followed by locoregional treatment, or locoregional treatment followed by four cycles of equivalent adjuvant chemotherapy. In the French tradition, locoregional treatment usually consisted of very radical radiotherapy (54 Gy with a boost to 75–80 Gy for responders) followed by surgery if persistent tumour was detected. At a median follow-up of 54 months,

a statistically significant survival difference was reported in favour of the primary chemotherapy group (86% versus 78% 5-year survival, $p = 0.04$), with a similar non-significant trend in favour of metastatic disease-free rates (73% versus 68%, $p = 0.09$). Sixty-five per cent of patients had an objective clinical response after four cycles of chemotherapy. The 5-year actuarial local control rates were 73% for primary versus 81% for postoperative adjuvant chemotherapy (no significant difference). The authors note, however, that patients in the neoadjuvant group received 80.6% of the planned doxorubicin dose whereas patients in the adjuvant arm received 77.6% of the planned dose ($p = 0.02$). A subsequent update of this trial, not yet published, has no longer indicated a survival difference.

In a Russian trial[29] from 1985 to 1990, 271 patients with operable breast cancer (stage IIB–IIIA) were randomized to receive either combination chemotherapy consisting of thiotepa 20 mg i.m. on days 1, 3, 5, 7, 9 and 11, methotrexate 40 mg/m^2 i.v. on days 1 and 8, and 5-fluorouracil 500 mg/m^2 i.v. on days 1 and 8 (TMF regimen), for one to two cycles plus radiotherapy, or preoperative radiotherapy alone. After preoperative treatment all patients underwent mastectomy and complete axillary lymph node resection, followed by four to six courses of TMF according to the number of courses received preoperatively. In the chemotherapy plus radiotherapy arm, 69% of patients responded with 12% complete clinical responses and 29% complete pathological responses. In the radiotherapy-only arm, 57% of patients responded with 6% complete clinical responses and 19% complete pathological responses. There was no significant difference in overall survival (86% versus 78% respectively), but the authors report a difference in 5-year disease-free survival of 81% in the chemotherapy plus radiotherapy arm and 72% in the radiotherapy-only arm ($p = 0.04$).

In 1990, Danforth and colleagues[30] initiated a prospective randomized trial comparing dose-intensive chemotherapy given either preoperatively or postoperatively to patients with stage II breast cancer. The chemotherapy consisted of five 21-day cycles of 5-fluorouracil (400 mg/m^2 on days 1–3), folinic acid (500 mg/m^2 on days 1–3, doxorubicin (15 mg/m^2 on days 1–3) and cyclophosphamide (600 mg/m^2 on day 1) (FLAC) + GM-CSF 5 µg/kg s.c. on days 4–18. The doxorubicin and cyclophosphamide doses were escalated at each cycle to achieve an absolute neutrophil count of less than 500 µl for 3–5 days. Hormone receptor-positive patients were treated with tamoxifen at the completion of therapy. Locoregional treatment consisted of mastectomy or segmentectomy with axillary lymph node dissection and radiotherapy, according to patient preference. With a median follow-up of 33 months there were five distant and one local recurrence in the postoperative arm and one death as a result of primary ovarian cancer, and no local recurrences in the preoperative arm.

PROGNOSTIC AND PREDICTIVE FACTORS

Primary chemotherapy has both advantages and disadvantages over more traditional approaches in terms of prognosis and prediction of response to therapy. Its major disadvantage is that pre-treatment axillary node status is unknown; in addition, accurate histological grading is difficult on needle biopsy material and is unavailable on fine-needle aspirate. Balanced against this, the primary itself offers a potentially important measure of chemosensitivity both clinically and perhaps through surrogate biological markers of prognosis and response prediction.

Tumour response

Several groups have reported that initial tumour response to chemotherapy predicts survival. In the cumulative Milan studies, Bonadonna et al[8] reported that all but one of the eleven patients who achieved pathological complete remissions remained disease free at the time of reporting; in addition, patients who achieve a good partial remission had a 5-year disease-free survival rate of 63%, compared with 31% for those achieving only a minor response. Scholl et al[31] found that patients achieving a greater than 50% tumour regression after two cycles of chemotherapy had a 5-year survival rate of 87%, compared with 79% for those failing to achieve this degree of response ($p = 0.16$). Ferrière et al[32] reported a correlation between tumour response and outcome in 329 patients (but only 188 potentially operable, the rest having locally advanced/inflammatory disease) treated with primary chemotherapy for stage II or III breast cancer between 1982 and 1991, using a combination of doxorubicin, vincristine, cyclophosphamide and 5-fluorouracil (AVCF). Kaplan–Meier estimates demonstrated significantly increased overall survival for patients achieving complete remission compared with those who did not. At 5 years, 83% of complete responders were still alive compared with 71% of other patients; estimated 10-year survival figures were 78% and 51%, respectively ($p < 0.05$). The same group had previously noted that patients who were oestrogen- and progesterone-receptor positive achieved higher objective response rates and that response was higher after six cycles of chemotherapy than after three.

Calais et al,[33] in a series of 158 patients, reported metastatic relapses occurring in 15% of responders to chemotherapy compared with 39% of non-responders ($p < 0.02$), with 5-year actuarial survival higher for responders than for non-responders ($p < 0.03$).

Hortobagyi et al,[34] in a mixed series of 174 patients with both operable and inoperable locally advanced breast cancer, also found that response correlated with prognosis. Five-year survival rates for stage IIIA patients achieving complete remission was 93% and for those achieving partial remission 78% (not significant); for stage IIIB patients the respective figures were 88% for complete responders, 44% for partial responders and 24% for non-responders ($p = 0.01$).

The achievement of high response rates, and in particular complete remissions, has proved an essential prerequisite for improved treatment outcome in diseases where chemotherapy is relatively successful, as discussed earlier. This raises a key question relating to response and treatment outcome for primary chemotherapy in breast cancer. Is response merely an indicator of a biologically predetermined prognostic grouping, or a predictive measurement of treatment outcome that can be manipulated with improved therapies? Will improved response rates, and in particular improved complete remission rates, with more active treatment lead to improved survival? These are central issues for primary chemotherapy and require appropriately constructed randomized trials as discussed below.

Nodal status

In the NSABP B-18 trial, 41% of patients had involved axillary nodes after primary chemotherapy compared with 58% of patients randomized to receive adjuvant chemotherapy after surgery.[26] This suggests an influence of primary chemotherapy on micrometastatic nodal involvement, but the prognostic significance awaits follow-up survival data. The achievement of complete remission on primary chemotherapy appeared to predict involved axillary nodes in this trial; 71% of patients achieving complete clinical remission had negative nodes on histological resection. It is also worth noting that pathological lymph node involvement after primary chemotherapy was the most important prognostic indicator in multivariate analysis in an MD Anderson study of patients with locally advanced breast cancer.[35]

Bonadonna et al[8] reported that 60% of patients have involved axillary nodes after resection and their review stated that the extent of axillary node status was an important prognostic factor; further details were not given.

Botti et al[36] reported on a prospective study of 56 consecutive patients receiving high-dose, anthracycline-based, primary chemotherapy for large but potentially resectable breast cancer; in a multivariate analysis at a median follow-up period of 36 months, they also found that the only independent predictor of relapse was the number of involved metastatic nodes posttreatment.

Scholl et al[28] found that *clinically* involved nodes preoperatively carried a decreased chance of survival with a relative risk of 2.7 (95%CI = 1.3–5.3).

Tumour size and response to chemotherapy

There is disagreement in the literature about the interrelationship of tumour size, response and outcome. Bonadonna et al[8] showed an inverse relationship; the complete remission rate was 50% for patients with tumours less than 2 cm in size, 38% in those with tumours 2–4 cm and only 18% in patients with tumours over 4 cm in size. In contrast, others have reported no clear-cut association between initial tumour size and response to chemotherapy.[10,34,36]

Tumour size is of established prognostic survival significance in conventional approaches to breast cancer management, and this appears to hold true in primary chemotherapy studies where the issue has been assessed. Scholl et al[31] reported that large tumour size was associated with increased risk of metastatic recurrence rate, with a relative risk for T3 tumours of 2.02 (95%CI = 1.2–3.4). Khayat et al[37] likewise found clinical tumour size to be a significant prognostic indicator in a multivariate Cox analysis ($p = 0.0001$).

AGE AND MENSTRUAL STATUS

Most groups who have examined this issue have shown no significant influence of age or menopausal status on response to chemotherapy or survival. As an exception, Scholl et al[31] reported that patients younger than 35 years had an increased risk of metastatic recurrence with a relative risk of 2.46 (95%CI = 1.2–5.0). Jacquillat et al[9] reported tumour response to be inversely related to age; complete remissions were achieved in 18% of patients less than 50 years old compared with 37% of patients over 50

($p = 0.007$). This did not translate, however, into survival differences between the two groups.

Biological parameters

Primary chemotherapy also offers the important possibility of biological studies on the primary tumour *after* treatment to increase our understanding of mechanisms of response and chemoresistance.

At the Royal Marsden, study has been made of apoptotic index (AI), proliferation (Ki-67) and Bcl-2 protein expression in the primary cancer of 40 patients immediately before infusional ECF (epirubicin, cisplatin and 5-fluorouracil) chemotherapy and in 20 of these with residual tumour at the completion of six courses of treatment. The implication in this study was that the residual tumour was, by definition, chemoresistant.

Thirteen patients (65%) showed a greater than 50% reduction in proliferation as measured by Ki-67 after chemotherapy. Eleven patients (55%) showed a greater than 50% reduction in AI after chemotherapy; median pre-treatment AI was 0.6% and post-treatment 0.2%. Of patients 65% were positive for Bcl-2 before treatment. After chemotherapy five of seven patients previously negative for Bcl-2 became strongly positive; median pre-treatment Bcl-2 score was 56% before compared with 80% afterwards. These data suggest the hypothesis that apoptosis and proliferation are closely related in vivo and that the phenotype of reduced apoptosis and proliferation, along with increased Bcl-2, is associated with breast cancer cells resistant to cytotoxic chemotherapy.

In a separate type of study apoptotic index was compared before and 24 hours after infusional ECF chemotherapy to give a measure of the immediate effects of chemotherapy on apoptosis. Apoptotic index was increased by more than 50% in 7 of 13 such patients (54%) with a median pre-treatment AI of 0.75% compared with a post-treatment AI of 1.1%. This study provides the first direct clinical evidence that apoptosis is induced by chemotherapy, and offers the intriguing possibility that this might relate to response and subsequent treatment outcome[38] These studies demonstrate the enormous potential for the primary chemotherapy model in studying the underlying mechanisms of chemotherapy effects on human tumours.

PRIMARY ENDOCRINE THERAPY

Several preoperative chemotherapy studies have included the use of tamoxifen, and there is a simple rationale for this: earlier trials in metastatic disease have shown that combined chemoendocrine therapy has a higher response rate than chemotherapy alone[39] Primary endocrine therapy in its own right is an important tool in clinical research; the underlying rationale is the same as for chemotherapy with the advantage of minimal toxicity.

In initial experience at the Royal Marsden Hospital 42 patients were treated with primary endocrine therapy (38 received tamoxifen 20 mg daily and 4 received the luteinizing hormone-releasing hormone (LHRH) analogue leuprorelin in a dose of 7.6 mg by monthly depot injection) between 1985 and 1988. Patients were selected simply on the criterion of being over the age of 50. Twenty achieved a partial response (47%) with one achieving a complete remission (2%). In addition four further patients (10%) had a minor response and 16 (38%) had stable disease for at least 4 months. Only two (5%) progressed during the first 2 months of treatment.[40]

The Edinburgh group reported 61 patients treated with initial endocrine therapy (five premenopausal patients treated with surgical oophorectomy and seven with the LHRH analogue goserelin (Zoladex), 11 postmenopausal women with tamoxifen 20 mg orally daily or aminoglutethimide 500 mg with 40 mg hydrocortisone acetate and 10 patients with aromatase inhibitors). The first 36 of these patients were treated independently of ER status, but in this group no patient with an ER concentration of less than 20 fmol/mg showed significant regression and two-thirds of these progressed; subsequently primary endocrine therapy was reserved only for patients with ER of 20 fmol/mg or more. Twenty-four of 61 patients (39%) had significant tumour regression and all responding tumours had an ER concentration of 20 fmol/mg or more. The median time taken to achieve half tumour volume was 44 days (range 3–150 days) and only one tumour achieved complete clinical regression. Response occurred in 24 of 46 ER-positive patients (52%).

Tamoxifen was first evaluated as initial treatment of breast cancer in elderly women over 70 years of age in the early 1980s; it was shown to be very active with a response rate of 73%.[41] In a subsequent randomized trial involving 116 patients aged 70 or over, randomized either to primary tamoxifen or to surgery, Gazet et al[42] showed no difference in either time to progression or survival between the two treatments. Indeed there was a non-significant trend towards a decreased risk of local recurrence and a delay in the development of distant metastases in patients treated with primary tamoxifen. This trial had a large proportion of patients with T3/T4 tumours. In a trial of similar design, involving 135 patients aged over 70, Robertson et al showed no significant difference in survival between the two groups (mortality rate for metastatic breast cancer was 11% for tamoxifen and 15% for mastectomy). In this trial, however, there was a 43% local failure rate in the tamoxifen-alone arm at 3 years of follow-up.[43] In a large Cancer Research Campaign trial, 381 women over 70 years old were randomized to optimal surgery or tamoxifen 40 mg alone. At a median follow-up of 34 months, there was no significant difference in survival or quality of life between the two groups, but significantly more patients had local relapse after tamoxifen alone than in the surgical arm (23% versus 8%).[44]

These randomized trials in elderly patients urge caution in using primary endocrine therapy as a substitute for surgery but nevertheless indicate that there may be benefit in using this approach before surgery. Currently, a pilot feasibility trial of tamoxifen given either preoperatively 3 months before surgery or as adjuvant treatment following surgery is being carried out at the Royal Marsden. The long-term aim is towards a large multi-centre trial of similar design to assess whether there is a benefit in: (1) downstaging and more conservative surgery and (2) survival.

PROBLEMS RELATING TO PRIMARY CHEMOTHERAPY

Diagnosis

In primary chemotherapy diagnosis is made either by incisional needle biopsy or by fine-needle aspiration. There are advantages and disadvantages to each. The authors' own practice has been to use needle biopsy. The procedure is simple and well tolerated with a local anaesthetic. It virtually excludes the risk of a false-positive diagnosis, and allows differentiation between invasive and in situ carcinoma. Accurate histological grading is difficult, but it nevertheless provides a fairly detailed and representative histological evaluation with opportunities for immunohistochemical staining.

In contrast fine-needle aspiration is a quick and simple form of diagnosis, and is easier than needle biopsy for small tumours. With good cytological back-up the risk of false positivity is very low.[45] A current problem is the difficulty in differentiating between invasive and in situ cancers. Histological grading is obviously unavailable, although attempts are being made to define a cytological grading system of prognostic significance. In addition, immunocytochemistry linked to flow cytometric techniques is being developed to provide prognostic biological data.[46,47]

Axillary node status

Lack of prognostic data relating to pathological axillary node status has been raised as one of the major criticisms of primary chemotherapy. The counter-argument is that chemotherapy is increasingly indicated irrespective of nodal involvement, particularly in younger patients with large tumours; tumour size is of course an important and readily available prognostic factor in itself. The additional aim must be to develop immunohistochemical and immunocytochemical markers of prognosis which can be linked to tumour size.

In this context, it is important to note that the main issue is not so much to identify markers of very high risk but to identify those of low risk. Clinically, the long-term aim is to exclude those patients with very good prognosis who are unlikely to require any form of adjuvant medical treatment at all (a minority, excluding screen-detected patients). We are optimistic that this challenge should be surmountable, particularly when small tumour size is taken into account. Other patients (the majority) who would merit some form of adjuvant medical treatment anyway would immediately become eligible for primary medical therapy trials if their tumours were large; current randomized trials will determine whether there is also survival benefit that would translate to patients with smaller tumours.

Monitoring response to treatment (clinical, mammography, ultrasonography)

Clinical measurement represents the standard approach to response assessment in primary chemotherapy. Precise measurement is difficult and subject to considerable interobserver variation; on the other hand, the high degree of chemosensitivity seen in most patients usually presents little difficulty in defining broad categories of response (partial response, complete remission).

Mammography was used to assess response in addition to clinical examination by Semiglazov et al[29] and they found a higher complete remission rate (35%) using this method than with clinical examination alone (12%). In the Royal Marsden experience, however, mammography is a very inaccurate way of quantifying response; mammographic changes can be observed in most patients, but the irregularity of architectural distortion and the persistence of microcalcification make accurate measurement difficult.

The role of ultrasonography has been studied at the Royal Marsden to try to predict pathological

remissions, but with only limited success. In a series of 52 patients who had follow-up ultrasonography, 31 (60%) achieved complete clinical remission but in only five of these was the post-treatment ultrasonic scan normal. For the rest, there was a consistent finding of a residual mass lesion or diffusely echogenic tissue, although 10 such patients had no residual disease pathologically. The use of colour Doppler signal aided prediction. Five of six patients with clinical complete remission and positive colour Doppler had residual invasive cancer or in situ cancer on histology whereas 7 of 12 with Doppler-negative mass lesions on ultrasonography had a pathologically complete remission.[48]

Newer techniques, including dynamic enhanced magnetic resonance imaging, are now being studied to assess response. This technique measures the changes in signal intensity as contrast agents diffuse into the tumour extravascular space. It is sensitive to capillary permeability, stromal consistency and capillary density, and is therefore sensitive to the same factors that are responsible for tumour growth. It may therefore offer an accurate means of monitoring treatment non-invasively and evaluating residual disease.

The role of surgery following primary chemotherapy

As previously described, the group at the Royal Marsden has already produced data suggesting that infusional chemotherapy may achieve higher clinical complete remission rates than conventional chemotherapy. As this approach develops, it is likely that the use of new drugs (e.g. the taxoids) and more intensive chemotherapy will continue this trend of high complete clinical remissions. Providing radical radiotherapy is used after chemotherapy, then the intriguing question is raised of whether these patients require surgery at all. Caution is required here; it is clear from all published trials that complete clinical remissions in most patients do not translate into complete pathological remissions, and residual microscopic disease within the breast is still found at surgery. Whether this microscopic residuum requires surgery or could just as easily be controlled with radiotherapy is unknown. It is the authors' view that the role of surgery following complete clinical remission after primary chemotherapy can only be determined in a randomized trial; currently such a trial is being piloted at the Royal Marsden.

PRIMARY CHEMOTHERAPY: THE NEXT GENERATION OF TRIALS

One of the most important questions in primary chemotherapy concerns the relationship between response (including complete remission) and survival. This relates to a central problem with adjuvant chemotherapy trials, which lack a surrogate endpoint for survival (or disease-free survival) and thus take many years to produce results. This inherent delay slows therapeutic progress; in addition it creates difficulties in assessing promising new agents at an early stage in their development in adjuvant therapy programmes. The key question with primary chemotherapy is therefore whether the early endpoint of improved response rate (or complete remission rate) will predict the late endpoint of improved survival.

The fact that responders in general have a better survival than non-responders, in currently published trials of primary chemotherapy, does not in any way answer this question; as described earlier, such response rates could simply reflect inherent biological characteristics associated with favourable prognosis. Randomized trials are required, and these could be of two types.

In the first, treatment A is compared with treatment B in the hope that different response rates will translate into differences in survival. One such trial is already been conducted at the Royal Marsden Hospital, comparing infusional ECF chemotherapy with conventional AC chemotherapy. This type of trial design allows the early introduction of new agents or novel therapies (infusional or high-dose chemotherapy, for example) into the experimental arm, with the potential for relating initial response to subsequent survival in the two arms. The potential limitation of this type of trial is that it fails to take advantage of the individual tumour as an in vivo measure of responsiveness to chemotherapy.

A second, but rather more complicated, trial design addresses this latter problem. Here, patients achieving a very good response to treatment A continue on this; others with only minor responses are randomized either to continue with treatment A after a predetermined number of courses or to switch to treatment B. In initial trials using CMF chemotherapy, the authors noted four such patients who went on to achieve excellent clinical regression with second-line doxorubicin. This trial design addresses the question of whether such second-line responses, as determined by the chemosensitivity of the individual tumour, translate into survival.

This latter type of trial would be greatly enhanced by the development of early biological predictors of chemotherapy responsiveness; these would allow a much earlier change of therapy than reliance on clinical response. The authors' studies, investigating changes in apoptosis determined by fine-needle aspirate and flow cytometry 24 hours after chemotherapy, are an approach to this challenge.

CONCLUSIONS

It is already well established that primary chemotherapy can achieve significant tumour regressions in the great majority of patients with early breast cancer; for those with initially large tumours mastectomy can frequently be avoided as initial therapy. Well-documented follow-up data on the long-term risk of local recurrence in comparison with initial mastectomy are still required to make a full assessment of this approach.

In addition, long-term comparative survival data are required from randomized trials. So far, none has shown primary chemotherapy to have a detrimental survival effect, and some are hinting at the intriguing possibility that primary chemotherapy has in effect a survival advantage, as predicted by experimental tumour models. Against this background, the key question of whether improved response rates translate into improved survival also requires answering. If so, then our overall strategy for the management of breast cancer will require complete re-thinking. In such circumstances, biological markers of good prognosis would be required, based on fine-needle aspirate and immunocytochemistry, to determine which patients do *not* require chemotherapy and/or endocrine therapy. For the rest, primary medical treatment would become the norm, irrespective of initial tumour size, using the tumour as an in vivo model of individual chemosensitivity so that treatment could be optimized for the individual patient. In addition, primary chemotherapy would offer an important test bed for new drug development at a much earlier stage than is currently offered by an adjuvant chemotherapy strategy.

REFERENCES

1. Halsted WS. The results of operations for the cure of cancer of the breast performed at The Johns Hopkins Hospital from June, 1889 to January, 1894. *Johns Hopkins Hosp Rep* 1894–1895; **4**:297–350.

2. Leroy d'Etiolles JJJ. Une lettre de M. Leroy d'Etiolles sur l'extirpation des tumeurs cancereuses. *Bull Acad Med* 1867; **9**:454–8.

3. Paget J. Statistiek van den kanker (Cancer Statistics). *Ned Weekl Geneesk* 1852; **2**:275, 410.

4. Christian MC, McCabe MS, Korn EL, Abrams JS, Kaplan RS, Friedman MA. The National Cancer Institute audit of the National Surgical Adjuvant Breast and Bowel Project Protocol B-06. *N Engl J Med* 1995; **333**:1469–74.

5. Haagensen CD, Bodian C. A personal experience with Halsted's radical mastectomy. *Ann Surg* 1984; **199**:143–50.

6. Forrest AP, Levack PA, Chetty U, et al. A human tumour model. *Lancet* 1986; **ii**:840–2.

7. Anderson ED, Forrest AP, Hawkins RA, et al. Primary systemic therapy for operable breast cancer. *Br J Cancer* 1991; **63**:561–6.

8. Smith IE, Jones AL, O'Brien MER, et al. Primary medical (neo-adjuvant) chemotherapy for operable breast cancer. *Eur J Cancer (Part A)* 1993;**29**:592–5.

9. Bonadonna G, Valagussa P, Zucali R, Salvadori B. Primary chemotherapy in surgically respectable breast cancer. *CA Cancer J Clin* 1995; **45**:227–43.

10. Jacquillat C, Weil M, Baillet F, et al. Results of neoadjuvant chemotherapy and radiation therapy in the breast conserving treatment of 250 patients with all stages of infiltrative breast cancer. *Cancer* 1990; **66**:119–29.

11. Chollet P, Belembaogo E, Cure H, et al. Four year results of neoadjuvant chemotherapy for 148 operable breast cancer [abstract]. *Proc Annu Meet Ams Soc Clin Oncol* 1993; **12**:A157.

12. Lara FU, Zinser JW, Castaneda N, Ramirez MT, Maafs E, Perez VM. Neoadjuvant (NA) chemotherapy (CT) with cisplatin (P), doxorubicin (A) and cyclophosphamide (C) (PAC) in stage II–III breast cancer (BC) [abstract]. *Proc Annu Meet Am Soc Clin Oncol* 1995; **14**:A179.

13. Di Blasio B, Cocconi G, Boni C, et al. Primary chemotherapy in operable breast carcinoma (BC). A prospective randomized trial comparing CMF with an anthracycline-containing regimen (CMFEV) [abstract]. *Proc Annu Meet Am Soc Clin Oncol* 1996; **15**:A169.

14. Jones AL, Smith IE, O'Brien MER, et al. Phase II study of continuous infusional 5FU with epirubicin and cisplatin (infusional ECF) in patients with metastatic and locally advanced breast cancer: an active new regimen. *J Clin Oncol* 1994; **12**:1259–65.

15. Smith IE, Walsh G, Jones A, et al. High complete remission rates with primary neoadjuvant infusional chemotherapy for large early breast cancer. *J Clin Oncol* 1995; **13**:424–9.

16. Bernardo G, Plastina M, Bernardo A, Strada MR, Bottero G, Betta PG. Neoadjuvant chemotherapy (cyclophosphamide, epirubicin and fluorouracil) plus G-CSF for operable breast cancer [abstract]. *Proc Annu Meet Am Soc Clin Oncol* 1995; **14**:A201.

17. Charrier S, Brain E, Cure H, et al. Neoadjuvant chemotherapy in breast cancer. High pathological response rate induced by intensive anthracycline-based regimen [abstract]. *Proc Annu Meet Am Soc Clin Oncol* 1995; **14**:A218.

18. Simpson-Herren L, Sanford AH, Holmquist JP. Effects of surgery on the cell kinetics of residual tumor. *Cancer Treat Rep* 1976; **60**:1749–60.

19. Fisher B, Saffer EA, Rudock C, et al. Presence of a growth stimulating factor in serum following

primary tumour removal in mice. *Cancer Res* 1989; **49**:1996–2001.

20. Fisher B, Saffer EA, Rudock C, et al. Effect of local or systemic treatment prior to primary tumour removal on the production and response to a serum growth stimulating factor in mice. *Cancer Res* 1989; **49**:2002–4.

21. Reading H, Monaghan P, Ormerod M, et al. Detection of micrometastases in patients with primary breast cancer. *Lancet* 1983; **ii**:1271–3.

22. Porro G, Menard S, Tagliabue E, et al. Monoclonal antibody detection of carcinoma cells in bone marrow biopsy specimens from breast cancer patients. *Cancer* 1988; **61**:2407–11.

23. Ross AA, Cooper BW, Lazarus HM, et al. Detection and viability of tumor cells in peripheral blood stem cell collections from breast cancer patients using immunocytochemical and clonogenic assay techniques. *Blood* 1993; **82**:2605–10.

24. Goldie JH, Coldman AJ. A mathematical model for relating the drug sensitivity of tumours to their spontaneous mutation rate. *Cancer Treat Rep* 1979; **63**:1727–33.

25. Fisher B, Rockette H, Robidoux A, et al. Effect of preoperative therapy for breast cancer in locoregional disease. First report of NSABP B-18 [abstract]. *Proc Am Soc Clin Oncol* 1994; **13**:64.

26. Powles TJ, Hickish TF, Makris A, et al. Randomized trial of chemoendocrine therapy started before or after surgery for treatment of primary breast cancer. *J Clin Oncol* 1995; **13**: 547–52.

27. Mauriac L, Durand M, Avril A, Dilhuydy J-M. Effects of primary chemotherapy in conservative treatment of breast cancer patients with operable tumours larger than 3 cm. *Ann Oncol* 1991; **2**:347–54.

28. Scholl SM, Fourquet A, Asselain B, et al. Neoadjuvant versus adjuvant chemotherapy in premenopausal patients with tumors too large for breast conserving surgery: preliminary results of a randomized trial. *Eur J Cancer* 1994; **30A**:645–52.

29. Semiglazov VF, Topuzov EE, Bavli JL, et al. Primary (neoadjuvant) chemotherapy and radiotherapy compared with primary radiotherapy alone in stage IIb–IIIa breast cancer. *Ann Oncol* 1994; **5**:591–5.

30. Danforth D, Jacobson J, O'Shaughnessy J, et al. Effect of preoperative chemotherapy on axillary lymph node metastases in stage II breast cancer: a prospective randomized trial [abstract]. *Proc Annu Meet Am Soc Clin Oncol* 1995; **14**:A213.

31. Scholl SM, Pierga JY, Asselain B, et al. Breast tumour response predicts local and distant control as well as survival. *Eur J Cancer* 1995; **12**:1969–75.

32. Ferrière JP, Assier I, Cure H, et al. Primary chemotherapy in breast cancer: correlation between tumour response and patient outcome [abstract]. *Proc Am Soc Clin Oncol* 1996; **15**:84.

33. Calais G, Berger C, Descamps P, et al. Conservative treatment feasibility with induction chemotherapy, surgery, and radiotherapy for patients with breast carcinoma larger than 3 cm. *Cancer* 1994; **74**:1283–8.

34. Hortobagyi GN, Ames FC, Buzdar AU, et al. Management of stage III primary breast cancer with primary chemotherapy, surgery and radiation therapy. *Cancer* 1988; **62**:2507–16.

35. McCready DR, Hortobagyi GN, Kau SW, Smith TL, Buzdar AU, Balch CM. The prognostic significance of lymph node metastases after preoperative chemotherapy for locally advanced breast cancer. *Arch Surg* 1989; **124**:21–5.

36. Botti C, Vici P, Lopez M, Scinto AF, Cognetti F, Cavaliere R. Prognostic value of lymph node metastases after neoadjuvant chemotherapy for large-sized operable carcinoma of the breast. *J Am Coll Surg* 1995; **181**:202–8.

37. Khayat D, Weil M, Auclerc G, et al. Clinical relevance of tumor regression (TR) in neoadjuvant (neoadj) chemotherapy (chemo) in breast cancer (BC) revisited [abstract]. *Proc Annu Meet Am Soc Clin Oncol* 1994; **13**:A99.

38. Ellis PA, Smith IE, Salter J, et al. Preoperative/noeadjuvant chemotherapy for early breast cancer induces apoptosis [abstract]. *Proc Am Soc Clin Oncol* 1996; **15**:112.

39. ANZ Breast Cancer Trials Group. A randomised trial of post-menopausal patients with advanced breast cancer comparing endocrine and cytotoxic therapy given sequentially or in combination. *J Clin Oncol* 1986; **4**:186–93.

40. Mansi JL, Smith IE, Walsh G, et al. Primary medical therapy for operable breast cancer. *Eur J Cancer Clin Oncol* 1989; **25**:1623–7.

41. Preece PE, Wood RAB, Mackie CR, Cushieri A. Tamoxifen as initial sole treatment of breast cancer in elderly women: a pilot study. *BMJ* 1982; **284**:869–70.

42. Gazet J-C, Markopoulos CH, Ford HT, et al. Prospective randomised trial of tamoxifen versus surgery in elderly patients with breast cancer. *Lancet* 1988; **i**:679–81.

43. Robertson JFR, Todd JH, Ellis IO, Elston CW,

Blamey RW. Comparison of mastectomy with tamoxifen for treating elderly patients with operable breast cancer. *BMJ* 1988; **297**:511–14.

44. Bates T, Riley DL, Houghton J, et al. Breast cancer in elderly women: a Cancer Research Campaign trial comparing treatment with tamoxifen and optimal surgery with tamoxifen alone. *Br J Surg* 1991; **78**:591–4.

45. Hammond S, Keyhani-Rofagha S, O'Toole RV. Statistical analysis of fine needle aspiration cytology of the breast: a review of 678 cases plus 4265 cases from the literature. *Acta Cytol* 1987; **31**:276–80.

46. Brotherick I, Lennard TWJ, Cook S, et al. Use of biotinylated antibody DAKO-ER 1D5 to measure oestrogen receptor on cytokeratin positive cells obtained from primary breast cancer cells. *Cytometry* 1995; **20**:74–80.

47. Pollice AA, McCoy JP, Shackney SE, et al. Sequential paraformaldehyde and methanol fixation for simultaneous flow cytometric analysis of DNA, cell surface proteins, and intracellular proteins. *Cytometry* 1992; **13**:432–44.

48. Seymour MT, Moskovic EC, Walsh G, Trott P, Smith IE. Ultrasound assessment of residual abnormalities following primary/neoadjuvant chemotherapy for breast cancer. *Br J Cancer* 1997; in press.

7

Conventional adjuvant chemotherapy

Gianni Bonadonna, Pinuccia Valagussa

CONTENTS • **International overview** • **Long-term results in individual trials** • **Newer strategies of chemotherapy administration** • **Controversial issues** • **Conclusions**

Throughout most of this century, early breast cancer was believed to be a locoregional disease best managed by extensive surgery, sometimes followed by adjuvant regional radiotherapy. The underlying theory was that breast cancer spread first by direct extension into contiguous tissue and, then, by an orderly progression through the lymphatic circulation, to the rest of the body.[1] Therefore, extensive locoregional treatment could achieve cure, catching all the cells before they could infiltrate locally or break through the nodal filter.

Major conceptual challenges to the halstedian hypothesis did not appear until the 1960s. The seminal studies by Fisher and co-workers[2,3] revealed that regional lymph nodes were of biological rather than anatomical importance, and the observed findings led to the conclusion that the lymphatic and blood vascular systems were so interrelated that it was impractical to consider them as independent routes of neoplastic dissemination. It also became apparent that micrometastases existed at the time of diagnosis in many patients,[4,5] and that extensive locoregional treatment could possibly achieve cure only in a minority of women not harbouring such micrometastases.

The early concepts regarding the potential value of chemotherapy as an adjunct to surgery originated during the late 1950s in the laboratory, where an inverse relationship between the size of a tumour and its curative response to cytotoxic drugs was documented.[6,7] In ensuing years, investigators at the Southern Research Institute,[8,9] working with murine systems, provided the cardinal principles on the kinetics of tumour cells by use of effective anti-cancer drugs and determined, quantitatively, the optimal approaches to surgery plus chemotherapy.

The National Surgical Adjuvant Breast and Bowel Project (NSABP) started the first clinical trial to evaluate the role of systemic adjuvant chemotherapy in operable breast cancer in 1958.[10] Single-agent chemotherapy was administered perioperatively, i.e. during and for a short period after operation, with the intent that it would destroy tumour cells disseminated as a result of breast cancer surgery. Although treatment outcome demonstrated an improvement in both relapse-free and overall survival in premenopausal women with node-positive tumours, the overall results were considered as disappointing, based on the expectations that all patients would be cured. Albeit disappointing, these findings provided the initial evidence that the natural history of breast cancer could be perturbed by adjuvant drug therapy.

The concepts underlying systemic adjuvant therapy were introduced into full-scale clinical trials in cancer in the 1970s. A forerunner of adjuvant therapy was the recognition of the possible complementary therapeutic action of different modalities when chemotherapy was first introduced. Subsequently, the demonstration of successful application of various treatment modalities directed against the early stages of Wilms' tumour led to the concept of combined modality treatment.

Also modern adjuvant systemic therapy for high-risk breast cancer was pioneered during the early 1970s, and during the past two decades an enormous body of information was generated; the consistency of therapeutic findings has resulted in a profound revolution in the approach, management and evaluation of breast cancer.[11]

INTERNATIONAL OVERVIEW

The first two modern randomized studies using adjuvant chemotherapy in node-positive patients were activated in 1971[12] and 1973,[13] respectively. Early and intermediate results showed a consistent benefit in terms of relapse-free survival in favour of the treated groups, whereas the benefit in overall survival was less clearly evident, at least during the first years. The publication of the early results raised both hopes and controversies, and was followed by a large number of trials on adjuvant systemic therapy in operable breast cancer. Unfortunately, most of the trials were relatively small and the encouraging or discouraging results they achieved could result from chance alone. For this reason, in 1985 the Early Breast Cancer Trialists' Collaborative Group pooled the data from all available prospective, randomized, clinical trials of adjuvant systemic therapy for operable breast cancer and performed an overview, or meta-analysis. The methodology used and the very large number of available patients provided much greater statistical power than could be achieved from any individual clinical trial.[14] Therefore, the overview was able to establish that adjuvant chemotherapy and adjuvant endocrine therapy (tamoxifen in post-menopausal or ovarian ablation in pre-menopausal patients) produced significant reductions in the annual odds of death and recurrence compared with no adjuvant systemic therapy.

In 1990, an updated follow-up of all trials activated before 1985 was completed and the 10-year findings were published in 1992.[15] Results from the trials of polychemotherapy (i.e. chemotherapy with more than one drug for more than one month) versus no chemotherapy confirmed a statistically significant benefit for the treated group in terms of both relapse-free and overall survival. Table 7.1 summarizes the essential results, from both direct and indirect comparisons.

The reported findings warrant a few important considerations. The first is that the same reduction in the annual odds of an event in two patient subsets at different baseline risk (i.e. the risk after locoregional treatment alone) does not translate into the same absolute benefit. Let us consider that a 30% reduction in the annual odds of disease recurrence is produced by adjuvant systemic therapy. In a subset of patients whose baseline risk of disease recurrence is greater than 40% at 10 years, this reduction will yield an approximate absolute benefit of 12%. By contrast, if the baseline risk is 10–20%, the same reduction will yield an approximate absolute benefit of 4%.[15]

Another issue of concern in interpreting the findings from a meta-analysis is the reasonableness of the calculation of average effect. When the studies being pooled are similar with regard to the therapy delivered, patient population and data quality, then averaging the results makes sense and it is quite valuable for detecting moderate treatment effects. Often, however, the studies will differ with regard to the therapeutic interventions compared. Even if two studies plan to employ the same modality (i.e. polychemotherapy), they may vary in terms of classes of agents used, duration of treatment and doses of drugs actually delivered, and especially methods of follow-up and evaluation. In these situations, it must be recognized

Table 7.1 Essential findings from the international overview on chemotherapy trials		
	Typical reduction (% ± s.d.) in annual odds of	
	Recurrence or prior death	Death from any cause
Polychemotherapy, any age	28 ± 3	17 ± 3
<50 years, premenopause	36 ± 5	25 ± 6
<50 years, postmenopause	37 ± 19*	NA
50–59 years, premenopause	25 ± 9*	23 ± 9*
50–59 years, postmenopause	29 ± 5	13 ± 7
60–69 years	20 ± 5	10 ± 6
≥70 years	NA	NA
Polychemotherapy alone vs nil, any age	27 ± 3	18 ± 4
<50 years	37 ± 5	27 ± 6
≥50 years	22 ± 4	14 ± 5
Polychemotherapy plus TAM vs TAM, any age	28 ± 6	5 ± 9*
<50 years	32 ± 16*	−6 ± 23*
≥50 years	26 ± 5	10 ± 7
CMF regimens	32 ± 4	22 ± 5
CMF with other drugs	23 ± 6	10 ± 7
Other regimens	25 ± 5	12 ± 6

s.d., standard deviation; NA, not assessed because of small number of patients; TAM, tamoxifen; CMF, cyclophosphamide, methotrexate, fluorouracil.
* Statistically unstable results with s.d. ≥9.

that average results may not be representative of the components making up the average.

Another important finding in the 1992 overview is that, although the meta-analysis demonstrated that polychemotherapy was most effective in women under 50 years of age (i.e. premenopausal patients), benefits were also demonstrated in postmenopausal patients under 70 years of age, i.e. in all age groups with sufficient patients for analysis (Table 7.1). The different magnitude of the effect between pre- and postmenopausal women has been ascribed by some authors to result primarily from an ovarian suppression-mediated mechanism because many premenopausal women became amenorrhoeic, either temporarily or permanently, while on drug therapy. However, it is unlikely that all of the benefit obtained by chemotherapy in premenopausal patients is achieved through a hormonal mechanism. In fact, there is a significant, albeit smaller, benefit of polychemotherapy in postmenopausal patients. Moreover, it is also unlikely that the two modes of treatment work through the same mechanism: the overview indicated that additional benefit can be achieved when ovarian ablation is added to chemotherapy[15] and salvage ovarian ablation was able to induce a similar therapeutic palliation in women previously untreated with adjuvant chemotherapy, as well as in patients who became amenorrhoeic following adjuvant CMF (cyclophosphamide, methotrexate and 5-fluorouracil).[16] In addition, the large experience of the Milan Cancer Institute has confirmed an impact of CMF, independent of patient age, with the exception of women over 60 years of age, who, either by protocol design or because of protocol violations, received lower doses of the three drugs.[17] Downward dose adjustments for anticipated toxicity in older patients could have also been performed in other chemotherapy trials analysed in the overview and this may have largely affected therapeutic results.[18] Of note, recent trials in which the same drug doses were planned and administered regardless of patient age have indeed failed to achieve dissimilar benefit in pre- versus postmenopausal women.

LONG-TERM RESULTS IN INDIVIDUAL TRIALS

The 20-year results of the first CMF trial carried out at the Milan Cancer Institute in node-positive breast cancer have recently been published.[19] Briefly, both relapse-free and overall survival remained significantly superior in women given adjuvant CMF than in patients treated with surgery alone (Table 7.2). The time to relapse was 83 months after CMF, compared with 40 months in the control group, and the maximum recurrence rate occurred during the first 3 years after surgery; from this time on, the difference between the two treatment arms remained about the same for subsequent years. This observation indicated that the early findings could predict the late outcome with sufficient accuracy and suggested that micrometastases included very aggressive cell lines that are mostly resistant to cytotoxic chemotherapy. Most probably, full or almost full doses of chemotherapy, as delivered in this trial, are sufficient to kill most (at times all) drug-sensitive tumour cells, whereas early and late relapses are the result of the overgrowth of primary resistant tumour cells. The median overall survival was 137 versus 104 months,

Table 7.2 Twenty-year results of the first CMF study performed at the Milan Cancer Institute

	Control group (%)	CMF group (%)
Relapse-free survival	25*	32*
Total first relapse	73	64
Locoregional alone	15	13
Contralateral breast	4	7
Distant	54	44
Overall survival	23**	34**

Adjusted relative risk:
*0.65 (95% confidence interval 0.51–0.83), $p < 0.001$.
**0.76 (95% confidence interval 0.60–0.97), $p = 0.03$.

respectively, and the two curves started diverging only after the seventh year from starting adjuvant therapy.

The results of the CMF programme confirmed the importance of nodal extent, because there was a consistent inverse relationship between number of involved lymph nodes and treatment outcome. As previously reported, in this trial the significant achievements in premenopausal women were not duplicated in postmenopausal patients. When results were broken down according to age groups, only women over 60 years of age failed to achieve benefit from adjuvant chemotherapy.[17] Of note, by protocol design, this patient subset received CMF at reduced doses.[18] It is worth mentioning that the 20-year analysis of this trial also confirmed the previously reported prognostic importance of received dose rate: regardless of nodal extent and menopausal status, women receiving full or almost full doses of the planned drug therapy fared significantly better than patients receiving low-dose chemotherapy.[18,19]

These findings were also supported by recent data from a prospective randomized trial by the Cancer and Leukemia Group B.[20]

The cumulative incidence of first relapse according to anatomical site is also given in Table 7.2. The main therapeutic effect of adjuvant CMF was to reduce the incidence of distant metastases (10 percentage point difference at 20 years between women who received CMF and those who did not). These data are strikingly different from those reported by investigators from the International (Ludwig) Breast Cancer Study Group (IBCSG) who found that, compared with less effective adjuvant therapy, more effective systemic treatments predominantly acted by reducing the risk of first relapse in soft tissue from 36% to 18% at 10 years, with little effect on the incidence of other sites of relapse.[21] The reason for such a different outcome is not clear. It is notable that, in their study performed in premenopausal women with one to three positive axillary nodes,[22] these investigators documented a higher frequency of bone metastases after CMF plus low-dose prednisone (CMF-p) (17%) than in patients treated with CMF alone (7%), the incidence of other sites of disease recurrence being similar for both treatment groups.

The favourable effect of adjuvant CMF has also been confirmed in a more recent study performed in node-negative and oestrogen receptor-negative breast cancer.[23] At 12 years from locoregional treatment, 71% of patients given adjuvant CMF remained disease free as compared with 48% of women in the control group ($p = 0.008$). Treatment outcome after CMF was unrelated to tumour size, grade and proliferative activity, and both pre- and postmenopausal patients benefited from adjuvant chemotherapy.

Another important issue in adjuvant trials is the optimal duration of treatment. Various randomized studies have addressed this question and the more mature of them have been analysed in the overview.[15] Overall, a longer treatment duration (usually 12 or more cycles of polychemotherapy) failed to achieve significant benefit as compared with a shorter (generally six cycles) duration of the same regimen. The

experience of the Milan Cancer Institute, in which a randomized study testing 12 versus 6 cycles of adjuvant CMF was activated in 1975,[24] is displayed graphically in Figures 7.1 and 7.2. The 18-year analysis confirms previous observations on the lack of an additional effect from a treatment prolonged over six-monthly cycles. Conceptually, these findings indicate that the drug-sensitive tumour cells can be controlled, if not eradicated, within the first cycles of the same chemotherapy, leaving tumour-resistant cells as the major obstacle to curing most patients with micrometastases. Practically, relatively short-term chemotherapy means an improved cost–benefit ratio, i.e. decreased acute and probably delayed toxicity and financial costs. Even if the optimal duration of adjuvant chemotherapy has not yet been entirely clarified, since trials testing three to four cycles versus six cycles of the same regimen reported contradictory results, both the overview and individual trials have clearly demonstrated that

Table 7.3 Long-term results of chemotherapy trials from the International Breast Cancer Study Group (median follow-up: 13 years)

	Disease-free survival (%)	Overall survival (%)
Premenopause, 1–3 nodes		
CMF vs	52	65
CMF-p	49	59
Premenopause, >3 nodes		
CMF-p vs	24	33
CMF-p + Ox	24	38
Postmenopause, ≤ 65 years		
Surgery alone vs	14*	32**
CMF-p + TAM vs	35	48
p + TAM	25	36

p, low-dose continuous prednisone; Ox, surgical oophorectomy; TAM, tamoxifen for 1 year.
*$p < 0.0001$; **$p = 0.01$.

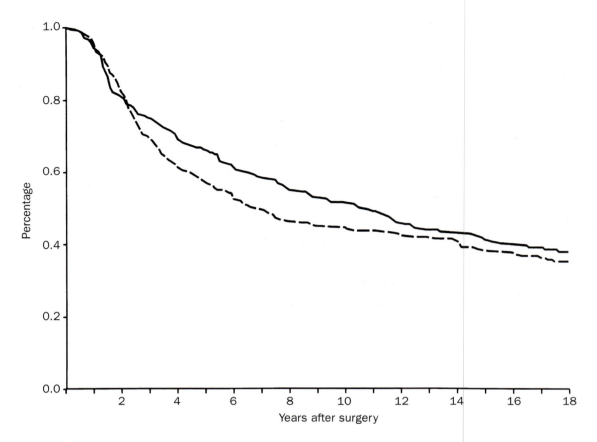

Figure 7.1 Eighteen-year relapse-free survival from the randomized study testing 6 (—) vs 12 (– – –) cycles of standard CMF performed at the Milan Cancer Institute. No statistically significant differences were detected.

one cycle of perioperative chemotherapy is definitely inferior to six cycles of the same drug combination.[15]

The long-term results of the studies activated in 1978 by the IBCSG have recently been published.[22] The essential findings from the chemotherapy trials are shown in Table 7.3. Briefly, the addition of continuous low-dose prednisone to standard CMF failed to improve treatment outcome. Of concern, as previously mentioned, is the greater incidence of bone metastases, possibly caused by a negative interaction between prednisone and the growth-inhibiting compounds, which was documented in the subset of patients with one to three

positive nodes treated with CMF-p. In high-risk premenopausal women with more than three positive axillary nodes, the addition of surgical oophorectomy failed overall to improve disease-free and total survival. A subset analysis revealed a modest benefit, which appeared beyond 4 years of follow-up, limited to patients with oestrogen receptor-positive tumours. The trial carried out in postmenopausal women who were 65 years or younger, was the first to identify a significant advantage for the chemo-endocrine therapy, compared with endocrine therapy alone or with no adjuvant treatment. These results are in line with the findings from the overview[15] showing a significant reduction

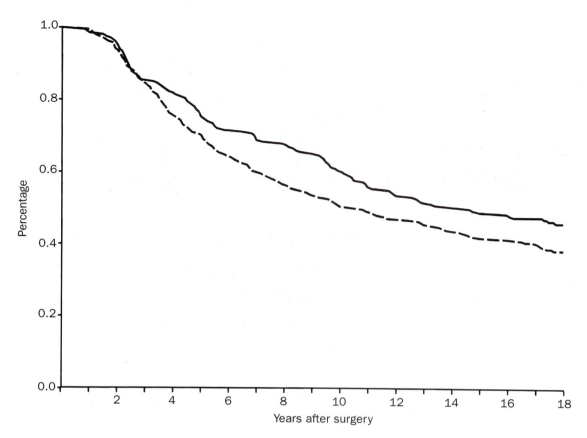

Figure 7.2 Eighteen-year overall survival from the randomized study testing 6 (—) vs 12 (– – –) cycles of standard CMF performed at the Milan Cancer Institute. A trend ($p = 0.052$) favouring the six-cycle regimen was documented.

in the annual odds of recurrence ($26 \pm 5\%$) and death ($10 \pm 7\%$) when polychemotherapy plus tamoxifen was compared with tamoxifen alone.

NEWER STRATEGIES OF CHEMOTHERAPY ADMINISTRATION

Both individual trials and the international overview have clearly established that adjuvant CMF significantly prolongs relapse-free and overall survival. In addition, direct and indirect comparisons in the overview indicated that CMF was superior to single-agent chemotherapy and no worse than its variants in which other pharmacological compounds were either substituted or added (see Table 7.1). Several other trials have compared the simultaneous administration of adjuvant chemotherapy and endocrine treatment with chemotherapy alone. Individual results are somehow contradictory and, despite the overview indicated an additional reduction in the annual odds of recurrence and death favouring chemoendocrine therapy,[15] no firm conclusions can be drawn as yet. In fact, presently available results rely heavily on menopausal status, oestrogen receptor status and types of treatments delivered.

Although moderate, the reductions in the

odds of recurrence and death achieved with the first generation of adjuvant chemotherapy trials are worth while, considering the many thousands of women treated world wide for operable breast cancer. Based on the previously reported findings, adjuvant treatment of 100 000 women could well prevent, or substantially delay, an additional 10 000 deaths. Nevertheless, these results are far from satisfactory and the efforts of the research community are directed to the search of more effective chemotherapeutic regimens. Innovative ways of administering old drugs have been prospectively explored during recent years, and most of the current activity in the field of conventional chemotherapy has concerned dosing and scheduling.

Role of dose intensity

The concept that dose is a critical factor in achieving higher cell kill by chemotherapy has long been recognized in animal models.[9] Animal models, however, do not provide for reduced dosage or delay as a result of toxicity, and optimal treatment can be determined by treating beyond lethal toxicity. This is not possible in humans in whom attempts to define optimal treatments have resulted in a plethora of schedules, combinations and schemes to reduce doses and delay treatments. These schemes have obscured dose–response relationships until 1985, when, after a retrospective analysis of received doses of adjuvant CMF,[18] there was progressively widespread interest in the subject of dose intensity of cancer chemotherapy. Dose intensity is a mathematical concept developed by Hryniuk and Bush,[25] consisting of the amount of drug administered per unit time; for a single drug regimen it may be expressed simply as milligrams per square metre of body surface per week, regardless of the schedule used.

Wood and co-workers, from the Cancer and Leukemia Group B (CALGB), published their experience, in 1994, on the disease-free and overall survival of 1572 women with breast cancer treated with one of three dose levels of CAF (cyclophosphamide, doxorubicin [Adriamycin], fluorouracil) chemotherapy.[20] Patients were randomly allocated to receive low, intermediate or high doses of therapy (Table 7.4). The low-dose arm represented half as much drug treatment over 4 months as the high-dose arm; the intermediate-dose arm delivered the same total amount of chemotherapy as in the high-dose arm but over a prolonged (i.e. 6 months) period of time. At 5 years, the low-dose arm yielded a significantly worse outcome, in terms of both relapse-free and overall survival, than the other two arms. No statistically significant difference was detected between the high- and intermediate-dose arm, despite a trend favouring the high-dose arm. These data suggest the possibility of a dose–intensity or a dose–threshold effect of the drug regimen used.

The French Adjuvant Study Group (FASG) has recently reported, in an abstract form, the results of two prospective studies testing the role of dose intensity and duration of chemotherapy in node-positive breast cancer. In the first trial premenopausal women were randomized to receive three different schedules of FEC (fluorouracil, epirubicin, cyclophosphamide) chemotherapy (Table 7.4). In one arm the classic doses of the three drugs, with epirubicin at 50 mg/m², were delivered for six cycles; in a second arm the same doses were delivered for three cycles; in the remaining arm three cycles were also delivered, but the dose of epirubicin was increased to 75 mg/m².[26] The univariate analysis failed to reveal a statistically significant difference in terms of relapse-free and overall survival, but a multivariate analysis demonstrated a significant difference ($p = 0.031$) in the relapse-free survival, favouring the six-cycle regimen. A subsequent study was conducted using the same six-cycle regimen with epirubicin at 50 mg/m² versus a three-cycle regimen with epirubicin at 100 mg/m². Eligible patients were those under 65 years of age with more than three positive nodes or with one to three positive nodes and negative oestrogen receptors.[27] The 3-year analysis showed a significant difference ($p = 0.02$) in the relapse-free survival favouring

Table 7.4 Selected randomized trials attempting to define the role of total dose and dose intensity

Research group	Drug regimen (doses in mg/m²)	Interval (days)	No. of cycles	Comments
CALGB[20]	C (600) A (60) F (600)	28	4	At 5 years, the low-dose
	vs			arm yielded a significantly
	C (400) A (40) F (400)	28	6	worse outcome. No significant
	vs			differences were detected
	C (300) A (30) F (300)	28	4	between the other two arms
FASG[26]	F (500) E (50) C (500)	21	6	At 5 years, the multivariate
	vs			analysis detected a significant
	F (500) E (50) C (500)	21	3	difference favouring the
	vs			six-cycle arm in terms of
	F (500) E (75) C (500)	21	3	relapse-free survival
FASG[27]	F (500) E (50) C (500)	21	6	At 3 years, a significant
	vs			improvement of relapse-free
	F (500) E (100) C (500)	21	3	survival was achieved in the arm with E 100
NSABP[28]	A (60) C (600)	21	4	At 3 years, no benefit
	vs			from the higher doses
	A (60) C (1200)	21	2	of C was documented
	vs			
	A (60) C (1200)	21	4	

C, cyclophosphamide; A, doxorubicin (Adriamycin); F, fluorouracil; E, epirubicin.
All drugs delivered intravenously on day 1, with the exception of F in the study by CALGB where it was given on days 1 and 8.

the three-cycle arm with epirubicin at 100 mg/m², but no differences were documented in the overall survival.

The NSABP reported the initial results of study B-22 in which 2092 women with node-positive breast cancer were randomly assigned to receive AC (doxorubicin and cyclophosphamide) chemotherapy with three different dose levels of cyclophosphamide.[28] All patients received 60 mg/m² of the anthracycline for four cycles, whereas the doses of cyclophosphamide were 600 mg/m² for four cycles versus 1200 mg/m² for two cycles versus 1200 mg/m² for four cycles, drug treatment being administered every 21 days. The 3-year analysis failed to detect a benefit from the higher doses of the alkylating agent.

Overall, these studies suggest that, provided established drug regimens are delivered at full dose and on time, modest increases in dose may have little impact on final treatment outcome and confirm that clinical trials involve more complexity than any mathematical model may encompass and probably tolerate. The important lesson from these studies is that the doses of the drugs combined in an effective regimen should not be arbitrarily reduced. Not only does lowering the doses not prevent side effects, but, most importantly, final treatment outcomes are adversely affected.

Role of anthracyclines

Anthracyclines (i.e. doxorubicin and epirubicin) are among the most active agents for the treatment of metastatic breast cancer.[29] Doxorubicin-containing regimens have been introduced in the adjuvant setting since 1973, through a prospective non-randomized study performed at the MD Anderson Institute in Houston.[30] Subsequently, several prospective trials were activated comparing anthracycline-containing with non-anthracycline-containing regimens, but consistent evidence for the superiority of the anthracycline combinations was not confirmed. This, at least in part, can be the result of the low dose of the anthracycline administered in some of the earlier trials.

One of the largest modern studies comparing AC for four cycles versus standard CMF for six-monthly cycles was carried out by the NSABP group in node-positive patients.[31] The two regimens yielded similar treatment outcome, but the AC regimen was preferred, by patients and nurses alike, because of its shorter duration and better tolerance. Another recent study compared dose-intensive CEF (cyclophosphamide, epirubicin and fluorouracil) against CMF in premenopausal women with node-positive breast cancer.[32] After a median follow-up of 37 months, an improved relapse-free survival was reported for CEF-treated patients (71% vs 62%, $p = 0.05$), whereas survival rates were superimposable in both treatment arms. A troublesome finding in this study was the occurrence of four cases of secondary leukaemia, all documented in the epirubicin group and within a median of 18 months from study entry. The fact that alkylating agents can induce acute leukaemia, especially when combined with radiotherapy, has long been recognized.[33] More recently, topoisomerase II inhibitors have also been reported potentially to induce secondary leukaemia, usually with a typical 11q23 translocation. A description of all the long-term side effects from systemic drug treatment is given in Chapter 13 by Armand et al.

Most of the studies so far activated with an anthracycline-containing regimen have integrated doxorubicin or epirubicin into a classic combination regimen, in which all the drugs are usually given simultaneously and recycled over time to allow haematological recovery. It is well known that, to avoid overlapping toxicity from the different drugs used in a combination, a compromise in the dose of each single agent is necessary, thus resulting in a dose level that is less than the permissible single-agent dose. Both retrospective[25] and prospective evaluations have demonstrated that doxorubicin is capable of exhibiting a rising dose–response relationship within the usual dose range. It is therefore plausible that the lack of a clear advantage for the anthracycline regimens may, at least in part, be ascribed to the suboptimal dose of these agents when integrated in a combination of drugs. This is particularly worrisome in light of the recent findings by Muss et al[34] who reported that the significant dose–response effect for the CAF regimen[20] was influenced by the level of expression of *c-erbB-2*. Should these findings be confirmed by other investigators, then over-expression of this oncogene may help in selecting patients who are more likely to benefit from adequate doses of adjuvant doxorubicin.

Sequential non-cross-resistant chemotherapy

An alternative to the simultaneous administration of various agents in a single combination is to deliver them in sequences of drug regimens. In the setting of adjuvant chemotherapy for breast cancer, this approach has been tested in a study activated 15 years ago in a CALGB trial[35] which compared CMF plus vincristine and prednisone (CMFVP) for 14 months with CMFVP for 8 months followed by 6 months of VATH (vinblastine, doxorubicin, thiotepa and the androgen fluoxymesterone). The sequential regimen (CMFVP → VATH) was able to achieve a superior treatment outcome limited to patients with more than three positive axillary nodes.

In the attempt to circumvent, in part, the phenomenon of primary drug resistance, adjuvant trials with sequential chemotherapy were designed in the early 1980s at the Milan Cancer

Institute. As a result of the clinical non-cross-resistance of CMF and doxorubicin, the sequential administration of these two regimens was tested in two different patient subsets. Doxorubicin was always delivered intravenously at the dose of 75 mg/m^2 every 3 weeks for four courses. To avoid non-compliance problems with oral cyclophosphamide,[18] all the three drugs in the CMF regimen were delivered intravenously and recycled every 21 days.[36,37]

In women with one to three positive nodes, twelve courses of CMF were randomly compared with eight courses of the same combination, followed by four courses of doxorubicin.

The aim of the study was to assess whether the anthracycline was able to overcome drug resistance, possibly induced by a 6-month treatment with CMF.[24] The recently updated 10-year results confirmed the previous findings[36] on the inability of the sequential CMF → A regimen to improve both relapse-free (57% vs 59%) and overall survival (75% vs 75%) over CMF alone. It is notable that adequate delivery of drug doses failed to affect treatment outcome between pre- and postmenopausal women.

In patients with more than three positive nodes, the sequential administration of A → CMF was randomly tested against the alternating delivery of the same regimens

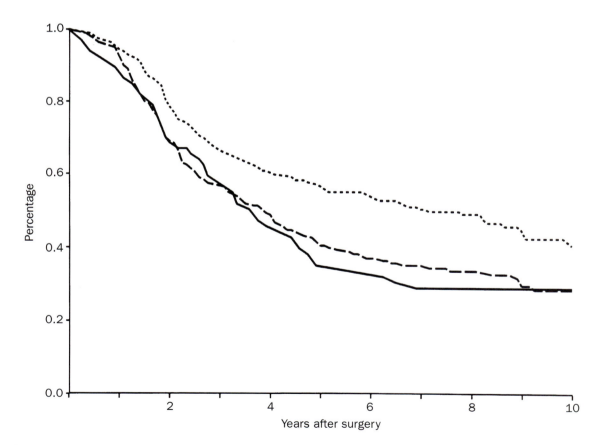

Figure 7.3 Milan Cancer Institute experience with adjuvant chemotherapy in women with over three nodes involved. In a prospective randomized study, sequential A → CMF (.....) obtained a significantly superior relapse-free survival ($p = 0.002$) compared with the alternating administration of the same drug regimens (– – –). The last curve (—) reports the previous experience with 12 monthly cycles of standard CMF in a similar patient subset.

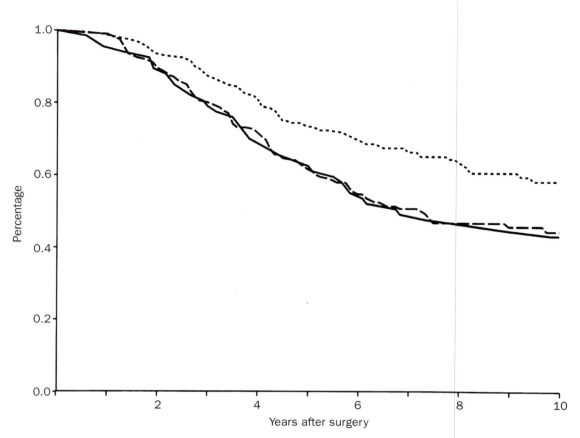

Figure 7.4 Milan Cancer Institute experience with adjuvant chemotherapy in women with over three nodes involved. In a prospective randomized study, sequential A → CMF (·····) obtained a significantly superior overall survival ($p = 0.002$) compared with the alternating administration of the same drug regimens (– – –). The last curve (—) reports the previous experience with 12 monthly cycles of standard CMF in a similar patient subset.

(CMF/A). The 10-year results[37] confirmed that treatment outcome was significantly superior for patients who received the sequential A → CMF regimen compared with those given the alternating chemotherapy (relapse-free survival 42% vs 28%, $p = 0.002$; overall survival 58% vs 44%, $p = 0.002$). With the only variation being the drug sequence, the median duration of relapse-free survival was almost doubled after sequential A → CMF (86 months) compared with CMF/A (47 months). Despite the introduction of the anthracycline agent, the

alternating schedule produced results that were closely comparable with those achieved with classic CMF alone (Figures 7.3 and 7.4). The results achieved with A → CMF in a poor-risk subset could probably be explained by use of full dose size, dose intensity and density, and the sequence of administration of the two regimens. Overall, treatment duration, total drug dose and total received dose intensity were comparable in the two treatment arms. Total treatment duration required 33 weeks; however, in the sequential plan the four cycles of doxorubicin were administered within 9 weeks whereas in the alternating plan they were spread over 27 weeks. Thus, in the sequential arm the dose intensity of anthracycline administration (namely, its administration at full dose and on time) was significantly increased and by itself could account for the superiority of the cross-over treatment. The observation that the inverse sequence of administration (CMF → A) failed to improve treatment outcome in women with one to three positive nodes confirms that the type of drug sequence is important; further studies on this topic could provide more biological insights into the design of optimal regimens in the adjuvant treatment of breast cancer.

New agents

Navelbine, paclitaxel and docetaxel are promising new agents with demonstrated efficacy against advanced breast cancer (see Chapter 21). Among these agents, paclitaxel has already been introduced in the adjuvant setting. Based on the previously mentioned successful experience with A → CMF[37] and on the preliminary results of a pilot study with doxorubicin followed by dose-dense cyclophosphamide,[38] investigators from the Memorial Sloan–Kettering Cancer Center in New York have activated a pilot study in which doxorubicin was followed by paclitaxel and then cyclophosphamide, with three cycles of each drug given every 2 weeks at maximum tolerated dose level and with granulocyte colony-stimulating factor (G-CSF) support.[39] Although early promising results were reported, this sequential regimen had marked haematological toxicity: up to 44% of the patients needed hospital admission during doxorubicin treatment, 24% while receiving paclitaxel and 42% while receiving cyclophosphamide.

Other research groups have also recently activated prospective randomized trials including paclitaxel. In node-positive breast cancer, the Intergroup study compares three different doses of doxorubicin (60 vs 75 vs 90 mg/m^2) plus concomitant cyclophosphamide (600 mg/m^2) every 3 weeks followed by either four cycles of paclitaxel (175 mg/m^2) or no further chemotherapy. A similar study with doxorubicin and cyclophosphamide followed by paclitaxel has been activated by the NSABP (B-28). The Milan Cancer Institute is presently coordinating a multicentre European study in patients with breast cancer measuring over 2 cm at diagnosis in which postoperative A → CMF is being compared with A plus concomitant paclitaxel (T) followed by CMF; in a third arm of the study, AT followed by CMF are delivered before surgery as a primary chemotherapy regimen.[40]

CONTROVERSIAL ISSUES

Timing of chemotherapy and sequencing with radiotherapy

Data from animal models suggest that early initiation of adjuvant chemotherapy is important to achieve optimal therapeutic results. In most clinical trials, adjuvant chemotherapy was planned to start within 4–6 weeks of breast cancer surgery, and retrospective analyses of some of these studies attempting to define the optimal time to start treatment have reported conflicting results.

One large prospective trial designed to assess this issue was carried out by the IBCSG.[41] Patients were randomly allocated to receive one cycle of intravenous CMF immediately after surgery (perioperative chemotherapy) versus no immediate adjuvant systemic therapy. On confirmation of pathological axillary stage, cases of node-positive breast cancer were allocated to either the one single cycle of chemotherapy already applied or six conventionally timed cycles of standard CMF or to both perioperative and conventionally timed chemotherapy. All patients with node-negative tumours received no additional systemic therapy. Treatment outcome in node-positive patients revealed a statistically significant advantage, in terms of both relapse-free and overall survival, favouring both arms of prolonged chemotherapy over one single cycle of perioperative chemotherapy. However, no advantage was detected by the earlier initiation of adjuvant CMF (perioperative plus conventionally timed chemotherapy) over conventionally timed CMF (i.e. started within 3–4 weeks of surgery). Also a recently published overview of randomized trials of perioperative polychemotherapy failed to detect a statistically significant difference in overall survival between earlier versus conventional initiation of adjuvant treatment.[42] However, women allocated to receive perioperative chemotherapy had a significantly lower risk of local disease recurrence ($p < 0.0001$), whereas the difference in distant metastases was of borderline significance ($p = 0.052$).

Limited information is available about the efficacy of adjuvant chemotherapy started beyond the conventional 6 weeks after surgery. This is indeed an important issue, considering that today many more patients are treated with breast-conserving surgery and postoperative radiotherapy. In a retrospective analysis, Recht et al[43] at the Joint Center for Radiation Therapy in Boston reported that the 5-year actuarial rate of local failure, among 252 patients who started radiotherapy within 16 weeks of their breast surgery, was 5% compared with 28% among 34 patients who did not start postoperative irradiation until more than 16 weeks after breast-conserving surgery. In this case series, a delay of more than 16 weeks before starting irradiation occurred preferentially in women with extensive nodal involvement. In this patient subset, adjuvant chemotherapy preceded irradiation in the attempt to decrease the risk of distant metastases. Conflicting findings were subsequently reported by other investigators. The overall results from these studies are, however, somewhat difficult to interpret for several reasons: their retrospective nature, limited numbers of patients in many case series, various follow-up times, and different definition of critical intervals.

Recently, Recht et al[44] reported the 5-year analysis of a prospective trial in 244 women at substantial risk of distant micrometastases. After breast-conserving surgery, patients were randomly assigned to receive a 12-week course of chemotherapy either before or after radiotherapy. Overall, treatment outcome was not significantly different between the two treatment groups. A higher risk of local recurrence was detected in the chemotherapy-first group (14% vs 5%) whereas a higher risk of distant metastases was documented in the radiotherapy-first group (32% vs 20%), the difference in the pattern of first site of disease relapse being of borderline statistical significance ($p = 0.07$). It is notable that overall survival favoured the chemotherapy-first group (81% vs 73%, $p = 0.11$). Another important piece of information from this prospective trial was a significant ($p < 0.01$) difference in the median dose of chemotherapy delivered, which was lower in the radiotherapy-first group.

The results of this study[44] cannot be extrapolated to other regimens, especially those requiring 6 or more months to complete the chemotherapy programme. Nevertheless, they are important from many aspects. In the sequencing of adjuvant chemotherapy and radiotherapy, the issue of local disease control seems less controversial because, as also reported in this case series, it does not affect overall survival, at least for the first 5 years. Moreover, locoregional irradiation, such as that delivered in this study, adversely affects the administration of optimal doses of chemotherapy and, consequently, reduces the beneficial effects of drug treatment against distant micrometastases.

Another point of concern in the appropriate sequence of chemotherapy and radiotherapy is the growing use, in an adjuvant setting, of full doses of powerful drugs, such as doxorubicin and paclitaxel, which could have an undesirable toxic effect when delivered concomitantly with or immediately after irradiation. In addition, further changes in the management of early breast cancer, namely primary or neoadjuvant chemotherapy, are within view and will be of much greater importance to the conventional sequencing of treatment modalities.[40,45]

Use of haemopoietic growth factors

Prospective trials[20] have confirmed the findings from retrospective analyses[18,19,25] that, within the narrow ranges of doses that can be delivered without haemopoietic growth factor support, dose is an important variable in treatment outcome. However, as doubling the dose of cyclophosphamide failed to improve therapeutic results,[28] some investigators have designed pilot studies to test the possibility of increasing the dose intensity of known drug regimens through different schedules of administration.

In conventional regimens, myelosuppression is the most important factor limiting either the delivery of higher doses of some drugs or the possibility of shortening the intervals between treatment cycles. The recent introduction into clinical practice of some haemopoietic colony-stimulating growth factors (CSFs) has proved that it is possible to reduce the haematological toxicity of some of the standard drug regimens. Consequently, CSFs have been used in pilot studies of conventional adjuvant chemotherapy to test the feasibility of higher dose-intensity regimens. Although most of these trials, published mainly in abstract form, reported that higher drug doses or shorter intervals between cycles were devoid of major toxicities, no therapeutic results are as yet available which demonstrate that dose-intense regimens can indeed improve treatment outcome over full-dose standard polychemotherapy. Consequently, in current clinical practice, CSFs must be delivered only following the recommendations of the American Society of Clinical Oncology.[46]

Who should not be treated with adjuvant chemotherapy?

The large body of information available through the international overview[15] has clearly demonstrated that the relative reduction in risk of recurrence and death is fairly constant among all groups of patients with varying baseline prognosis. However, as previously mentioned, the absolute benefit (i.e. the absolute percentage difference between treated and untreated patients) is closely related to the baseline prognosis.

For many years, and even currently, the most powerful prognostic indicator remained the axillary nodal status. Consequently, consensus was easily reached about the benefit of adjuvant systemic therapy for women with involved axillary nodes, whereas there is still considerable controversy about the proper treatment for women with node-negative breast cancer in whom the overall risk of disease relapse is about 20–30% 10 years after surgery.

Over the past two decades, several factors have been identified in the attempt to define patients who should or should not receive adjuvant systemic therapy (see Chapter 3). For most of these factors, each of which has prognostic significance in univariate analysis, to have a role in clinical decision-making, they must still be demonstrated in multivariate analysis to add significantly to the information obtained from the established factors or to be powerful enough to replace them.

A third generation of these factors, which have still not been well defined, attempts to predict benefit or lack of benefit of specific therapies. For example, there is little doubt that in women with oestrogen 'receptor-poor' (negative or <10 fmol/mg) tumours, the effect of tamoxifen is of much less benefit than in patients with oestrogen receptor-positive tumours.[15] The fact that age and menopausal status are in themselves important predictors of specific treatment response is less clearly established. Apart from women over 70 years of age, only a minority of whom have been enrolled into prospective studies of adjuvant chemotherapy, both the international overview[15] and modern effective regimens[20,36,37] have clearly demonstrated that postmenopausal patients can also benefit significantly from adjuvant chemotherapy, provided that they are given full or almost full doses of the planned drugs.

Recently, retrospective analyses have reported that c-erbB-2 expression can predict for response to specific types of adjuvant systemic therapy. Investigators from the IBCSG[47] have observed that methotrexate-containing adjuvant chemotherapy was more effective in patients with c-erbB-2-negative tumours than in women whose tumours over-expressed this oncogene. A similar effect, namely resistance to treatment for tumours over-expressing this oncogene, was also reported in patients treated with adjuvant tamoxifen. In another retrospective analysis carried out in a case series allocated to receive three different dose intensities of CAF chemotherapy, investigators from the Cancer and Leukemia Group B[34] found that higher doses of the doxorubicin-containing regimen were more effective than lower doses in *c-erbB-2*-positive tumours. However, dose intensity did not appear to have an impact on *c-erbB-2*-negative tumours.

Although intriguing, the above-mentioned findings, as well as preliminary analyses on the potential ability of p53 and other molecular factors to predict for treatment responsiveness, still need confirmation and validation through well-designed prospective studies. No less important for most of these variables, it is mandatory to have standardization of laboratory techniques and appropriate definition of cut-off values so that results are reproducible across different case series.

It must be recognized that women with non-invasive breast cancer, as well as those with a minimal risk of disease relapse (e.g. <10% at 10 years), are not candidates for routine adjuvant systemic therapy. For all the remaining patients who elect not to participate in (or are ineligible for) clinical trials, selection of specific modalities of systemic adjuvant treatment still remains controversial, despite the numerous Breast Cancer Conferences which have attempted to reach a consensus. Apart from women with node-negative breast cancer associated with oestrogen receptor-positive and well-to-moderately differentiated tumours, and older (i.e. >70 years of age) women, there are no reasons at present to withhold chemotherapy treatment in any patient subset at moderate-to-high risk of disease relapse, unless clearly dictated by medical contraindications. Adjuvant chemotherapy can be combined with endocrine therapy in certain subgroups (e.g. postmenopausal women and older premenopausal patients with oestrogen receptor-positive tumours). However, despite the suggestions from the international overview,[15] individual studies have not entirely clarified the extent of the additional benefit of the combined chemoendocrine treatment or the

appropriate timing of endocrine therapy (concomitant with or subsequent to chemotherapy) and its optimal duration (2 vs 5 vs >5 years).

In individual cases, it is essential to determine the presence and severity of coexistent morbid conditions, as well as their influence on the selection of therapy. Adjuvant chemotherapy is not reasonable in patients with severe cardiovascular disease (especially if the regimen contains anthracycline drugs) or in women with other severe organ dysfunctions or major immune deficiencies. In older patients with a long-term survival expectancy, adjuvant chemotherapy is not contraindicated, provided full drug doses are delivered. Lowering the doses does not reduce the side effects of the drugs but will compromise the efficacy of treatment.

By making appropriate use of the available information on established prognostic factors, clinicians should be able to quantify the potential benefits of the treatment options. As a result of the many remaining open questions on the optimal adjuvant systemic therapy, patients should be encouraged to participate in ongoing clinical trials activated by all major cooperative groups and cancer centres all over the world. It remains of utmost importance to inform each individual breast cancer patient accurately and openly about the available alternatives, the potential risk and the expected benefits. The patient's own perceptions of the cost–benefit ratio should be strongly considered in decision-making.

CONCLUSIONS

The primary therapy of resectable breast cancer was initiated about a century ago on the principle of centrifugal disease spread along anatomical pathways. Studying the biology of the disease has resulted in the abandonment of the belief that breast cancer always spread sequentially from the primary sites to the nearest draining lymph nodes and then systematically. The adoption of the concept that some cancers may invade the bloodstream early to form micrometastases became very helpful in developing several forms of multidisciplinary strategies. The new biological model was followed by success when correctly applied through prospective randomized trials; these, in turn, were capable of generating new biological concepts, pharmacological strategies and clinical approaches.

The multidisciplinary strategy has contributed towards the emphasis on the complexity of breast cancer, namely the heterogeneity of the primary tumour.[48] Tumour heterogeneity has become the major prognostic determinant of treatment selection and outcome, and remains the major stumbling block to the cure of a large fraction of patients, even when optimal treatment is delivered.

Available clinical results are far from optimal and clinicians must still face many failures. However, reductions in the risk of recurrence and death, as reported by individual trials as well as by the international overview, can well prevent or significantly delay hundreds of thousands of deaths. In a population-based study, Olivotto et al[49] sought to evaluate the effects of adjuvant therapy on survival after a diagnosis of breast cancer, by looking at survival rates over three separate periods of time: 1976 when no adjuvant systemic therapy was delivered; 1980 when adjuvant chemotherapy was delivered to node-positive premenopausal women; and 1984 when chemotherapy was administered to high-risk, node-negative, premenopausal patients and tamoxifen to high-risk, postmenopausal women. The analysis reveals that survival improvements for the two patient subsets occurred at different times: for premenopausal patients improvements began with the 1980 cohorts; for postmenopausal women improvements were only seen in the 1984 cohorts. The authors suggested that these changes were caused by the effects of the introduction of adjuvant systemic therapy into clinical practice. Although their conclusions may be challenged on a number of fronts (e.g. uncertainty that all patients actually received systemic therapy, increasing use of mammography screening), this report is encouraging and certainly suggests that results of positive adjuvant trials can be generalized to the population at large.

Improvements in therapeutic results can now be achieved by the delivery of optimal drug dose intensity and the sequential administration of given non-cross-resistant agents. Our own promising and provocative results with doxorubicin followed by CMF have already started a revision of prior concepts about optimal delivery of single drugs or combinations of drugs. New drugs such as the taxanes hold promises of becoming effective new cytotoxic regimens in the treatment of early breast cancer, but it will take a few years to be appropriately tested in prospective randomized studies. Another area of investigation is represented by the so-called 'biochemical modulation', that is, the development of strategies that favourably alter the interaction of conventional therapeutic agents with their target endpoints in both malignant and non-malignant cells. Therapeutic results achieved in metastatic breast cancer with fluorouracil and folinic acid, combined with other cytotoxic drugs, warrant an appropriate test of their efficacy in an adjuvant setting. High-dose chemotherapy with autologous bone marrow transplantation or reinfusion of peripheral blood progenitor cells should be further pursued and refined within the context of controlled clinical trials. Last, but not least, chemotherapy and endocrine therapy are not mutually exclusive but, rather than competing for given patient subsets, they should become effective partners. Considering steroid receptor heterogeneity, the combined treatment of cytotoxic drugs and hormone manipulations seems rational and has already shown some additive effect.[15] The concomitant administration of both modalities may result in an antagonistic effect as a consequence of their specific mode of action.[50] Therefore, in our opinion, an attractive working hypothesis would be to deliver them sequentially. Relatively short intensive chemotherapy should be given first to kill rapidly proliferating tumour cells, and tamoxifen should then be delivered for appropriate prolonged periods of time to increase further the long-term disease-free status.

Current results on biological response

modifiers, namely BCG, levamisol and interferons, have so far yielded disappointing results.[15] Other modern biological therapies seem to have the promise of adding new dimensions to the therapy of breast cancer, but they still need appropriate testing in advanced breast cancer.

In conclusion, treatment findings accumulated over the last quarter of this century indicate that modern adjuvant chemotherapy is not a fugitive venture and, if properly administered, less toxic than anticipated. Therefore, adjuvant chemotherapy has a definite role in the treatment of primary breast cancer. Both laboratory and clinical results provided biological and therapeutic models which were very helpful in developing contemporary multidisciplinary strategy and more effective polydrug regimens.

Having confirmed on clinical grounds that, in many patient subsets, operable breast cancer is predominantly a microdisseminated disease, the strategic role of drug therapy should now open the possibility of generating new innovative trials aimed at increasing the cell kill of these distant micrometastases. One such opportunity may be provided by the use of effective preoperative drug regimens in high-risk patients.

REFERENCES

1. Halsted WS. The results of radical operations for the cure of carcinoma of the breast. *Ann Surg* 1907; **46**:1–19.
2. Fisher B. Laboratory and clinical research in breast cancer: a personal adventure. The David A. Karnofsky Memorial Lecture. *Cancer Res* 1980; **40**:3863–74.
3. Fisher B. The evolution of paradigms for the management of breast cancer: a personal perspective. *Cancer Res* 1992; **52**:2371–83.
4. Fisher B, Fisher ER. The interrelationship of hematogenous and lymphatic tumor cell dissemination. *Surg Gynecol Obstet* 1966; **122**:791–8.
5. Schabel FM. Concepts for systemic treatment of micrometastases. *Cancer* 1975; **35**:15–24.
6. Martin DS, Fugman RA. A role for chemotherapy as an adjuvant to surgery. *Cancer Res* 1957; **17**:1098–101.
7. Martin DS, Fugman RA, Stolfi RL, Hayworth PE. Solid tumor animal model therapeutically predictive for human breast cancer. *Cancer Chemother Rep* 1975; **5**:89–109.
8. Skipper HE, Schabel FM Jr. Tumor stem cell heterogeneity: implication with respect to the classification of cancers by chemotherapeutic effect. *Cancer Treat Rep* 1984; **68**:43–61.
9. Schabel FM, Griswold DP, Corbett TH, et al. Increasing the therapeutic response rates to anticancer drugs by applying the basic principles of pharmacology. *Cancer* 1984; **54**:1160–7.
10. Fisher B, Ravdin RG, Ausman RK, et al. Surgical adjuvant chemotherapy in cancer of the breast: results of a decade of cooperative investigation. *Ann Surg* 1968; **168**:337–56.
11. Bonadonna G. Evolving concepts in the systemic adjuvant treatment of breast cancer. *Cancer Res* 1992; **52**:2127–37.
12. Fisher B, Carbone P, Economou SG, et al. L-Phenylalanine mustard (L-PAM) in the management of primary breast cancer: a report of early findings. *N Engl J Med* 1975; **292**:117–22.
13. Bonadonna G, Brusamolino E, Valagussa P, et al. Combination chemotherapy as an adjuvant treatment in operable breast cancer. *N Engl J Med* 1976; **294**:405–10.
14. Early Breast Cancer Trialists' Collaborative Group. Effects of adjuvant tamoxifen and cytotoxic therapy on mortality in early breast cancer: an overview of 61 randomized trials among 28,896 women. *N Engl J Med* 1988; **319**:1681–92.
15. Early Breast Cancer Trialists' Collaborative Group. Systemic treatment of early breast cancer by hormonal, cytotoxic, or immune therapy. 133 randomised trials involving 31 000 recurrences and 24 000 deaths among 75 000 women. *Lancet* 1992; **339**:1–15, 71–85.
16. Valagussa P, Brambilla C, Zambetti M, Bonadonna G. Salvage treatments in relapsing resectable breast cancer. *Recent Results Cancer Res* 1989; **115**:69–76.
17. Bonadonna G, Valagussa P. The contribution of medicine to the primary treatment of breast cancer. *Cancer Res* 1988; **48**:2314–24.
18. Bonadonna G, Valagussa P. Dose–response effect of adjuvant chemotherapy in breast cancer. *N Engl J Med* 1981; **304**:10–15.
19. Bonadonna G, Valagussa P, Moliterni A, et al. Adjuvant cyclophosphamide, methotrexate, and fluorouracil in node-positive breast cancer. The results of 20 years of follow-up. *N Engl J Med* 1995; **332**:901–6.

20. Wood WC, Budman DR, Korzun AH, et al. Dose and dose intensity of adjuvant chemotherapy for stage II, node-positive breast carcinoma. *N Engl J Med* 1994; **330**:1253–9.

21. Goldhirsch A, Gelber RD, Price KN, et al. Effect of systemic adjuvant treatment on first sites of breast cancer relapse. *Lancet* 1994; **343**:377–81.

22. Castiglione-Gertsch M, Johnsen C, Goldhirsch A, et al. The International (Ludwig) Breast Cancer Study Group Trials I-IV: 15 years of follow-up. *Ann Oncol* 1994; **5**:717–24.

23. Zambetti M, Valagussa P, Bonadonna G. Adjuvant cyclophosphamide, methotrexate and fluorouracil in node negative and estrogen receptor-negative breast cancer. Updated results. *Ann Oncol* 1996; **7**:481–5.

24. Tancini G, Bonadonna G, Valagussa P, et al. Adjuvant CMF in breast cancer: comparative 5-year results of 12 versus 6 cycles. *J Clin Oncol* 1983; **1**:2–10.

25. Hryniuk W, Levine MN. Analysis of dose intensity for adjuvant chemotherapy trials in stage II breast cancer. *J Clin Oncol* 1986; **4**:1162–70.

26. Bremond A, Kerbrat P, Fumoleau P, et al. Five year follow-up results of a randomized trial testing the role of the dose intensity and duration of chemotherapy in node positive premenopausal breast cancer patients [abstract]. *Proc Am Soc Clin Oncol* 1996; **15**:113.

27. Bonneterre J, Rochè H, Bremond A, et al. A randomized trial of adjuvant chemotherapy with FEC 50 vs FEC 100 for node-positive operable breast cancer: early report [abstract]. *Proc Am Soc Clin Oncol* 1996; **15**:104.

28. Dimitrov N, Anderson S, Fisher B, et al. Dose intensification and increased total dose of adjuvant chemotherapy for breast cancer: findings from NSABP B-22 [abstract]. *Proc Am Soc Clin Oncol* 1994; **13**:64.

29. Harris JR, Hellman S, Henderson IC (eds) *Breast Diseases*, 2nd edn. Philadelphia, PA: JB Lippincott, 1991.

30. Buzdar AU, Gutterman JU, Blumenschein GR, et al. Intensive postoperative chemoimmunotherapy for patients with stage II and stage III breast cancer. *Cancer* 1978; **41**:1064–75.

31. Fisher B, Brown AM, Dimitrov NV, et al. Two months of doxorubicin–cyclophosphamide with and without interval reinduction therapy compared with 6 months of cyclophosphamide, methotrexate, and fluorouracil in positive-node breast cancer patients with tamoxifen-nonresponsive tumors: results from the National Surgical Adjuvant Breast and Bowel Project B-15. *J Clin Oncol* 1990; **8**:1483–96.

32. Levine M, Bramwell V, Bowman D, et al. CEF vs CMF in premenopausal women with node positive breast cancer [abstract]. *Proc Am Soc Clin Oncol* 1995; **14**:103 .

33. Valagussa P, Bonadonna G. Carcinogenic effects of cancer treatment. In: *Oxford Textbook of Oncology* (Peckham M, Pinedo H, Veronesi U, eds). Oxford: Oxford University Press, 1995: 2348–58.

34. Muss HB, Thor AD, Berr DA, et al. *C-erbB-2* expression and response to adjuvant therapy in women with node-positive breast cancer. *N Engl J Med* 1994; **330**:1260–6.

35. Perloff M, Norton L, Korzun AH, et al. Advantage of an adriamycin combination plus halotestin after initial cyclophosphamide, methotrexate, 5-fluorouracil, vincristine and prednisone (CMFVP) for adjuvant therapy of node-positive stage II breast cancer [abstract]. *Proc Am Soc Clin Oncol* 1986; **5**:70.

36. Moliterni A, Bonadonna G, Valagussa P, et al. Cyclophosphamide, methotrexate, and fluorouracil with and without doxorubicin in the adjuvant treatment of resectable breast cancer with one to three positive axillary nodes. *J Clin Oncol* 1991; **9**:1124–30.

37. Bonadonna G, Zambetti M, Valagussa P. Sequential or alternating doxorubicin and CMF regimens in breast cancer with more than three positive nodes. Ten-year results. *JAMA* 1995; **273**:542–7.

38. Hudis C, Legwohl J, Crown T, et al. Feasibility of adjuvant dose-intensive cyclophosphamide with G-CSF after doxorubicin in women with high risk stage II/III resectable breast cancer [abstract]. *Proc Am Soc Clin Oncol* 1992; **12**:55 .

39. Hudis C, Seidman A, Baselga J, et al. Sequential adjuvant therapy with doxorubicin/paclitaxel/cyclophosphamide for resectable breast cancer involving four or more axillary nodes. *Semin Oncol* 1995; **22** (suppl 15):18–23.

40. Bonadonna G. Current and future trends in the multidisciplinary approach for high-risk breast cancer: the experience of the Milan Cancer Institute. *Eur J Cancer* 1996; **32A**:209–14.

41. The Ludwig Breast Cancer Study Group. Combination adjuvant chemotherapy for node-positive breast cancer: inadequacy of a single perioperative cycle. *N Engl J Med* 1988; **319**:677–83.

42. Clahsen PC, Van de Velde C, Goldhirsch A, et al.

An overview of randomized perioperative poly-chemotherapy trials in women with early breast cancer. *J Clin Oncol* 1996: in press.

43. Recht A, Come SE, Gelman RS, et al. Integration of conservative surgery, radiotherapy, and chemotherapy for the treatment of early-stage, node-positive breast cancer. Sequencing, timing and outcome. *J Clin Oncol* 1991; **9:**1662–7.

44. Recht A, Come SE, Henderson IC, et al. The sequencing of chemotherapy and radiation therapy after conservative surgery for early-stage breast cancer. *N Engl J Med* 1996; **334:**1356–61.

45. Bonadonna G, Valagussa P, Zucali R, Salvadori B. Primary chemotherapy in surgically resectable breast cancer. *CA Cancer J Clin* 1995; **45:**227–43.

46. American Society of Clinical Oncology. Recommendations for the use of hematopoietic colony-stimulating factors: evidence-based clinical practise guidelines. *Blood* 1994; **12:**2471–508.

47. Gusterson BA, Gelber RD, Goldhirsch A, et al. Prognostic importance of *c-erbB-2* expression in breast cancer. *J Clin Oncol* 1992; **10:**1049–56.

48. Heppner GH. Tumor heterogeneity. *Cancer Res* 1984; **44:**2259–65.

49. Olivotto IA, Bajdik CD, Plenderleith IH, et al. Adjuvant systemic therapy and survival after breast cancer. *N Engl J Med* 1994; **330:**805–10.

50. Osborne CK, Kitten L, Arteaga CL. Antagonism of chemotherapy-induced cytotoxicity for human breast cancer cells by antiestrogens. *J Clin Oncol* 1989; **7:**710–17.

8

Conventional adjuvant hormonal therapy

Kathleen I Pritchard

CONTENTS • Background • Rationale • Adjuvant ovarian ablation • Adjuvant tamoxifen • Other adjuvant endocrine therapies • Conclusions

BACKGROUND

Ovarian ablation was first used by Beatson[1] before the turn of the century and proved useful in shrinking widespread breast cancer. Around the same time, Schinzinger suggested that oophorectomy be done before or at the time as mastectomy in order to 'involute' the breast thus 'containing tumour cells'.[2] The subsequent development of methods for radiation ovarian ablation led others to suggest that radiation castration after radical mastectomy might prevent or postpone the development of metastatic disease.[3] A series of small trials of adjuvant ovarian ablation were subsequently carried out, but the small size of the studies, poor study design, lack of sophisticated methodology for analysis and the apparently minimal effects seen in these trials led to a loss of interest in this modality, which was then overshadowed by the promising early results of adjuvant chemotherapy in the mid-1970s.[4,5]

By the early 1980s, however, it was apparent that combination chemotherapy was also limited in its effects. Chemotherapy, at least as given at that time, seemed to provide little improvement for postmenopausal women and, even in the premenopausal population, it was

not a panacea. In turn, the more widespread availability of measurements of estrogen receptors (ERs) and progesterone receptors (PRs), and the development of several new hormonal agents,[6,7] encouraged a re-examination of adjuvant endocrine therapy. Early in its use, it became obvious that adjuvant tamoxifen, particularly in postmenopausal patients, had an effect that was not dissimilar from that of adjuvant combination chemotherapy in premenopausal women, at least in terms of relapse-free survival. With this conceptual shift to the use of adjuvant endocrine therapy in postmenopausal women, there was renewed interest in ovarian ablation in the premenopausal population. The development, in 1984, of the Early Breast Cancer Trialists' Collaborative Group (EBCTCG), a consortium of investigators interested in examining adjuvant hormonal and chemotherapy trials using the meta-analysis or overview technique, led to a re-examination of the entire area of adjuvant therapy. It was really the results of this first overview analysis that finally made it clear that tamoxifen in postmenopausal women and ovarian ablation in premenopausal women had consistent and significant effects on both relapse and overall survival.[8]

RATIONALE

In women with metastatic breast cancer, ablative or additive endocrine therapies produce response rates of 30% in unselected patients, close to 50% in women with ER-positive tumors and up to 80% in women with ER, PR-positive tumors.[9,10] In contrast, fewer than 5–10% of ER-negative or ER- and PR-negative tumors will respond to hormonal manipulations.[9,10] Response rates are proportional to the levels of hormone receptor measured.[10,11] Receptor levels measured in primary tumors correspond quite closely to levels measured in recurrent disease, at least in the absence of intervening hormonal therapy.[12] Thus, the receptor status of the primary tumor probably represents that of any occult metastases left after primary surgery quite accurately, and so it would seem likely that adjuvant endocrine therapy of any type would prove most effective in women with high ER and PR levels at the time of primary surgery.

ADJUVANT OVARIAN ABLATION

Trials of adjuvant ovarian ablation versus no other systemic therapy

After the proposal of adjuvant oophorectomy by Schinzinger,[2] over 20 trials of various types of ovarian ablation, with or without the addition of prednisone, were carried out. Many of these trials, however, were done before the era of randomized clinical trials and before the widespread availability of ER or PR measurements.

The first trials of ovarian ablation consisted mainly of series of patients from single institutions, often with historical, non-matched, non-randomized controls. Furthermore, information was seldom present on such now well-appreciated prognostic factors as nodal status.[13] In spite of the problems with these early studies, however, most suggested some advantage in favor of ovarian ablation. A little later, several studies were carried out using surgical or radiation castration, with matched but non-randomized control groups.[14–18] Some of these also suggested a degree of benefit for patients who received ovarian ablation,[16,18] although others found neither benefit nor detriment.[14,15,17]

As randomized controlled clinical trials came into more common usage, several prospective randomized trials of ovarian ablation have been carried out (Table 8.1).[19–28]

Trials of ovarian ablation plus chemotherapy versus the same chemotherapy used alone

In addition to the randomized studies of ovarian ablation versus no further systemic therapy, there are at least five trials in which women were randomized to receive ovarian ablation by either surgery or radiation in addition to systemic therapy, versus the same systemic therapy used alone (Table 8.2). These trials in general began somewhat later and, as a result, only two of them have been published in individual form,[29,30] although three others have provided updated information to the Oxford overview process.

Trials of medical ovarian ablation or suppression

At the time of the 1995 Oxford overview update, four trials in which premenopausal women were randomized to receive or not to receive medically induced ovarian suppression were registered (Table 8.3). No data were available for the 1995 overview analysis from any of these trials, and no results have as yet been published. The overall results of all of these trials have been summarized best in the recent overview analysis of ovarian ablation just published in *The Lancet*[31] and summarized below.

EBCTCG or Oxford overview of ovarian ablation in early breast cancer: the 1995 update

In 1995, the EBCTCG based in Oxford sought information about every patient who had been

Table 8.1 Randomized trials of ovarian ablation versus no systemic therapy

Trial	Ovarian treatment (Gy)	Accrual period	Randomized <50 years	>50 years	Data available	Published (Ref.)
Paterson (Christie)	4.5	1948–50	178	11	Yes	Yes (19)
Nissen-Meyer (Norwegian)	10	1957–63	151	195	Yes	Yes (20)
Nevinny (Boston)	Surgery	1961*		143	No	Yes (26)
Ravdin (NSABP)	Surgery	1961–7	184	0	Yes	Yes (21)
Bryant and Weir (Saskatchewan)	Surgery	1964–74	255	124	Yes	Yes (25)
Meakin and Hayward (Princess Margaret Hospital, Toronto)	20†	1965–72	349	430	Yes	Yes (22,23) 24
Ontario Cancer Research and Treatment Foundation	15	1968–77	9	323	Yes	Yes (27)
CRFB Cancer Agency	9/14	1971–6	1	51	Yes	Yes (28)
Bradford RI	Surgery	1974–85	42	9	Yes	No
Subtotal (except Nevinny)		1948–85	1169	1143	Yes	

NSABP, National Surgical Adjuvant Breast Project; RI, Radiotherapy Institute; CRFB, Centre Regionale François Baclesse.
*143 patients were randomized but there are no individual patient data available on accrual period, age distribution or outcome.
†Stratum 1: control vs 20 Gy.

Table 8.2 Randomized trials of ovarian ablation plus chemotherapy versus chemotherapy alone

Trial	Ovarian treatment (Gy)	Common systemic therapy	Accrual period	Randomized <50 years	>50 years	Data available	Published (Ref.)
Bradford RI	Surgery	M + TT	1974–85	38	5	Yes	No
Toronto–Edmonton Study Group	15 +P	CMF† (some ±TT)	1978–88	241	56	Yes*	No
Ragaz BCCA Vancouver	16 +P	CMF	1979–85	111	23	Yes*	Yes (29)
IBCSG/Ludwig II	Surgery	CMF + P	1978–81	281	75	Yes*	Yes (30)
SWOG 7827B	Surgery	CMFVP	1979–89	262	52	Yes*	No
Subtotal			1974–89	933	211		

RI, Radiotherapy Institute; IBCSG, International Breast Cancer Study Group; BCCA, British Columbia Cancer Agency; SWOG, South West Oncology Group.
*Estrogen receptors available only in these trials
†First patients were cross-randomized to receive or not to receive immunotherapy with oral BCG (Bacillus Calmette–Guèrin).
IT, immunotherapy; F, 5-fluorouracil; TT, thiotepa; C, cyclophosphamide; V, vincristine; M, methotrexate; P, prednisone.

in any randomized trial of ovarian ablation or suppression versus control that had been started before 1990 for the purpose of an updated overview or meta-analysis. Data were available for 12 of the 13 known studies assessing ovarian ablation by radiation or surgery, but not for any of the four known studies assessing ovarian suppression by drugs, all of which started after 1980. As menopausal status was not consistently defined across these trials, the main analysis of the 1995 Oxford overview has been carried out in women aged under 50, as has been done in the past.[8,32–34] Although the overview attempted to analyze results according to ERs, these measurements were only available in the later trials – those of ovarian ablation plus chemotherapy versus the same chemotherapy alone.

Effects in women under 50

The 1995 overview analysis[31] reports the results from 2102 women aged less than 50 when randomized. At the time of the 1995 analysis, there had been 1130 deaths and an additional 153 recurrences in these women. The analysis shows that 15-year survival showed a highly significant improvement among those allocated to ovarian ablation (52.4% vs 46.1%: difference = 6.3% ± s.d. 2.3; $p = 0.001$) (Figure 8.1a). Recurrence-free survival was even more significantly improved (45% vs 39%: difference = 6.0% ± s.d. 2.3; $p = 0.0007$) (Figure 8.1b).

The numbers of events in the study, although large, are too small for really reliable subgroup analyses. In addition, attempts to analyze the results in node-negative versus node-positive women are heavily confounded by the fact that

Table 8.3 Randomized trials of medical ovarian ablation							
Trial	Ovarian treatment (Gy)	Common systemic therapy	Accrual period	Randomized <50 years	>50 years	Data available	Published (Ref.)
CRC under 50s	Goserelin	± Tam	1987–SR	972	0	No	No
FNCLCC France	Triptorelen or goserelin	FAC or FEC	1989–SR	746	120	No	No
SE Sweden	Goserelin	± Tam	1989–SR	191	0	No	No
ECOG EST 5188	Goserelin	FAC ± Tam	1989–94	1382	155	No	No
Subtotal			1987–	3291	275		

F, 5-fluorouracil; C, cyclophosphamide; V, vincristine; A, adriamycin (doxorubicin); E, epirubicin; SR, still randomizing patients; Tam, tamoxifen; CRC, Cancer Research Campaign, FNCLCC, Federation Nationale de Centres de Lutte Contre le Cancer, Institut Gustave Roussy; SE, south-east; ECOG, Eastern Cooperative Oncology Group.

almost all of the node-negative women were entered into trials of ovarian ablation versus no therapy, whereas almost all of the node-positive women were entered into trials of chemotherapy plus ovarian ablation versus the same chemotherapy given alone. Thus, the relative effectiveness of ovarian ablation with respect to nodal status could only be assessed, in the overview, in those ovarian ablation trials in which chemotherapy was not given. In the trials of ovarian ablation alone versus no other systemic therapy, however, proportional risk reductions for node-positive and node-negative women appeared similar, although the absolute risk reduction was not significantly greater for node-positive women. For both recurrence-free and overall survival, there was a significant improvement within both node-negative ($p = 0.01$ for recurrence; $p = 0.01$ for survival) and node-positive ($p = 0.0002$ for recurrence; $p = 0.0007$ for survival) subgroups of women

receiving ovarian ablation (Figure 8.2a and 8.2b).

Estrogen receptor measurements on the primary tumor were available for four of the five trials in which women were randomized to receive chemotherapy plus ovarian ablation versus the same chemotherapy used alone. Among the 194 women with ER-poor primary tumors, there was no apparent benefit to the addition of ovarian ablation in terms of recurrence-free or overall survival. Among the 550 women with ER-positive primary tumors, however, the addition of ovarian ablation appeared beneficial for both recurrence-free survival (odds reduction = 13% ± s.d. = 11; non-significant [NS]) and overall survival (odds reduction 17% ± s.d. = 13; NS), but these differences were not statistically significant.

Analyses were done to examine the degree of benefit provided by ovarian ablation added to cytotoxic chemotherapy, in comparison to its benefit when given in the absence of cytotoxic

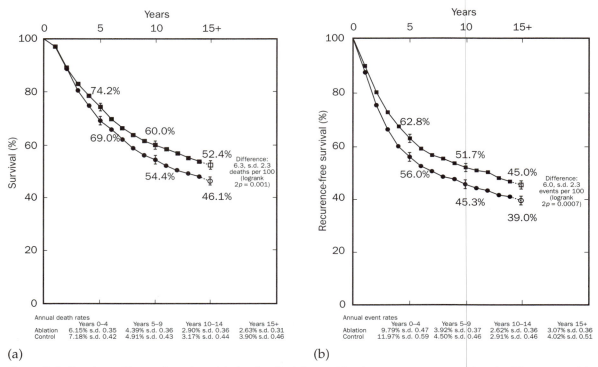

Figure 8.1 Absolute effects of ovarian ablation in all trials combined among women aged under 50 at entry. (a) Overall survival and (b) recurrence-free survival for 2102 women aged under 50, when randomized between ovarian ablation (■) and control (●). Bars indicate standard deviations (s.d.).

chemotherapy. The proportional improvement in annual odds of recurrence in women in the absence of chemotherapy was 25% ± s.d. = 7 ($p = 0.0005$), whereas the proportional improvement in annual odds of recurrence in the presence of chemotherapy was only 10% ± s.d. = 9 ($p > 0.1$, NS).[31] Similarly, the proportional improvement in annual odds of death was 24% ± s.d. = 7 ($p = 0.0006$) in the absence of chemotherapy, but only 8% ± s.d. = 10 ($p > 0.1$; NS) in the presence of chemotherapy. As a result of the small numbers of deaths, however, it is difficult to tell whether these differences are actually reliable. Furthermore, formal statistical testing using tests for heterogeneity, although known to lack power, do not confirm a significant difference between the effects of ovarian ablation in the presence and those in the absence of chemotherapy.

Effects in women over 50
In the 1995 overview analysis, data were available on 1354 women aged 50 or over who were randomized to receive or not to receive ovarian ablation. Most of these would have been peri or postmenopausal. There was only a small and non-significant improvement in survival and recurrence-free survival in this subset. By year 15 after randomization, there were 3.1% (± s.d. = 2.6; NS) fewer recurrences or deaths per 100 women allocated to ovarian ablation. There were 32% alive without recurrence in the ovarian ablation group versus 28.9% in the controls (NS) and 36.9% alive overall in the ovarian ablation group versus 34.5% of controls (NS).

Late effects and effects on non-breast cancer deaths
The late effects of ovarian ablation can be clearly examined in this overview analysis.

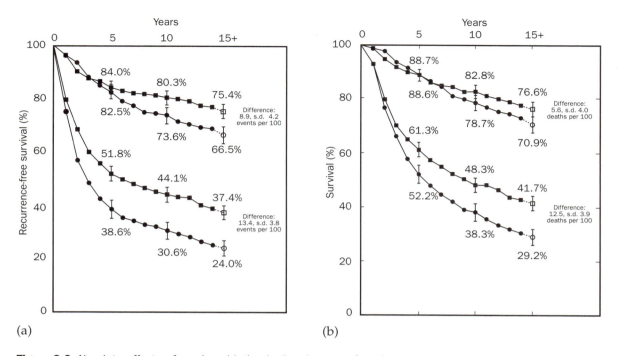

(a) (b)

Figure 8.2 Absolute effects of ovarian ablation in the absence of routine chemotherapy in all trials combined among women aged under 50 at entry. (a) Recurrence-free survival and (b) overall survival for 473 node-negative and 696 node-positive women who were aged under 50 when randomized between ovarian ablation (■) and control (●) in the trials, or parts of trials, where cytotoxic therapy was not routinely used. Among node-negative women, in years 0–4 there were 28 deaths out of 1170 person-years in the ablation group versus 25/1037 in the controls (annual death rates: 2.4%, s.d. 0.5 versus 2.4%, s.d. 0.5); in years 5–9 there were 15/1030 versus 21/884 (1.5%, s.d. 0.4 versus 2.4%, s.d. 0.5); in years 10–14 there were 12/931 versus 15/779 (1.3%, s.d. 0.4 versus 1.9% s.d. 0.5); and in years 15+ there were 33/1580 versus 43/1309 (2.1%, s.d. 0.4 versus 3.3%, s.d. 0.5). Among node-positive women, the corresponding values are: years 0–4, 166/1620 versus 134/997 (10.3%, s.d. 0.8 versus 13.4%, s.d. 1.2); 5–9, 55/1077 versus 37/577 (5.1%, s.d. 0.7 versus 6.4%, s.d. 1.1); 10–14, 29/870 versus 23/426 (3.3%, s.d. 0.6 versus 5.4%, s.d. 1.1); and 15+, 40/1151 versus 28/491 (3.5%, s.d. 0.6 versus 5.7%, s.d. 1.1). All *p* values are 2-sided and were calculated by the logrank method.

Most of the patients in these trials were randomized before 1970 and for most survivors there is follow-up information going beyond 1990. Thus, there is a large amount of information available beyond year 15 of follow up. Even during this later time period, the annual death rates for all women in the overview remain lower among those who were originally allocated to ovarian ablation (2.6% ± s.d. = 0.3) than among the controls (3.9% ± s.d. = 0.5). Thus, the effects of ovarian ablation appear to persist long after the

women underwent this procedure.

The overview also attempted to study cause-specific mortality. Among women under 50 who died without any record of a distant recurrence of their breast cancer, 116 were classified as having died of non-breast cancer causes. Taking into account the fact that those allocated to ovarian ablation survived longer, and were therefore at more prolonged risk of death from other causes, there was then no significant difference between the treatment groups in terms of vascular deaths (22/922 in the ovarian ablation group vs 20/824 in the controls) in trials for which data were provided. Similarly, there was no difference in non-breast cancer, non-vascular deaths (44/929 vs 30/824) or all non-breast cancer deaths.

Second breast primaries

An attempt was made to look at the incidence of contralateral breast cancer, but there was insufficient information to examine this issue. Thirty contralateral breast cancers were recorded as the first event among 712 women allocated to ovarian ablation, compared with 32 of 679 women in the control arm in trials for which data were provided.

1995 overview summary

In summary, the overview confirms suggestions from individual trials that ovarian ablation in premenopausal women provides a small, but statistically significant, benefit in terms of recurrence-free and overall survival. This benefit appears similar for node-positive and node-negative women. There appears to be some degree of benefit both in the presence and in the absence of chemotherapy, although the degree of benefit in the presence of chemotherapy is not statistically significant. Although the degree of benefit appears larger when ovarian ablation is given in the absence than in the presence of chemotherapy, this appearance is not fully confirmed by formal statistical testing, because tests of heterogeneity suggest no significant difference between the effects of ovarian ablation in the two situations. From the few trials for which ER measurements are available, the effect of ovarian ablation appears to be significant in those women with ERs in their tumors and not significant in those without. The numbers available to examine this issue are, however, very small. Similarly, it is difficult to draw firm conclusions regarding non-breast cancer deaths or the incidence of second primary breast cancers. There is, however, no obvious difference in the incidence of non-cancer deaths in those randomized to ovarian ablation.

Relationship between amenorrhea and response to chemotherapy

The results outlined above suggest that ovarian ablation may not be as effective when it is added to chemotherapy as it is when given alone. An obvious explanation of this could involve the degree of ovarian suppression provided by chemotherapy. The incidence of amenorrhea has been reported from several trials of cytotoxic chemotherapy in premenopausal women and ranges from 40% to 90%.[35–40] Several investigators have attempted to examine whether chemotherapy acts through ovarian ablation, by trying to correlate the effectiveness of chemotherapy with amenorrhea in women within each randomized trial. Three investigators have found that women who develop amenorrhea have a longer disease-free and/or overall survival,[35–37] but three others have not found this relationship.[38–40] These conflicting data suggest that, although more investigation is required, it may well be that part of the explanation for the better effects of cytotoxic chemotherapy in younger or premenopausal women is that a medical castration is achieved in many of these women.[35–37] Clearly, however, this effect does not explain the entire action of cytotoxic chemotherapy in this setting.[38–40] Thus, it is probable that the results of the Oxford overview, in which ovarian ablation does not appear to add as much for women who are also receiving cytotoxic chemotherapy, may relate to the fact that the cytotoxic chemotherapy is already carrying out castration even in the non-ovarian ablation control groups in these trials.

Comparability of ovarian ablation to chemotherapy

Very few studies exist comparing chemotherapy directly to ovarian ablation. One small study by the Scottish Cancer Trials Breast Group[41] compared adjuvant ovarian ablation with combination chemotherapy using cyclophosphamide, methotrexate and 5-fluorouracil (CMF) in premenopausal women with pathologic stage II breast cancer. In this group, ovarian ablation was comparable in its effects to CMF, in terms of both disease-free and overall survival, for the entire group of women randomized. When one divided the patients by ER positivity and negativity, however, it seemed that ovarian ablation produced a substantially better effect in ER-positive women, whereas chemotherapy produced a substantially better effect in ER-negative women. It is worth noting that the CMF given in this study was not particularly dose intensive, and that more aggressive or intensive types of chemotherapy, such as the classic Bonadonna regimen[5] given in full doses or the newly reported CEF regimen[42] which appears to be superior to classic Bonadonna CMF, may provide more substantial effects and thus, presumably, be superior to ovarian ablation used alone. This sort of indirect conclusion is somewhat unsatisfactory, however, and it is to be hoped that more direct comparisons of ovarian ablation and chemotherapy will be carried out in the future in order to delineate their relative roles in premenopausal women further.

Equivalence of ovarian medical suppression and surgical or radiation ovarian ablation

Although a number of the newer trials outlined above are now substituting medical ovarian ablation for radiation or surgical ablation, the equivalence of this treatment or indeed the equivalence of ovarian ablation by surgery and by radiation is unclear.

Ovarian irradiation has been assumed to produce an effect similar to that of surgical oophorectomy. There are considerable data, however, to suggest that after ovarian irradiation, depending on the dose and dose schedule and the age of the patient, ovarian function may not be totally destroyed. For example, in the study of Nissen-Meyer and others, 13% of the women castrated by irradiation resumed menses at some later date.[20] Similarly, in the study of Meakin and others,[22] 3.3% of women receiving 20 grays (Gy) to the ovaries in five fractions resumed menstruation over subsequent years (7% of those over 45 at the time of therapy). Thus, ovarian irradiation may not produce the complete and permanent ablation that is presumably achieved by surgery. In spite of this there seems no obvious difference between the results of ovarian ablation and surgical ablation in the various individual trials or in the Oxford overview analysis.

Similarly, medical ablation with drugs such as goserelin (Zoladex) is assumed to be equivalent to surgical oophorectomy. The luteinizing hormone-releasing hormone (LHRH) agonist, goserelin, has been shown to suppress ovarian function and to produce clinical responses in pre- and perimenopausal women with advanced breast cancer; these responses are similar to those previously reported for other hormonal therapies in phase I and II trials.[43–46] This has recently been confirmed in a randomized study comparing goserelin to ovarian ablation in premenopausal women with metastatic disease.[47] In ongoing adjuvant trials, however, the LHRH analogs are given for periods of time that range from 2 to 5 years. Depending on the age of the patients involved, 5 years of an LHRH analog may take them through the time when they would normally reach a physiologic menopause, but, in younger women, the discontinuation of the LHRH analog would usually lead to resumed ovarian function because the endocrine effects of these analogs are reversible; the menses also usually return within 1–2 months of discontinuing the therapy.[48] Presumably, the length of the ovarian suppression will affect its efficacy as adjuvant therapy, perhaps in a similar way to the effects demonstrated with varying lengths of tamoxifen treatment.[49,50] The relative importance of length of treatment in this setting has been poorly studied to date and still needs to be clarified in future trials.

Effects of ovarian ablation on other body systems

It is well recognized that premature ovarian ablation can have deleterious effects on the cardiovascular and skeletal systems.[51,52] Whether this assumes a major role in terms of comparing competing risks of death with the risk of dying from breast cancer has not, however, been clearly established. Certainly, the most updated information from the Oxford overview does not suggest any strong trend towards increased cardiac or non-breast cancer deaths in the women randomized to receive ovarian ablation. The difficulty of establishing cause of death, particularly in a meta-analysis setting in which information is obtained retrospectively from multiple centres, may, however, obscure a relatively small or even a moderately large effect on deaths from other causes. Alternatively, the competing risk of death from breast cancer may be so high that it greatly outweighs any effect on deaths from other causes. In particular, deaths related to increased osteoporosis will not be as frequent as those from breast cancer, nor will they occur until the patients have had 20–30 years of follow-up after ovarian ablation. Cardiac deaths may be of greater concern in that they are both more common and occur at younger ages, but to date increased cardiac deaths have not been demonstrated in any individual study or in the overview analysis. Further data concerning these long-term risks of death still have to be collected.

Conclusions and future directions

It seems clear that ovarian ablation has a small but significant effect on disease-free and overall survival in premenopausal women, particularly those with positive ERs. This effect appears significant and fairly similar in both node-positive and node-negative women, although it appears to have a greater absolute effect in those with positive nodes. The effect appears to be more dramatic when ovarian ablation is used alone than when it is given in the presence of cytotoxic chemotherapy. The indirect comparisons of treatment effects in different circumstances, i.e. node-negative versus node-positive, or ovarian ablation in the presence versus in the absence of chemotherapy, have, however, to be interpreted with more caution than the results obtained from direct comparisons within each randomized trial and from the summaries of those direct comparisons obtained in the overview. Much additional follow-up information will be available on each of these individual trials over the next 5–10 years and for the next cycle of the overview which will occur in the year 2000. For example, one Chinese trial of ovarian ablation which started in 1991 has already randomized more than 3000 premenopausal women. In addition, there are over 3000 women in the recent trials of ovarian suppression with LHRH agonists. A large study comparing tamoxifen plus ovarian ablation as adjuvant therapy versus tamoxifen plus ovarian ablation at the time of recurrence is also taking place in Vietnam (Richard Love, personal communication). These trials will add considerable additional information to what is already available.

It would still be useful, however, to undertake further large randomized trials assessing the additional effects of ovarian ablation in the presence of cytotoxic chemotherapy, as well as the additional effects of cytotoxic chemotherapy in the presence of ovarian ablation, and for further assessment of the effects of both or either of these modalities in the presence of prolonged tamoxifen therapy. Such trials could be designed as three-way comparisons of ovarian ablation versus cytotoxic chemotherapy versus both, which could add data in each of the areas that researchers might wish to examine further. Until further information becomes available, however, there is insufficient information to conclude that ovarian ablation is useful in premenopausal women with positive ERs, in whom it produces effects comparable to those of CMF-type chemotherapy in that setting. Although there is a far larger body of data establishing the role of CMF or comparable types of chemotherapy in the premenopausal setting, certainly enough data exist to suggest that ovarian ablation might be used as an alternative in ER-positive women for whom chemotherapy is either unacceptable or unsuitable for whatever reason. In the meantime, it is necessary to await further data before recommending ovarian ablation as a routine alternative to chemotherapy in any group of premenopausal women, or before recommending it for routine addition to chemotherapy in that setting.

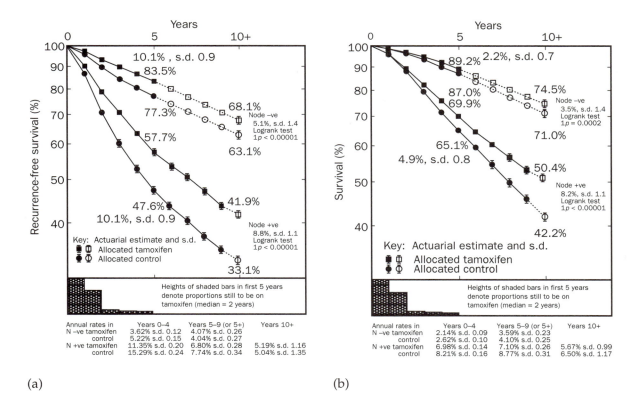

Figure 8.3 (a) Recurrence (all ages) and (b) mortality (all ages) in tamoxifen trials. (Reprinted with permission from *Lancet* 1992; **339:**1–15, 71–85.)

ADJUVANT TAMOXIFEN

Tamoxifen has been evaluated extensively in the adjuvant setting, especially in post-menopausal node-positive women[53–66] but also in premenopausal[53,55,56,63,65–68] and node-negative women.[41,53–56,63,66,67,69,70] Over 40 prospective randomized trials of adjuvant tamoxifen have been carried out, either comparing tamoxifen with placebo or no systemic therapy[55–67,69] or comparing tamoxifen plus cytotoxic therapy with cytotoxic therapy alone.[53,58,62,64,65,68,71–82]

Oxford overview analysis

These trials of tamoxifen are similar in their outcomes, and have probably been best summarized in the EBCTCG overview analyses.[8,32–34] The data in *The Lancet* in 1992 represent the most updated published results from this collaboration, but additional data were obtained and analyzed in September of 1995 and will be published in detail in 1997. The overview demonstrates, as of course do many of the individual trials that contribute to it, that tamoxifen prolongs both disease-free and overall survival in the entire group of women studied. The EBCTCG then carried out a series of subgroup analyses. As the overall data set is so large, many of these subanalyses are very powerful.

Effects of tamoxifen by nodal status

When all women randomized to trials of tamoxifen versus no tamoxifen, with or without chemotherapy, are examined, it is possible to demonstrate a reduction in recurrence of 5.1% ± s.d. = 1.4 ($p < 0.00001$) for node-negative and 8.8% ± s.d. = 1.1 ($p < 0.0001$) for node-positive women (Figure 8.3a). Survival benefits are 3.5 ± s.d. = 1.4 ($p = 0.0002$) and 8.2% ± s.d. = 1.1 ($p = 0.00001$) for node-negative and node-positive women, respectively (Figure 8.3b).

Effects in women receiving chemotherapy versus those not receiving chemotherapy

This analysis suggests that the overall effects of tamoxifen tend to be somewhat less in the presence than in the absence of chemotherapy, but this apparent interaction is not significant and tamoxifen produces highly significant ($p < 0.00001$) recurrence and mortality ($p < 0.001$) reductions in both circumstances. When the effects of tamoxifen given in the presence of chemotherapy are analyzed within the under-50 and over-50 subgroups, however, a slightly different picture emerges. Although tamoxifen given in the presence of chemotherapy in older women clearly prolongs both recurrence-free ($p < 0.0001$) and overall ($p < 0.001$) survival, it does not significantly prolong either disease-free or overall survival in the younger women in the presence of chemotherapy, although there is a trend towards benefit, particularly for recurrence[33,34] (EBCTCG, 1995, personal communication).

Effects in ER-positive versus ER-negative women

It is also clear from analyses done within the Oxford overview that, although the role of ER status in predicting response to adjuvant tamoxifen has been controversial, there are now a great many data to suggest that tamoxifen is of substantially more benefit in patients who have ER-positive tumors, and particularly those who have high levels of ER. Women with high ER levels have a substantially greater reduction in recurrence than those who have ER-poor tumors.[33,34] Although the published information on mortality from the 1992 analysis[33,34] shows only a trend towards a greater reduction in mortality in highly ER-positive women, the subsequent 1995 analyses of these data confirm a substantially

increased mortality benefit in highly ER-positive women (EBCTCG, personal communication).

Effects in women over and under 50

In women over 50 and/or postmenopausal, tamoxifen provides a substantial reduction in the annual odds of recurrence (about 30% ± s.d = 3%), a highly significant reduction in odds of recurrence of about one-third in comparison to that in women not receiving tamoxifen.[33,34] Similarly, women aged 50 or over and/or postmenopausal have an approximately 20% reduction in the annual odds of death (± s.d. = 5%);[33,34] once again, there is a highly significant but slightly smaller reduction in odds of death of about one-fifth in comparison to that in women not receiving tamoxifen.

In women under 50, the effects of tamoxifen as adjuvant therapy are somewhat less clear. Recurrence is substantially reduced in women under 50 who are given tamoxifen ($p = 0.009$).[33,34] Mortality is not, however, significantly reduced in this group.[33,34] Subsequent subset analyses in younger women tend to suggest that tamoxifen alone may provide a stronger effect on recurrence and mortality than tamoxifen given in the setting of chemotherapy (EBCTCG, personal communication). As a result of the relatively small numbers of premenopausal women randomized to tamoxifen alone in the 1990 overview analysis, however, it is difficult to be certain that this is the case. More updated analyses of these data, including a much larger number of women randomized to tamoxifen alone versus no treatment as part of the node-negative trials, will be published by the Oxford overview group as a result of their 1995 analyses, which are currently being prepared for publication.

Duration of tamoxifen

In general, in the overview, the trials in which patients receive tamoxifen for an average of more than 2 years tend to show that longer duration of tamoxifen produces a greater benefit than shorter duration (tests for heterogeneity between the different lengths of tamoxifen show results of $p < 0.001$ [recurrence] and $p = 0.02$ [mortality]). Caution must be taken in interpreting these

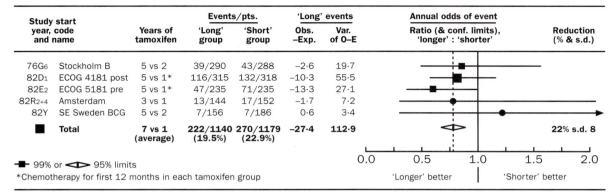

Figure 8.4 Recurrence (all ages): longer versus shorter periods of tamoxifen. (Reprinted with permission from *Lancet* 1992; **339:**1–15, 71–85.)

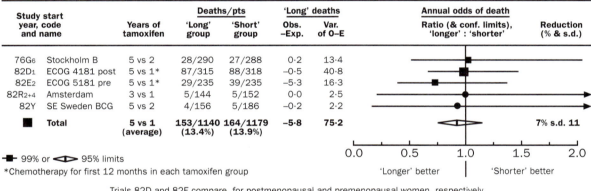

Figure 8.5 Mortality (all ages): longer versus shorter period of tamoxifen. Each trial is described by one line of information – code number (the first two digits of which show the year the trial began), name, treatment schedule, crude results, and statistical analysis. Any restrictions on eligibility to node negative (N−), receptor positive (ER+), postmenopausal (PO), or premenopausal status are given in italics. The analysis is chiefly based on calculation of logrank 'observed minus expected' events among the treatment-allocated patients. (In a trial where the treatment group has fared better than the control group, the quantity O-E must be negative, and vice versa.) For each separate trial O-E and its variance are both printed, and are used to estimate the odds ratio (treatment:control) and the 99% confidence interval for this odds ratio, which for that one trial are plotted as a black square and a horizontal line. The black square indicates that actual trial results, and the horizontal line indicates the range of odds ratios that could well have yielded such a result. (A trial involving many events yields a large black square and a short horizontal line.) The solid vertical line indicates an odds ratio of 1, i.e. no difference between treatment and control, so results to the left of this favour tamoxifen. The broken vertical line indicates the average risk reduction (25% for recurrence and 17% for mortality, in this example). To combine results unbiasedly from several trials, a grand total is constructed of one separate O-E from each trial. The overall variance of this grand total is likewise the sum of the separate variances, one per trial (and the standard deviation of the grand total is the square root of this overall variance). (Reprinted with permission from *Lancet* 1992; **339:**1–15, 71–85.)

results, however, because they represent indirect comparisons, i.e. comparisons of effects in one trial with those in another, rather than direct comparisons (comparisons of patients randomized within given trials). The overview also includes several studies in which women were actually randomized to receive longer versus shorter durations of tamoxifen. In the published overview, data for only five of these trials were available, but more than 20 such trials have been completed or are still ongoing across the world. The trials with data available at the time of the published overview analysis are shown in Figures 8.4 and 8.5, which represent recurrence (Figure 8.4) and mortality (Figure 8.5) in trials of longer versus shorter tamoxifen treatment. These studies demonstrate that, for the trials available at that time, longer tamoxifen duration showed a reduction in odds of recurrence of 22% (± s.d. = 8%), which is highly significant, but mortality was not significantly reduced (reduction = 7% ± s.d. = 11%).

Since this overview has been published, however, results from several individual randomized trials of duration of tamoxifen have also become available. These include the Spanish study of 2 versus 5 years of tamoxifen,[49] the Swedish study of 2 versus 5 years of tamoxifen[50] and the Cancer Research Campaign (CRC) study of 2 versus 5 years of tamoxifen (CRC, personal communication), all of which show a higher disease-free survival rate for women receiving 5 versus 2 years of tamoxifen. One of the three trials shows prolonged overall survival as well.[50] Paradoxically, published results now available from two trials of 5 years versus 10 years[83] and 5 years versus indefinite use of tamoxifen[84] show no real suggestion of benefit from the longer duration compared with 5 years of tamoxifen. The Scottish trial, which was completed as planned before analysis, shows a trend towards poorer results with indefinite tamoxifen, but this trend does not reach statistical significance (hazard ratio for events [relapse or death without relapse] is 1.27, confidence interval or CI = 0.87–1.85). There is a suggestion, however, that therapy for more than 5 years may increase the risk of endometrial cancer ($p = 0.064$).[84] The NSABP study, which was assessed with an interim analysis, shows a signif-

icantly higher recurrence rate, although not significantly more deaths; there is a trend towards both in the 10- versus the 5-year tamoxifen arm. As this is an interim analysis, however, the authors do not conclude that tamoxifen for 10 years is significantly worse. They have made power calculations which led them to close the 10-year arm of the trial, suggesting that it was extremely unlikely that 10 years of tamoxifen would be substantially better than 5.[83]

Thus, although a large amount of data remain to be analyzed, and further follow-up would be helpful, it appears that 5 years of tamoxifen provides more benefit than 2 years, but that treatment for more than 5 years may not be of additional benefit, at least on the basis of the data currently available. Currently, a group based in Oxford is conducting the ATLAS (Adjuvant Tamoxifen Longer Against Shorter) Trial; this is a large simple randomized trial in which patients are being randomized to 5 more years of tamoxifen after treatment with at least 2 years of tamoxifen, in settings in which the patient and/or the physician is uncertain whether tamoxifen should be continued. This level of uncertainty is decided by the individual clinician and patient according to local practice and local interpretations of the available data. Simple data on recurrence and survival are collected at yearly intervals in this study, so that large numbers of patients can be randomized without huge data collection expenses. It is hoped, in this way, to be able to demonstrate even a small benefit or detriment to longer versus shorter tamoxifen if there is one (Christine Davies, personal communication).

Role of tamoxifen given concurrently with chemotherapy

There has been some suggestion, particularly from the NSABP B09 Study,[72] but also from analyses in the Oxford overview, that tamoxifen given at the same time as chemotherapy, particularly in the younger or premenopausal patient group, may somehow be antagonistic to the effects of chemotherapy or vice versa. There are at least two possible explanations for this. Tamoxifen is, at least theoretically, a cytostatic drug, whereas chemotherapy works best against dividing cells. If tamoxifen were to stop cell division in a proportion of cells, then chemotherapy might be less effective. There is also evidence in in vitro and in vivo models[85-88] that tamoxifen may interfere with the action of certain cytotoxic drugs on tumor cells, at least in these artificial settings. This could be most apparent in the premenopausal group because it is in those patients that chemotherapy has the largest effects and, if inactivated, they could have its efforts decreased by the largest amount. Further analyses and studies are necessary to clarify these matters. For the time being, however, it seems that a policy of giving chemotherapy first, followed by tamoxifen, may be most prudent. Several major studies are currently ongoing that could help to clarify this matter.

One, a large intergroup study (ECOG, SWOG, NCCTG, CALGB and NCIC CTG) of more than 1400 postmenopausal, node-positive patients, has recently been completed and awaits analysis. In this study, women with ER- or PR-positive tumors were randomized to receive 5 years of tamoxifen alone, CAF (A, doxorubicin or Adriamycin) chemotherapy given for 6 months followed by 5 years of tamoxifen, or CAF chemotherapy given for 6 months starting together with 5 years of tamoxifen. This large study should help to determine whether concurrent or sequential timing of these drugs is important (Kathy Albain, personal communication). There are also at least three currently active trials that are studying this issue in the premenopausal setting. One, a National Cancer Institute of Canada Clinical Trials Group study, is randomizing premenopausal node-positive or high-risk node-negative patients who have completed 4 or 6 months of chemotherapy with AC, CMF or CEF (E, epirubicin) to receive subsequently 5 years of tamoxifen or 5 years of placebo (Vivien Bramwell, personal communication). A study of similar design is being carried out by the European Organization for Research and Treatment of Cancer (EORTC) in which node-positive or node-negative patients, who may be pre- or postmenopausal and of any ER status, are randomized, after chemotherapy of the usual local type, to receive or not to receive 3 years of subsequent tamoxifen (Martine Piccart, personal communication). An International Breast Cancer Study Group (IBCSG) trial is examining a similar

issue. In this study (IBCSG number 13), premenopausal node-positive women are randomized to receive or not to receive 5 years of subsequent tamoxifen after one of two types of chemotherapy (Aron Goldhirsch, personal communication). The results of these types of trials should be additionally helpful in clarifying the ideal timing of chemotherapy and tamoxifen.

Effect on second breast primaries

The results from randomized trials of tamoxifen versus observation also provide interesting results on the potential of tamoxifen as a preventive agent for breast cancer. Many of the trials included in the EBCTCG overview have data available on the occurrence of contralateral breast cancer in women allocated to tamoxifen in randomized trials.[8,32-34] Based on the occurrence of 122 contralateral breast cancers in 9128 tamoxifen-allocated women and 184 breast cancers in 9135 control patients, using life-table analysis a 39% reduction in risk for contralateral breast cancer was observed in this overview ($p < 0.0001$). The preventive effects tended to be greater in trials using longer duration of tamoxifen treatment, although this was not statistically significant. Reductions of risk were 26% for less than 2 years of tamoxifen treatment, 37% for 2 years of treatment and 53% for more than 2 years of treatment.[33,34] This preventive effect is also well summarized in a recent IARC (International Agency for Research in Cancer) monograph which discusses the anti-estrogens.[89]

Comparability of tamoxifen to ovarian ablation and chemotherapy

There have been no randomized trials comparing tamoxifen with ovarian ablation in the adjuvant setting in premenopausal women. There are, however, two published randomized studies of tamoxifen compared with oophorectomy in premenopausal women with metastatic disease,[90,91] and a meta-analysis of all of the available data examining ovarian ablation compared with tamoxifen in the metastatic setting is soon to be published.[92] These studies suggest that tamoxifen and ovarian ablation produce very similar effects in premenopausal women with metastatic disease. Thus, it would seem that tamoxifen use as an adjuvant in the premenopausal setting might be quite comparable to ovarian ablation, but this remains to be tested in future adjuvant trials.

There are also very few trials comparing tamoxifen with chemotherapy in this setting.[68] The few studies that there are suggest that tamoxifen may be equivalent or less effective, but this may well depend completely on the group of patients selected, their levels of ERs ± PRs and on the type, schedule and dose intensity of the chemotherapy being tested. Further studies comparing these two approaches are badly needed.

Effects of tamoxifen on other body systems

Tamoxifen in general is a minimally toxic drug. It has been documented to cause hot flushes in 10–20% of postmenopausal and as many as 60% of premenopausal women, and can also cause vaginal discharge or itching, mild nausea, and a variety of other relatively uncommon and generally transient effects.[67] Of more concern in the long term, there is a small but significant increase in the risk of development of endometrial cancer, at least when given in postmenopausal women. This degree of risk has been well summarized in a recent IARC monograph[93] which also stressed, however, that tamoxifen is clearly chemopreventive in reducing the risk of second menopausal malignancies.[89] In addition, there are recent data from the Tamoxifen Ophthalmologic Evaluation Study (TOES), an ophthalmologic study of a subset of women examined from the NSABP B14 trial, which suggests that patients receiving tamoxifen for 5 years or more have a somewhat increased incidence of posterior subcapsular lens opacities in comparison to those receiving placebo (National Institutes of Health, personal communication). These data are perhaps not surprising in view of the fact that tamoxifen has been known to produce cataracts in rats.

In addition, tamoxifen clearly has profound effects on other organ systems, including the endocrine system,[94] as well as causing changes in levels of antithrombin III, total cholesterol and low-density lipoprotein.[94–96] Perhaps related to these effects on lipid levels, at least two trials have shown tamoxifen-related reduction in deaths from myocardial infarction[97] or in hospitalizations for cardiovascular causes[98] in randomized trials of tamoxifen versus no therapy. Thus, tamoxifen may have some long-term beneficial effects other than those related to breast cancer recurrence and prevention of second primary breast cancers.

Conclusions and future directions

Thus, in summary, tamoxifen as adjuvant therapy appears to be useful for a wide variety of patients. It seems to have its greatest effect in women who are postmenopausal and have ER-positive tumors, particularly if the levels are high. It seems equally effective in node-positive and in node-negative women. Although most effective in older or postmenopausal women, it also provides some benefit in younger or premenopausal women. It seems to provide somewhat more benefit when given alone than when added to chemotherapy, and to be most beneficial when given for 5 years. There are, however, considerable data suggesting that shorter durations of tamoxifen are also useful, although perhaps not quite so much. It seems that additional tamoxifen after 5 years may not be of further benefit, but various trials require further follow-up and analysis in order to clarify this matter completely. Table 8.4 summarizes the situations in which tamoxifen is useful as adjuvant therapy and indicates those in which it would be considered standard.

OTHER ADJUVANT ENDOCRINE THERAPIES

A few trials of other endocrine modalities used as adjuvant therapy have been carried out. Prednisone, in particular, has been used in a number of adjuvant studies. As it is often combined with chemotherapy[99–101] or with other

Table 8.4 Current recommendations for adjuvant tamoxifen therapy		
Status	**Premenopausal**	**Postmenopausal**
Node positive ER and/or PR positive	May be additionally useful following chemotherapy	Standard therapy (additional chemotherapy may further reduce recurrence)
Node positive ER and PR negative	Not recommended	May be useful to a limited degree
Node negative ER and/or PR positive	Standard therapy or useful following chemotherapy	Standard therapy
Node negative ER and PR negative	Not recommended	May be useful to a limited degree

hormones such as tamoxifen,[102] however, its role is often unclear. There are three trials in premenopausal patients, two comparing CMF with CMF-P (P, prednisone)[37,74] and Meakin's study which compares ovarian irradiation, irradiation + prednisone and a no-treatment control arm. The studies of CMF versus CMF-P showed no advantage for the addition of prednisone, whereas Meakin's study showed a trend towards improvement with irradiation in all premenopausal women, but a statistically significant improvement in both disease-free and overall survival only for irradiation + prednisone in premenopausal women aged over 45 years.[23] Adrenalectomy seemed promising when used as adjuvant therapy in one small historically controlled trial in 17 postmenopausal women with four or more positive axillary nodes, but this approach has not been pursued because of the obvious morbidity of such major surgery.[103] A study of adjuvant aminoglutethimide was also abandoned because of considerable toxicity,[104] as was a small study of testosterone propionate.[105] The Copenhagen Breast Cancer Group's trial of adjuvant therapy in postmenopausal women showed a trend towards improved disease-free survival in diethylstilbestrol (DES)-treated, as

well as tamoxifen-treated, women in comparison to controls, although 42% of DES-treated patients discontinued treatment because of side effects.[106] Currently, a variety of randomized studies testing the new third-generation aromatase inhibitors, anastrozole (Arimidex), vorozole, exemestane and letrozole, in comparison to tamoxifen, after tamoxifen or concurrent with tamoxifen, are being undertaken. The extremely low toxicity of these new aromatase inhibitors will certainly lend them to more extensive investigation as adjuvant therapy.

CONCLUSIONS

Adjuvant endocrine therapy remains a cornerstone in the treatment of node-negative and node-positive women with breast cancer. Tamoxifen is still the drug of choice for both node-negative and node-positive ER- and/or PR-positive postmenopausal women whereas the role of additional chemotherapy remains to be fully clarified. Now, the newer aromatase inhibitors are being actively explored as alternatives or in addition to tamoxifen as adjuvant therapy in this same group of women.

In the meantime, ovarian ablation, by

surgery, radiation or medical castration, remains an alternative to chemotherapy in ER- and/or PR-positive premenopausal women but appears perhaps not to have quite the same magnitude of effect as the more aggressive combination chemotherapies now being used as adjuvants in this group. Adding ovarian ablation to chemotherapy in premenopausal women, although appearing promising in the earlier EBCTCG overview, now appears to add only minimal if any additional benefit in this group of women. The role of tamoxifen as an alternative to chemotherapy and/or ovarian ablation, or in addition to chemotherapy in the premenopausal group, remains to be more fully established. Additional trials comparing and refining the relative roles of ovarian ablation, tamoxifen and combination chemotherapy in these various groups of women are currently ongoing and their results will be awaited with considerable interest.

REFERENCES

1. Beatson GT. On the treatment of inoperable cases of carcinoma of the mamma: suggestions for a new method of treatment with illustrative cases. *Lancet* 1896; **ii:**104–7.
2. Schinzinger A. Ueber carcinoma mammae. *Verh Dtsch Ges Chir* 1889; **18:**28–9.
3. Taylor GW. Artificial menopause in carcinoma of the breast. *N Engl J Med* 1934; **211:**1138–40.
4. Fisher B, Carbone P, Economou SG, et al. L-Phenylalanine mustard (L-PAM) in the management of primary breast cancer: A report of early findings. *N Engl J Med* 1975; **292:**117–22.
5. Bonadonna G, Brusamolino E, Valagussa P, et al. Combination chemotherapy as an adjuvant treatment in operable breast cancer. *N Engl J Med* 1976; **294:**405–10.
6. Legha SS, Carter SK. Antiestrogens in the treatment of breast cancer. *Cancer Treat Rev* 1976; **3:**205–16.
7. Santen RJ, Samojik E, Lipton A, et al. Kinetic, hormonal and clinical studies with aminoglutethimide in breast cancer. *Cancer* 1977; **39:**2948–58.
8. Early Breast Cancer Trialists' Collaborative Group. Effects of adjuvant tamoxifen and of cytotoxic therapy on mortality in early breast cancer: An overview of 61 randomized trials among 28,896 women. *N Engl J Med* 1988; **319:**1681–92.
9. Osborne CK, Yochmowitz MG, Knight WA, McGuire WL. The value of estrogen and progesterone receptors in the treatment of breast cancer. *Cancer* 1980; **46:**2884–8.
10. Bloom ND, Tobin EH, Schreibman B, Degenshein GA. The role of progesterone receptors in the management of advanced breast cancer. *Cancer* 1980; **45:**2972–7.
11. Leclercq G, Heuson JC. Therapeutic significance of sex-steroid hormone receptors in the treatment of breast cancer. *Eur J Cancer* 1977; **13:**1205–15.
12. Allegra JC, Barlock A, Huff KK, Lippman ME. Changes in multiple or sequential estrogen receptor determinations in breast cancer. *Cancer* 1980; **45:**792–4.
13. Fisher B, Slack NH. Number of lymph nodes examined and the prognosis of breast carcinoma. *Surg Gynecol Obstet* 1970; **131:**79–88.
14. McWhirter R. Some factors influencing prognosis in breast cancer. *J Fac Radiol Lond* 1956; **8:**220–34.
15. Huck P. Artificial menopause as an adjunct to radical treatment of breast cancer. *N Z Med J* 1952; **51:**364–7.
16. Kennedy BJ, Mielke PW, Fortuny IE. Therapeutic castration versus prophylactic castration in breast cancer. *Surg Gynecol Obstet* 1964; **118:**524–40.
17. Alrich EM, Liddle HV, Morton CB. Carcinoma of the breast: Results of surgical treatment: Some anatomic and endocrine consideration. *Ann Surg* 1957; **145:**779–806.
18. Rennaes S. Prophylactic ovarian irradiation. *Acta Chir Scand* 1960; **266:**85–90.
19. Cole MP, Namer M, Lalanne CM (eds). A clinical trial of an artificial menopause in carcinoma of the breast. *Hormones and Breast Cancer*, 55th edn. Paris: INSERM, 1975:143–50.
20. Nissen-Meyer R, Namer M, Lalanne CM (eds). Ovarian suppression and its supplement by additive hormonal treatment. *Hormones and Breast Cancer*, 55th edn. Paris: INSERM, 1975:151–8.
21. Ravdin RG, Lewison EF, Slack NH, Gardner B, State D, Fisher B. Results of a clinical trial concerning the worth of prophylactic oophorectomy for breast carcinoma. *Surg Gynecol Obstet* 1970; **131:**1055–64.
22. Meakin JW, Allt WEC, Beale FA, et al. Ovarian irradiation and prednisone therapy following

surgery and radiotherapy for carcinoma of the breast. *Can Med Assoc J* 1979; **19**:1221–38.

23. Meakin JW, Hayward JL, Panzarella T, et al. Ovarian irradiation and prednisone therapy following surgery and radiotherapy for carcinoma of the breast. *Breast Cancer Res Treat* 1996; **37**: 11–19.

24. Meakin JW, Allt WEC, Beale FA, et al. Ovarian irradiation and prednisone following surgery and radiotherapy for carcinoma of the breast. *Br Cancer Res Treat* 1983; **3**:45–8.

25. Bryant AJS, Weir JA. Prophylactic oophorectomy in operable instances of carcinoma of the breast. *Surg Gynecol Obstet* 1981; **153**:660–4.

26. Nevinny HB, Nevinny D, Roscoff CB, Hall TC, Muench H. Prophylactic oophorectomy in breast cancer therapy. *Am J Surg* 1969; **117**:531–6.

27. Clarke EA, Fetterly JC, Ryan NC. The Ontario Cancer Treatment and Research Foundation Clinical Trial on the comparative effect of ovarian irradiation in carcinoma of the breast in the postmenopausal patient. In: *Treatment of Early Breast Cancer 1: Worldwide Evidence 1985–1990. A Systematic Overview of all Available Randomized Trials of Adjuvant Endocrine and Cytoxic Therapy* (Early Breast Cancer Trialists' Collaborative Group, eds). Oxford: Oxford University Press, 1990:106.

28. Delozier T, Juert P, Couette JE, et al. Ovarian irradiation in postmenopausal women with breast cancer and positive axillary nodes. In: *Treatment of Early Breast Cancer 1: Worldwide Evidence 1985–1990. A Systematic Overview of all Available Randomized Trials of Adjuvant Endocrine and Cytoxic Therapy* (Early Breast Cancer Trialists' Collaborative Group, eds). Oxford: Oxford University Press, 1990:114.

29. Ragaz J, Jackson S, Nilson K, et al. Randomized study of locoregional radiotherapy and ovarian ablation in premenopausal patients with breast cancer treated with adjuvant chemotherapy [abstract]. *Proc Am Soc Clin Oncol* 1988; **7**:12.

30. The International Breast Cancer Study Group. Late effects of adjuvant oophorectomy and chemotherapy upon premenopausal breast cancer patients. *Ann Oncol* 1990; **1**:30–5.

31. Early Breast Cancer Trialists' Collaborative Group. Ovarian ablation in early breast cancer: an overview of the randomized trials. *Lancet* 1996; **348**:1189–96.

32. Early Breast Cancer Trialists' Collaborative Group (eds). *Treatment of early breast cancer.* In: *Treatment of Early Breast Cancer 1: Worldwide Evidence 1985–1990. A Systematic Overview of all Available Randomized Trials of Adjuvant Endocrine and Cytoxic Therapy.* Oxford: Oxford University Press, 1990.

33. Early Breast Cancer Trialists' Collaborative Group. Systemic treatment of early breast cancer by hormonal, cytotoxic or immune therapy: 133 randomized trials involving 31,000 recurrences and 24,000 deaths among 75,000 women. *Lancet* 1992; **339**:1–15A.

34. Early Breast Cancer Trialists' Collaborative Group. Systemic treatment of early breast cancer by hormonal, cytotoxic, or immune therapy. *Lancet* 1992; **339**:71–85B.

35. Howell A, George WD, Crowther D, et al. Controlled trial of adjuvant chemotherapy with cyclophosphamide, methotrexate and fluorouracil for breast cancer. *Lancet* 1984; **2**:307–11.

36. Pourquier H, Van Scoy-Moscher MB (eds). The results of adjuvant chemotherapy are predominantly caused by the hormonal changes such therapy induces. *Medical Oncology. Controversies in Cancer Treatment.* Boston: Hall, 1981:83–9.

37. Ludwig Breast Cancer Study Group. Adjuvant combination chemotherapy with or without prednisone in premenopausal breast cancer patients with metastases in 1 to 3 axillary lymph nodes: A randomized trial. *Cancer Res* 1985; **45**:4454–9.

38. Bonadonna G, Valagussa P, DePalo G, Van Scoy-Moscher MB (eds). The results of adjuvant chemotherapy are predominantly caused by the hormonal changes such therapy induces. *Medical Oncology. Controversies in Cancer Treatment.* Boston: Hall, 1981:100–9.

39. Fisher B, Sherman B, Rockette H, Redmond C, Margolese R, Fisher ER. L-Phenylalanine mustard (L-PAM) in the management of premenopausal patients with primary breast cancer: Lack of association of disease-free survival with depression of ovarian function. *Cancer* 1979; **44**:847–57.

40. Rubens RD, Knight RK, Fentiman IS, et al. Controlled trial of adjuvant chemotherapy with melphalan for breast cancer. *Lancet* 1983; **1**:839–43.

41. Scottish Cancer Trials Breast Group. Adjuvant ovarian ablation versus CMF chemotherapy in premenopausal women with pathological stage II breast carcinoma: The Scottish trial. *Lancet* 1993; **341**:1293–8.

42. Levine M, Bramwell V, Bowman D, et al. A clinical trial of intensive CEF versus CMF in premenopausal women with node positive breast cancer [abstract]. *Proceedings of the 31st Annual*

Meeting of the American Society for Clinical Oncology 1995; **14**:103.

43. Kaufmann M, Jonat W, Kleeberg UR. Goserelin, a depot gonadotropin-releasing hormone agonist in the treatment of premenopausal patients with metastatic breast cancer. *J Clin Oncol* 1989; **7**:1113–19.

44. Kaufmann M, Jonat W, Schachner-Wunschmann E. The depot GnRH analogue goserelin in the treatment of premenopausal patients with metastatic breast cancer – a 5 year experience and further endocrine therapies. *Onkologie* 1991; **14**:22–30.

45. Blamey RW, Jonat W, Kaufmann M. Goserelin depot in the treatment of premenopausal advanced breast cancer. *Eur J Cancer* 1992; **28A**: 810–14.

46. Blamey RW, Jonat W, Kaufmann M. Survival data relating to the use of goserelin depot in the treatment of premenopausal advanced breast cancer. *Eur J Cancer* 1993; **29A**:1498.

47. Taylor CW, Green S, Dalton WS, et al. A multicenter randomized trial of Zoladex versus surgical ovariectomy in premenopausal patients with receptor positive metastatic breast cancer. *Breast Cancer Res Treat* 1995; **37**:31.

48. West CP, Baird DT. Suppression of ovarian activity by Zoladex depot (ICI 118 630), a long acting luteinizing hormone releasing hormone agonist analogue. *Clin Endocrinol* 1987; **26**: 213–20.

49. Gallen M, Alonso MC, Ojeda B, et al. Randomized multicentre trial comparing two different time-spans of adjuvant tamoxifen therapy (ATT) in women with operable node positive breast cancer [abstract]. *Proc Am Soc Clin Oncol* 1994; **13**:76.

50. Swedish Breast Cancer Cooperative Group. Randomized trial of 2 versus 5 years of adjuvant tamoxifen in postmenopausal early-stage breast cancer [abstract]. *Proc Am Soc Clin Oncol* 1996; **15**:126.

51. Colditz GA, Willett WC, Stampfer MJ. Menopause and the risk of coronary heart disease in women. *N Engl J Med* 1987; **316**:1105–10.

52. Knoweldon J, Buhr AJ, Dunbar O. Incidence of fractures in persons over 35 years of age: a report to the M.R.C. working party on fractures in the elderly. *Br J Prev Soc Med* 1964; **18**:130–41.

53. Palshof T, Carstensen B, Briand P. Adjuvant endocrine therapy in pre and postmenopausal women with operable breast cancer. *Rev Endocrinol Rel Cancer* 1985; **17**:43–50.

54. Wallgren A, Baral E, Carstensen B, et al. Should adjuvant therapy be given for several years in breast cancer? In: *Adjuvant Therapy of Breast Cancer V* (Salmon SE, Jones SE, eds). New York: Grune & Stratton, 1984:331–7.

55. Ribeiro GG, Swindell R. The Christie Hospital adjuvant tamoxifen trial – Status at 10 years. *Br J Cancer* 1988; **57**:601–3.

56. Nolvadex Adjuvant Trial Organization. Controlled trial of tamoxifen as a single adjuvant agent in management of early breast cancer. Analysis at eight years by the Nolvadex Adjuvant Trial Organization. *Br J Cancer* 1988; **57**:608–11.

57. Rose C, Andersen KW, Mouridsen HT. Beneficial effect of adjuvant tamoxifen in primary breast cancer patients with high oestrogen receptor values. *Lancet* 1985; **i**:16–19.

58. Goldhirsch A, Gelber RD. Adjuvant chemoendocrine therapy or endocrine therapy alone for postmenopausal patients: Ludwig studies III and IV. *Rec Res Cancer Res* 1989; **115**:153–62.

59. Cummings FT, Gray R, David TE, et al. Adjuvant tamoxifen treatment of elderly women with stage II breast cancer. A double blind comparison with placebo. *Ann Intern Med* 1985; **103**:324–9.

60. Pritchard KI, Meakin JW, Boyd NF, et al. Adjuvant tamoxifen in postmenopausal women with axillary node positive breast cancer: An update. In: *Adjuvant Therapy of Cancer V* (Salmon SE, ed.). Orlando, FL: Grune & Stratton; 1987:391–400.

61. Scottish Cancer Trials Breast Group. Adjuvant tamoxifen in the management of operable breast cancer: The Scottish trial. *Lancet* 1987; **ii**:171–5.

62. Senanayake F. Adjuvant hormonal chemotherapy in early breast cancer: Early results from a controlled trial. *Lancet* 1984; **ii**:1148–9.

63. Margreiter R, Steindorfer P, Hausmaninger H, et al. Adjuvant tamoxifen therapy for early breast cancer: A controlled clinical trial. *Rev Endocrinol Rel Cancer* 1985; **17**:117–21.

64. Bianco AR, Delrio G, DePlaudo S, et al. Adjuvant tamoxifen, singly or in combination with CMF, in the primary treatment of breast cancer. *Rev Endocrinol Rel Cancer* 1985; **17**:129–32.

65. Kaufmann M, Jarat W, Caffier H, et al. Adjuvant systemic risk adapted cytotoxic and tamoxifen therapy in women with node positive breast cancer. In: *Adjuvant Therapy of Cancer*

V (Salmon SE, ed.). Orlando, FL: Grune & Stratton, 1987:337–46.

66. CRC Adjuvant Breast Trial Working Party. Cyclophosphamide and tamoxifen as adjuvant therapies in the management of breast cancer. *Br J Cancer* 1988; **57:**604–7.

67. Fisher B, Costantino J, Redmond C, et al. A randomized clinical trial evaluating tamoxifen in the treatment of patients with node-negative breast cancer who have estrogen-receptor-positive tumors. *N Engl J Med* 1989; **320:**479–84.

68. Kaufmann M, Jonat W, Abel U. Adjuvant chemo and endocrine therapy alone or in combination in premenopausal patients (GABG Trial 1). *Recent Res Cancer Res* 1989; **115:**118–25.

69. Caffier H, Rotte K, Horner G. Adjuvant tamoxifen therapy in postmenopausal women with node-negative breast cancer. *Rev Endocrinol Rel Cancer* 1985; **17:**103–5.

70. Fisher B, Redmond C, Wickerham DL, et al. Systemic therapy in patients with node-negative breast cancer. A commentary based on two National Surgical Adjuvant Breast and Bowel Project (NSABP) clinical trials. *Ann Intern Med* 1989; **111:**703–12.

71. Fisher B, Redmond C, Wolmark N, Salmon SE (eds). Long term results from NSABP trials of adjuvant therapy for breast cancer. *Adjuvant Therapy of Cancer V*. Orlando: Grune & Stratton, 1987:283–95.

72. Fisher B, Redmond C, Brown A, et al. Adjuvant chemotherapy with and without tamoxifen in the treatment of primary breast cancer: 5 year results from the National Surgical Adjuvant Breast and Bowel Project Trial. *J Clin Oncol* 1986; **4:**459–71.

73. Taylor SG, Knuiman MW, Slepper LA, et al. Six year results of the Eastern Cooperative Oncology Group trial of observation versus CMFP versus CMFPT in postmenopausal patients with node-positive breast cancer. *J Clin Oncol* 1989; **7:**897–9.

74. Tormey DC, Gray R, Gilchrist KW, et al. Adjuvant chemohormonal therapy with cyclophosphamide, methotrexate, 5-fluorouracil, and prednisone (CMFP) or CMFP plus tamoxifen compared with CMF for premenopausal breast cancer patients. *Cancer* 1990; **65:**200–6.

75. Hubay CA, Gordon NH, Crowe JP, et al. Antiestrogen–cytotoxic chemotherapy and Bacillus Calmette–Guérin vaccination in stage II breast cancer: Seventy-two month follow-up. *Surgery* 1984; **96:**61–71.

76. Wallgren A, Baral E, Beling V, et al. Tamoxifen and combination chemotherapy as adjuvant therapy in postmenopausal women with breast cancer. *Rec Res Cancer Res* 1984; **96:**197–203.

77. Ingle JN, Krook JE, Schaid DJ, et al. Randomized trial in postmenopausal women with node positive breast cancer: Observation versus adjuvant therapy with cyclophosphamide, 5-fluorouracil, prednisone with or without tamoxifen. Results with seven year median follow up. In: *Adjuvant Therapy of Cancer VI* (Salmon SE, ed.). Philadelphia: WB Saunders, 1990:216–25.

78. Pearson OH, Hubay CA, Gordon NH, et al. Endocrine versus endocrine plus five day chemotherapy in postmenopausal women with stage II estrogen receptor-positive breast cancer. *Cancer* 1989; **64:**1819–23.

79. Fisher B, Redmond C, Legault-Poisson S, et al. Postoperative chemotherapy and tamoxifen compared with tamoxifen alone in the treatment of positive node breast cancer patients 50 years and older with tumors responsive to tamoxifen: Results from National Surgical Adjuvant Breast and Bowel Project B-16. *J Clin Oncol* 1990; **8:**1005–18.

80. Boccardo F, Rubagotti A, Bruzzi P, et al. Chemotherapy versus tamoxifen versus chemotherapy plus tamoxifen in node-positive, estrogen receptor-positive breast cancer patients: Results of a multicentre Italian study. *J Clin Oncol* 1990; **8:**1310–20.

81. Rivkin S, Green S, Metch B, et al. Adjuvant combination chemotherapy (CMFVP) vs tamoxifen (TAM) vs CMFVP + TAM for postmenopausal women with ER+ operable breast cancer and positive axillary lymph nodes: An Intergroup study. *Proc Am Soc Clin Oncol* 1990; **9:**24.

82. Jonat W, Kaufmann M, Abel U. Chemo or endocrine adjuvant therapy alone or combined in postmenopausal patients (GABG Trial 1). *Rec Res Cancer Res* 1989; **115:**163–9.

83. Fisher B, Dignam J, Wieand S, et al. Duration of tamoxifen (TAM) therapy for primary breast cancer: 5 versus 10 years (NSABP B-14) [abstract]. *Proc Am Soc Clin Oncol* 1996; **15:**113.

84. Stewart HJ, Forrest APM, Everington D, et al. Randomized comparison of 5 years of adjuvant tamoxifen with continuous therapy for operable breast cancer. *Br J Cancer* 1996; **74:**297–9.

85. Benz C, Moellekin B, Cadman E. RNA and estrogen receptor effects associated with tamox-

ifen-fluorouracil synergy in breast cancer. *Proc Am Assoc Cancer Res* 1983; **24:**173.

86. Jordan VC, Tormey DC, Clifton K, et al. Treatment of rat mammary cancer by combinations of tamoxifen and cyclophosphamide. *Proc Am Assoc Cancer Res* 1980; **21:**293.

87. Levine R, Lippman ME, Longo D, et al. Effects of estrogen and tamoxifen on dihydrofolate reductase in gene-amplified methotrexate resistant human breast cancer cells. *Proc Am Assoc Cancer Res* 1983; **24:**173.

88. Goldenberg GJ. The effect of diethylstilbestrol and tamoxifen on the cytocidal activity and uptake of Melphalan (M) in human breast cancer cells in vitro. *Proc Am Soc Clin Oncol* 1983; **2:**22.

89. IARC Monograph Working Group. Some Pharmaceutical Drugs. *IARC Monographs on the Evaluation of Carcinogenic Risks to Humans* 1996; **66:**274–8.

90. Ingle JN, Krook JE, Green SJ, et al. Randomized trial of bilaterial oophorectomy versus tamoxifen in premenopausal women with metastatic breast cancer. *J Clin Oncol* 1986; **4:**178–85.

91. Buchanan RB, Blamey RW, Durrant KR, et al. A randomized comparison of tamoxifen with surgical oophorectomy in premenopausal patients with advanced breast cancer. *J Clin Oncol* 1986; **4:**1326–30.

92. Crump M, Sawka CA, DeBoer G, et al. An individual patient-based meta-analysis of tamoxifen versus ovarian ablation as first line endocrine therapy for premenopausal women with metastatic breast cancer. *Br Cancer Res Treat* 1997; in press.

93. IARC Monograph Working Group. Some pharmaceutic drugs. *IARC Monographs on the Evaluation of Carcinogenic Risks to Humans* 1996; **66:**260–74.

94. Sunderland MC, Osborne CK. Tamoxifen in premenopausal patients with metastatic breast cancer: A review. *J Clin Oncol* 1991; **9:**1283–97.

95. IARC Monograph Working Group. Some pharmaceutical drugs. *IARC Monographs on the Evaluation of Carcinogenic Risks to Humans* 1996; **66:**303–4.

96. IARC Monograph Working Group. Some pharmaceutical drugs. *IARC Monographs on the Evaluation of Carcinogenic Risks to Humans* 1996; **66:**305–7.

97. McDonald CC, Stewart HJ. Fatal myocardial infarction in the Scottish adjuvant tamoxifen trial. *BMJ* 1991; **303:**435–7.

98. Rutqvist LE, Mattson A. Cardiac and thromboembolic morbidity among postmenopausal women with early stage breast cancer in a randomized trial of adjuvant tamoxifen. *J Natl Cancer Inst* 1995; **87:**645–51.

99. Taylor SG, Kalish LA, Olson JE, et al. Adjuvant CMFP versus CMFP plus tamoxifen versus observation alone in postmenopausal, node positive breast cancer patients: Three year results of an Eastern Cooperative Oncology Group Study. *J Clin Oncol* 1985; **3:**144–54.

100. Glucksberg H, Rivkin SE, Rasmussen S, et al. Combination chemotherapy (CMFVP) versus L-phenylalanine mustard (L-PAM) for operable breast cancer with positive axillary nodes: A Southwest Oncology Group study. *Cancer* 1982; **50:**423–34.

101. Tormey DC, Weinberg VE, Holland JF, et al. A randomized trial of five and three drug chemotherapy and chemoimmunotherapy in women with operable node positive breast cancer. *Clin Oncol* 1983; **1:**138–45.

102. Ludwig Breast Cancer Study Group. Randomized trial of chemo-endocrine therapy, endocrine therapy, and mastectomy alone in postmenopausal patients with operable breast cancer and axillary node metastasis. *Lancet* 1984; **i:**1256–60.

103. Dao TLK, Nemoto T, Chamberlain A, et al. Adrenalectomy with radical mastectomy in the treatment of high-risk breast cancer. *Cancer* 1975; **35:**478–82.

104. Coombes RC, Chilvers C, Smith IE, et al. Adjuvant aminoglutethimide therapy for post-menopausal patients with primary breast cancer: Progress report. *Cancer Res* 1982; **42:** 3415–91.

105. Prudente A. Post operative prophylaxis of recurrent mammary cancer with testosterone propionate. *Surg Gynecol Obstet* 1945; **80:**575–92.

106. Palshof T, Mouridsen HT, Daehnfeldt JL. Adjuvant endocrine therapy of primary operable breast cancer. Report on the Copenhagen breast cancer trials. *Eur J Cancer* 1980; **2:**183–7.

9

Locally advanced breast cancer

Gabriel N Hortobagyi, Aman U Buzdar

CONTENTS • Initial evaluation and monitoring of therapeutic response • Primary chemotherapy • Combined modality therapy • Breast-conserving therapy • Disease-free and overall survival • Results of combined modality therapy in inflammatory breast cancer • Current directions in research

Locally advanced breast cancer includes large tumors with or without regional lymph node involvement, or tumors of any size with massive involvement of axillary, subclavicular and/or supraclavicular lymph nodes.[1] Patients with internal mammary metastases also belong in this category. Historically, locally advanced breast cancer included patients in all subcategories of stage III breast cancer, as well as patients with metastatic disease limited to the ipsilateral supraclavicular area (stage IV).[2] Stage III breast cancer includes all primary tumors more than 5 cm in largest diameter and palpable regional lymph nodes (T3N1–3), tumors of any size with direct skin involvement regardless of lymph node involvement (T4a–d N0–3), or tumors of any size but with matted/fixed axillary lymph nodes or internal mammary lymph node involvement (T0–4 N2–3). Patients with T3N0M0 breast cancer (those with tumors larger than 5 cm, but without regional lymph node involvement) also belong to this category, although in the most recent version of the TNM classification these tumors were placed in stage IIb.[3] Inclusion in the locally advanced breast cancer category requires either the presence of technically unresectable breast cancer without evident distant metastasis, or such large tumors, or such extensive regional lymph node involvement, that surgical therapy (or local/regional therapy) has little bearing on long-term survival.

A special type of locally advanced breast cancer is inflammatory breast cancer (stage IIId).[4] This group of patients represents 1–2% of all newly diagnosed breast cancers; inflammatory breast cancer is defined by a clinical triad of signs, including erythema of the skin of the breast, edema of the skin of the breast (*peau d'orange*) and ridging, which is a reflection of engorged dermal lymphatics within the breast (Figure 9.1). Another condition for the diagnosis of inflammatory breast cancer is a short duration of symptoms/signs, reflecting rapid development and progression of this disease.[5] This last requirement is important to separate patients with indolent, neglected, locally advanced, breast cancers, which may have been present for several months or years before the patient sought medical attention, from those with true locally advanced disease. There is ongoing controversy about whether pathologic demonstration of dermal lymphatic involvement by tumor cells contributes to, or is a requirement for, the diagnosis of inflammatory breast carcinoma.[6–8] Retrospective studies with

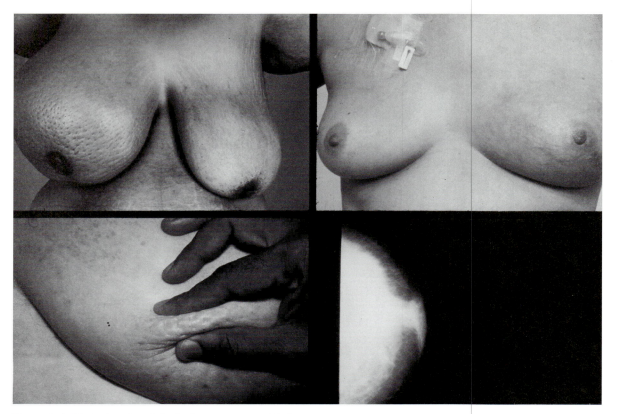

Figure 9.1 Clinical and radiological appearance of inflammatory breast cancer.

and without the inclusion of pathologic demonstration of dermal lymphatic involvement have demonstrated that the prognosis is equally poor for patients who have the clinical signs of inflammatory breast cancer.

More recently, the concept of locally advanced breast cancer has been extended to patients with large tumors in relation to the size of the breast.[9–11] Therefore, many stage II breast cancers that are clearly technically operable, but require a mastectomy, are now considered locally advanced.

For patients with locally advanced breast cancer who are technically operable (stage IIIA), a total mastectomy or a radical mastectomy was the treatment of choice for many decades. In fact, a classic Halsted radical mastectomy was systematized specifically to provide optimal local control to patients with locally advanced breast cancer.[12] For patients with technically inoperable, locally advanced, breast cancer (stage IIIB), including those with inflammatory breast cancer, primary radiotherapy to the breast, with or without preceding or subsequent total mastectomy, was the treatment of choice.[1] Numerous publications reviewing single-investigator or single-institutional experience with mastectomy only, radiotherapy only, or a sequential combination of mastectomy and radiotherapy for the treatment of locally

Table 9.1 Survival of patients with locally advanced or inflammatory breast carcinoma after single-modality and combined-modality therapies

Treatment	No. of patients	Percentage 5-year survivors
Locally advanced breast cancer		
Surgery only	2453	36
Radiotherapy only	2386	29
Surgery and radiotherapy	4249	33
Chemotherapy + surgery + radiotherapy	1923	63
Inflammatory breast cancer		
Surgery only	398	2
Radiotherapy only	334	3
Surgery and radiotherapy	142	5
Chemotherapy + surgery + radiotherapy	708	47

Numbers of patients and 5-year survival rates are derived from an overview of published studies included in a recent review.[1]

advanced and inflammatory breast cancer, demonstrated that these treatments were most ineffective in providing long-term control for advanced disease (Table 9.1).[1] More than 80% of patients treated only with local therapy died of distant metastasis within 10 years of diagnosis. Furthermore, when treated with individual regional therapies, local recurrence rate often exceeded 50%. The combination of surgery and radiotherapy, in either sequence, improved on local control rate without affecting long-term disease-free or overall survival rates. These studies have recently been reviewed elsewhere.[1] Therefore, it is clear that the major problem in locally advanced breast cancer is the development of micrometastases months or years before the diagnosis is made. As a corollary, the only way to make progress, in terms of disease-free and overall survival rates, is by developing effective systemic therapy for this disease.

The introduction of effective chemotherapies in the 1970s and 1980s provided another therapeutic alternative. Even before the systematic introduction of postoperative adjuvant chemotherapy for early-stage, high-risk, breast cancer, primary chemotherapy (also referred to as neoadjuvant or preoperative) was introduced for the management of patients with locally advanced breast cancer.[13,14] Numerous combined modality regimens were designed and tested in the 1970s. All of them had in common the introduction of systemic therapy (mostly chemotherapy, occasionally chemo-endocrine therapy) as the first and primary modality of treatment for patients with locally advanced and inflammatory breast cancer. The strategies used diverged after primary chemotherapy, because in some cases a mastectomy followed, whereas in others radiotherapy followed by a mastectomy, or additional systemic therapy, was the treatment of choice.

Locally advanced breast cancer is a heterogeneous group of tumor/regional node metastasis combinations. The prognostic subgroups are many, and the overall outcome of any therapeutic strategy depends, in part, on the composition of the group, although it is also influenced by the treatment strategy used. Five-year survival rates in historical studies that used a single modality of treatment varied between 0% and 60%. More recent series (including Surveillance Epidemiology and End Results Study (SEER) data) give higher survival rates, but the heterogeneity persists. As a result of such heterogeneity, randomized clinical trials have been difficult to institute and complete. Therefore, most of the information available to date, and that presented here, is based on prospective single-arm phase II studies.

INITIAL EVALUATION AND MONITORING OF THERAPEUTIC RESPONSE

Most locally advanced tumors are easy to detect and easy to measure. Therefore, for 70–80% of patients with locally advanced breast cancer, clinical evaluation is fairly accurate and appropriate to determine the extent of disease, and to measure response to systemic therapy or radiotherapy. The remaining 20–30% of patients have diffuse, poorly defined tumors. This is especially true for patients with inflammatory breast carcinoma. For these patients, clinical examination is usually inaccurate. For most patients, the addition of mammography and/or breast ultrasonography improves the accuracy of measuring tumor extent.[15–17] Mammographic evaluation is particularly important at baseline to evaluate both breasts, and to make sure that the overall extent of disease, including the determination of multiple foci of primary tumor, is determined. This information will be extremely helpful to the surgeon and the radiation oncologist later on in the course of management.

For patients with poorly defined extent of disease by clinical measurement, imaging is certainly the most accurate way of defining and monitoring the clinical course. Even with the combination of clinical examination, mammography and breast ultrasonography, there are a few patients whose tumors cannot be quantitated. The optimal management of these patients requires a multidisciplinary approach, and awaits better imaging techniques (such as magnetic resonance imaging, positron emission tomography, etc.). For all breast tumors biopsy confirmation of invasive breast cancer is necessary before treatment planning can proceed. Occasionally large tumors (>5 cm) may be entirely non-invasive, and local treatment alone would provide optimal therapy. Fine-needle aspiration can establish the presence of malignancy, but cannot differentiate between invasive and non-invasive breast cancer. Therefore, a core needle biopsy or an incisional biopsy is necessary to establish the presence of invasive breast cancer. In patients with palpable regional lymphadenopathy, the presence of malignant cells in fine-needle aspirates of both the primary tumor and the lymph node would, by definition, establish the presence of invasive disease.

PRIMARY CHEMOTHERAPY

Although there are multiple combination chemotherapy regimens of proven efficacy against metastatic breast cancer, most of the treatment regimens used for the management of locally advanced breast cancer included an anthracycline.[18] Numerous reports in which primary anthracycline-containing chemotherapy was used as the initial treatment demonstrated that 50–90% of patients with locally advanced breast cancer achieved a major objective regression of primary tumor and regional lymph node metastases.[18] Clinically complete responses were observed in 10–25% of these patients. In most studies, three to four cycles of primary chemotherapy were administered, although, in one, chemotherapy was continued until the achievement of maximum response to therapy.[19] This is an important issue, because in patients with metastatic breast cancer the median number of chemotherapy cycles to an objective regression (mostly partial remission) is three cycles, whereas that required to achieve a complete remission is five cycles. It is also known that some patients require as many as 10 cycles of chemotherapy to reach maximum response to therapy.

The study by Swain and collaborators demonstrated this to be true also for locally advanced breast cancer.[19] Some patients achieved maximum remission after one cycle, whereas others required more than 8 months of therapy to reach their maximum benefit. There did not seem to be a correlation between response and outcome in this particular study, suggesting that the prognostic significance of response at different times of follow-up might vary. On the other hand, if breast-conserving therapies are a major goal of treatment, then continuation of primary therapy until achieving the desired extent of tumor reduction might be an appropriate strategy. However, in several other clinical trials, complete response, especially pathologically confirmed complete response, correlated with markedly improved survival, compared with all other patients with lesser responses to primary chemotherapy.[20–22]

Clinical complete remission is not equivalent to pathologically determined complete remission.[1] The combination of physical examination and imaging improves on the accuracy of this evaluation. However, one-third of patients who are considered to have a complete remission by clinical examination and mammography will have residual invasive carcinoma in the surgical specimen. Conversely, about one-third of patients with no microscopic evidence of residual invasive carcinoma will be thought to have an incomplete response by clinical examination and imaging.

COMBINED MODALITY THERAPY

The combination of systemic and locoregional therapies provides optimal local control for patients with locally advanced breast cancer.[23]

Table 9.2 Local control rates in locally advanced breast cancer after combined modality therapy

Author (reference)	Treatment	No. of patients	Median follow-up (months)	IIB–IIIA/ IIIB–IV	Local control rate IIIA/B (%)
Valagussa[24]	CT + RT	72	120	NA	44
Valagussa[24]	CT + RT + CT	126	120	NA	56
Valagussa[24]	CTT + S + RT	79	120	NA	72
Buzdar[25]	CT ± S + RT	367	80+	148/219	93/74
Touboul[26]	CT + RT ± S	82	70	42/40	82
Pierce[27]	H/CT + RT ± S	76	64	48/59	88/79
Cardenas[28]	CT + S + RT	23	52	NA	78
Jacquillat[22]	CT + RT	98	40	30/68	87
Calais[29]	CT + S + RT	80	38	NA	94
Perloff[30]	CT + S/RT	113	37	36/77	63
Hobar[31]	CT + S ± RT	36	34	13/21	81
Conte[32]	CT + S ± RT	39	24	11/28	72
Aisner[33]	CT + S	27	24	–/27	59
Boyages[34]	CT + RT	35	24	8/27	71

CT, chemotherapy; RT, radiotherapy; S, surgery.

Furthermore, when multidisciplinary therapies are used, optimal local control can be obtained with less radical surgical excision or radiotherapy dose. Table 9.2 shows the local control rates in several published studies. It should be noted that in those multidisciplinary regimens where primary chemotherapy was followed by either surgery *or* radiotherapy, local control was obtained in 50–70% of patients. In those reports where both surgery *and* radiotherapy followed primary chemotherapy, local control appeared somewhat higher, in the 60–80% range.[18,35] There have been two prospective randomized trials that compared surgery and radiotherapy following induction chemotherapy.[36,37] These trials demonstrated that initial local control was similar for both modalities of treatment, and that there were no differences in survival regardless of which regional therapy was added to primary chemotherapy. Ultimately, local control was better, however, with surgical resection alone than with radiotherapy alone in both studies. One study compared primary chemotherapy followed by surgery with primary chemotherapy followed by surgery and radiotherapy.[38] No differences in outcome were detected between these two treatment modalities. However, only one cycle of preoperative chemotherapy was administered in this study, and the type and intensity of chemotherapy might have been substandard by today's criteria.

Another aspect of local control, in the context of multidisciplinary management, refers to long-term toxicity. As 30–50% of patients with locally advanced breast cancer survive beyond 5 years after multidisciplinary management, long-term toxicity becomes an important issue. After primary chemotherapy, a radical mastectomy is seldom, if ever, required to provide optimal tumor resection. Furthermore, if primary chemotherapy and surgical excision are used, then postoperative radiotherapy can be limited to standard doses with standard fractionation schedules, thus avoiding delayed radiation-related morbidities (rib and skin necrosis, etc.).[39] This is the major reason why the author's group has continued to use surgical resection for inflammatory breast cancer, in spite of the fact that surgical resection does not improve either local control or survival rates in these patients.[4] However, it spares them from the sequelae of high-dose radiotherapy.

BREAST-CONSERVING THERAPY FOR LOCALLY ADVANCED BREAST CANCER

As most patients with locally advanced breast cancer achieve a greater than 50% reduction in overall tumor burden after primary chemotherapy, it is apparent that many of them will undergo down-staging of their tumor. This implies that both the primary tumor and regional lymph node involvement will decrease sufficiently, so as to go from a higher tumor stage (TNM combination) to a lower tumor stage. In the experience of the authors' group this occurs in about 70% of patients. The major exception includes patients with tumor ulceration or skin edema (*peau d'orange*). In these patients, even complete disappearance of the primary tumor leaves behind visually (and often palpably) abnormal skin which precludes the down-staging from the T4 category.[40] In a number of patients in this subgroup of women, multiple biopsies or complete pathological evaluation fails to reveal residual tumor involvement in these breasts. For patients without skin involvement and with well-delimited disease, a major response to chemotherapy usually offers the option for breast-conserving therapy in a manner similar to that of patients with smaller tumors who have this option as first-line therapy for their disease.

For patients with initial skin involvement, or patients with poorly defined tumors even with the help of imaging, this becomes a more challenging proposition. The same criteria used to select patients with the T1N0 or T2 tumors for primary breast-conserving therapy were used to select patients for breast-conserving surgery after preoperative chemotherapy (Table 9.3). Initial experience, and that of others who have experience in this area, has demonstrated that this practice is safe and that local control rates are similar to what would be expected from smaller tumors subjected to breast-conserving treatments.[40–43] For the overwhelming majority of patients who are offered breast-conserving therapy after primary chemotherapy, the authors still prefer to excise residual tumor. This is, in part, a staging operation which provides prognostic information and, in part, it is performed with the purpose of removing all residual tumor, so that the dose of radiotherapy can be limited to one that does not result in long-term toxic effects.

Breast-conserving therapy for inflammatory breast cancer is more challenging. As skin changes often improve but do not disappear completely, it is difficult to direct the surgical excision to one single area of the breast. More than 60% of patients with inflammatory breast cancer have no palpable mass. Therefore, for most of these patients, if breast-conserving therapy is to be offered, then radiotherapy alone after primary chemotherapy is the only reason-

able option. To provide optimal local control, in the absence of assurance that there is no residual disease in the remaining breast, higher doses of radiotherapy are required, and these may result in chest wall and lung fibrosis, and other complications of high-dose radiotherapy.

DISEASE-FREE AND OVERALL SURVIVAL

The world overview of postoperative adjuvant chemotherapy and endocrine therapy demonstrated that the reduction in odds of recurrence and odds of death obtained with these adjuvant treatments was independent of the number of axillary lymph nodes involved, and/or the initial extent of disease (stage I, II or III).[44,45] Therefore, it is probably safe to assume that the efficacy of adjuvant systemic treatments for locally advanced breast cancer is similar (in relative terms) to that obtained in earlier stages of breast cancer. In fact, the few prospective randomized trials that have included patients with stage III breast cancer clearly demonstrate this to be the case.[46–48] Furthermore, prospective randomized trials that were restricted to patients with locally advanced or stage III breast cancer clearly demonstrated the benefit of adjuvant chemotherapy and endocrine therapy.[47,49,50] Unfortunately, some of these studies, like many of the earlier adjuvant chemotherapy and hormone studies, had insufficient numbers of patients registered (and, therefore, insufficient power) to achieve classic levels of statistical significance.

In recent years, several prospective randomized trials were implemented to determine whether preoperative or primary chemotherapy, in the context of combined modality therapy, is more effective than postoperative adjuvant chemotherapy for patients with locally advanced and high-risk primary breast cancer (Table 9.4).[21,53,56–59] Follow-up for many of these studies exceeds 5 years. Interim analyses have shown no disadvantage, in terms of relapse-free or overall survival rates, for primary or preoperative chemotherapy in any of these studies. In fact, two of these studies showed a modest (non-significant) advantage

---

Table 9.3 Criteria for selecting patients with locally advanced breast cancer for breast-conserving therapy after primary chemotherapy

1   Solitary primary tumor 4 cm or less in size, or two primary tumors within a sphere of less than 4 cm
2   Absence of multiple scattered malignant calcifications in the breast
3   No skin involvement
4   Tumor : breast size ratio small enough for a good cosmetic result
5   Clinically node-negative, or with small, mobile, low axillary nodes
6   Absence of extensive lymphatic involvement within the breast or the dermis
7   No contraindication for radiotherapy (i.e. collagen vascular disease)

Table 9.4 Prospective randomized trials that compare primary vs postoperative adjuvant chemotherapy for locally advanced breast cancer in the context of combined modality therapy

Author (reference)	Treatment	No. of patients	Median - follow-up (months)	Response rate (%)	Percentage disease-free	Percentage alive
Olsen[52]	Primary adjuvant	119	96	77	NA	19
				76	NA	19
Schaake-Koning[54]	Primary adjuvant	39	66	NA	24	37
		34		–	24	37
de Oliveira[55]	Primary adjuvant	81	120	NA	57	42
		90		–	53	40
Scholl[51]	Primary adjuvant	196	54	82	59	86
		194		NA	55	78
Semiglazov[53]	Primary adjuvant	137	53	69	86	86
		134		61	72	79
Ragaz[56]	Primary adjuvant	69	48	NA	57	69
		30		–	47	60
Rubens[57]	Primary adjuvant	12	40	50	50	50
		12		–	42	50
Pierga[58]	Primary adjuvant	200	36	64	68	93
		190		NA	66	86
Mauriac[9]	Primary adjuvant	133	34	63	80	95
		134		NA	79	88

NA, not applicable.

in disease-free survival in favor of primary chemotherapy,[56,58] and two additional studies showed a statistically significant survival benefit.[53,60] Although there are multiple theoretical reasons to believe that early institution of systemic therapy in patients with high-risk breast cancer might alter favorably the disease-free and overall survival of these patients, only well-designed prospective trials will demonstrate the worthiness of this hypothesis.

Retrospective analyses of large, single-institution trials compared with historical controls have also suggested a disease-free and overall survival benefit.[61] However, differences in staging technique, as well as differences in follow-up methodology, might make these analyses somewhat less compelling than the results of prospective randomized trials.

RESULTS OF COMBINED MODALITY THERAPY IN INFLAMMATORY BREAST CANCER

The clinical course of patients with inflammatory breast cancer treated with combined modality treatment, which includes primary chemotherapy, is dramatically different from what is derived from historical series, where patients were treated with surgery alone, radiotherapy alone or a combination of both regional treatments (reviewed in Jaiyesimi et al[4]). In the absence of chemotherapy, the historical series routinely showed a mortality rate that exceeded 90% in 2 years, and 95% in 5 years. In contrast, recent publications mostly show 5-year disease- or metastases-free survival rates in the 30–50% range.

Prognostic factors

In the older series of locally advanced breast cancer treated with regional therapy, it was evident that initial tumor burden, whether defined by the size of the primary tumor or the extent of lymph node metastases, represented the most important prognostic indicator. Secondary prognostic factors included hormone receptor status, and the kinetic parameters of the tumor, such as S-phase fraction. With currently used multidisciplinary regimens with primary chemotherapy, additional prognostic indicators become important. Although the initial stage retains weak prognostic value, the response to primary chemotherapy and the extent of residual disease *after* primary chemotherapy acquire primary importance.[62]

Biological correlates

Other factors that correlate with outcome include histological and nuclear grade,[63] thymidine labeling index, oncogene expression and the expression of other markers.[64–66] In the authors' experience, response to chemotherapy occurs with equal frequency in young and old patients, and in those with poorly and well-differentiated tumors. However, complete remissions are observed only in patients with moderately or poorly differentiated tumors, and not in those with well-differentiated tumors or low nuclear grade.[63] Although we have not evaluated this issue in patients treated with endocrine therapy, the converse might be true, because nuclear grade and degree of histological differentiation often correlate with hormone receptor expression.

The number of positive axillary nodes *after* primary chemotherapy appears to have the same prognostic value as in patients who receive primary surgical treatment.[62] Thus, as shown in Table 9.5, patients with locally

Table 9.5 Prognostic value of axillary lymph node involvement *after* preoperative chemotherapy[67]			
No. of positive nodes	No. of patients	Percentage disease free at 10 years	Percentage alive at 10 years
0	100	63	65
1–3	96	40	44
4–10	93	23	32
>10	34	9	9

advanced breast cancer and no residual lymph node involvement after preoperative chemotherapy have a 10-year survival of 65%, whereas those with 10 or more lymph nodes involved after primary chemotherapy have a 5-year disease-free survival rate of less than 5%. Therefore, as axillary lymph node status after primary chemotherapy can be used as a surrogate marker for disease-free and overall survival, postoperative systemic therapy could be selected based on the evaluation of lymph nodes. Using this hypothesis as a basis, it could be proposed that patients with many positive lymph nodes after chemotherapy ($\geq$10) should participate in novel investigational treatments, including dose intensification, or new cytotoxic agents, whereas patients with few or no involved lymph nodes could be treated optimally with standard chemotherapy and endocrine therapy regimens. Clinical trials to confirm this hypothesis are in progress.

CURRENT DIRECTIONS IN RESEARCH

Over the last decade, marked progress has been made in developing the field of dose intensification for cytotoxic therapy. The development of autologous bone marrow transplantation, and peripheral stem cell support, opened the doors of dose intensification for cytotoxic agents limited by myelosuppressive toxicity by a factor of 4–20, compared with the 20–50% increase in dose intensity before this technology developed. In addition, the development of hemopoietic growth factors (granulocyte colony- stimulating factor or G-CSF, granulocyte– macrophage CSF [GM-CSF], erythropoietin and others) improved the support mechanisms for myelosuppressed patients even further. Today autologous stem cell support with growth factor combinations allows the safe administration of highly dose-intensive cytotoxic regimens. A few pilot studies, in which dose-intensive chemotherapy has been used as intensification after combined modality treatment for patients with locally advanced breast cancer, have suggested higher disease-free survival rates than after standard dose therapies.[68] However, as these improvements may be based entirely on patient selection,[69] prospective randomized trials must be completed to corroborate these findings and exclude the influence of the selection process.

The last decade witnessed the development of several new, exciting and very active cytotoxic and hormonal agents. Among these, vinorelbine,[70] a new norvinblastine analog, the taxanes (paclitaxel and docetaxel),[71] gemcitabine[72] and the anthrapyrazoles (losoxantrone and teloxantrone)[73–75] are probably further along the clinical development path, and have demonstrated marked anti-tumor activity comparable to, or even exceeding, that of the anthracyclines, previously thought to be the most effective agents against breast cancer.[76,77] Several of these agents (vinorelbine, paclitaxel, docetaxel) are being tested as part of combinations or sequential therapy in the adjuvant or neoadjuvant therapy of high-risk primary breast carcinoma. The results of these clinical trials are awaited with great interest.

Occasional publications have reported on the efficacy of intra-arterial therapy for locally advanced breast cancer.[78–81] In some of these, single agent mitozantrone was used, whereas in others, combinations of mitomycin C, 5-fluorouracil and other agents have been employed. Although a high response rate was reported in most of these publications, some of which included not only locally advanced but locally recurrent breast cancer after radiotherapy, there is no evidence based on controlled trials that this approach is either more effective or less toxic than the standard combined modality treatments in use today.

There has been significant progress in the management of locally advanced breast cancer over the last few decades. Combined modality treatments based on primary or preoperative chemotherapy, with the judicious use of surgery, radiotherapy, adjuvant chemotherapy and endocrine therapy, have improved local control rates, quality of life, and probably disease-free and overall survival rates for many patients with locally advanced and inflammatory breast cancer. However, emphasis on early diagnosis, at stages where less complex treatments result in much higher overall cure rates, should be emphasized. The evaluation of novel treatment methods is a high priority in clinical research of these patients with locally advanced breast cancer.

REFERENCES

1. Hortobagyi GN, Buzdar AU. Locally advanced breast cancer: a review including the M.D. Anderson experience. In: *High-risk Breast Cancer* (Ragaz J, Ariel IM, eds). Berlin: Springer-Verlag, 1991:382–415.
2. Haagensen CD, Stout AP. Carcinoma of the breast. Criteria of inoperability. *Am Surg* 1943; **118**:859–66.
3. Anonymous. Breast. In: *Manual for Staging of Cancer* (Beahrs OH, Henson DE, Hutter RVP, Myers MH, eds). Philadelphia: JB Lippincott Co., 1988:145–50.
4. Jaiyesimi IA, Buzdar AU, Hortobagyi G. Inflammatory breast cancer: a review [review]. *J Clin Oncol* 1992; **10**:1014–24.
5. McBride CM, Hortobagyi GN. Primary inflammatory carcinoma of the female breast: staging and treatment possibilities. *Surgery* 1985; **98:** 792–7.
6. Robbins GF, Shah J, Rosen P, Chu F, Taylor J. Inflammatory carcinoma of the breast. *Surg Clin North Am* 1974; **54**:801–10.
7. Saltzstein SL. Clinical occult inflammatory carcinoma of the breast. *Cancer* 1974; **34**:382–8.
8. Lucas FV, Perez-Mesa C. Inflammatory carcinoma of the breast. *Cancer* 1978; **41**:1595–605.
9. Mauriac L, Durand M, Avril A, Dilhuydy JM. Effects of primary chemotherapy in conservative treatment of breast cancer patients with operable tumors larger than 3 cm. Results of a randomized trial in a single centre. *Ann Oncol* 1991; **2**:347–54.
10. Jacquillat C, Weil M, Auclerc G, et al. Neo-adjuvant chemotherapy in the conservative management of breast cancers – study on 205 patients. In: *Neo-adjuvant Chemotherapy* (Jacquillat C, Weil M, Khayat D, eds). London: John Libbey, 1986:197–206.
11. Bonadonna G, Veronesi U, Brambilla C, et al. Primary chemotherapy to avoid mastectomy in tumors with diameters of three centimeters or more. *J Natl Cancer Inst* 1990; **82**:1539–45.
12. Halsted WS. Results of operations for the cure of cancer of the breast performed at the Johns Hopkins Hospital from June, 1889 to January, 1894. *Ann Surg* 1894; **20**:497.
13. De La Garza JG, De La Huerta R, Torres R, Sanchez C. Different management of inflammatory breast carcinoma (chemo-RX-chemo) – experience in 18 cases during a 6 years period (1970–1976) [abstract]. *Proc Am Assoc Cancer Res* 1977; **18**:274.
14. DeLena M, Zucali R, Viganotti G, Valagussa P, Bonadonna G. Combined chemotherapy-radiotherapy approach in locally advanced (T_{3b}–T_4) breast cancer. *Cancer Chemother Pharmacol* 1978; **1**:53–9.
15. Fornage BD, Toubas O, Morel M. Clinical, mammographic, and sonographic determination of preoperative breast cancer size. *Cancer* 1987; **60**:765–71.
16. Sauven P, Grant R, Burn I. The role of mammography in the evaluation of advanced breast cancer treated by initial endocrine therapy. *Br J Surg* 1983; **70**:453–6.
17. Dershaw DD, Drossman S, Liberman L, Abramson, A. Assessment of response to therapy of primary breast cancer by mammography and physical examination. *Cancer* 1995; **75**:2093–8.
18. Hortobagyi GN. Multidisciplinary management of advanced primary and metastatic breast cancer [review]. *Cancer* 1994; **74** (suppl):416–23.
19. Swain SM, Sorace RA, Bagley CS, et al. Neoadjuvant chemotherapy in the combined modality approach of locally advanced nonmetastatic breast cancer. *Cancer Res* 1987; **47**:3889–94.
20. Feldman LD, Hortobagyi GN, Buzdar AU, Ames FC, Blumenschein GR. Pathological assessment of response to induction chemotherapy in breast cancer. *Cancer Res* 1986; **46**:2578–81.
21. Mauriac L, Durand M, Dilhuydy J-M, Avril A, and FBBGS. Randomized trial comparing induction chemotherapy to mastectomy for operable breast cancer larger than 3 cm [abstract]. *Breast Cancer Res Treat* 1992; **23**:181.
22. Jacquillat C, Baillet F, Weil M, et al. Results of a conservative treatment combining induction (neoadjuvant) and consolidation chemotherapy, hormonotherapy, and external and interstitial irradiation in 98 patients with locally advanced breast cancer (IIIA–IIIB). *Cancer* 1988; **61**:1977–82.
23. Fisher B, Anderson S. Conservative surgery for the management of invasive and noninvasive carcinoma of the breast: NSABP Trials. *World J Surg* 1994; **18**:63–9.

24. Valagussa P, Zambetti M, Bonadonna G, Zucali R, Mezzanotte G, Veronesi U. Prognostic factors in locally advanced noninflammatory breast cancer. Long-term results following primary chemotherapy. *Breast Cancer Res Treat* 1990; **15**:137–47.

25. Buzdar, AU, Singletary SE, Booser DJ, et al. (eds). Combined Modality Treatment of Stage III and Inflammatory Breast Cancer: M.D. Anderson Cancer Center Experience. *Surgical Oncology Clinics of North America*, Vol. 4, WB Saunders: Philadelphia 1995:715–34.

26. Touboul E, Lefranc JP, Blondon J, et al. Multidisciplinary treatment approach to locally advanced non-inflammatory breast cancer using chemotherapy and radiotherapy with or without surgery. *Radiother Oncol* 1992; **25**:167–75.

27. Pierce LJ, Lippman M, Ben-Baruch N, et al. The effect of systemic therapy on local–regional control in locally advanced breast cancer. *Int J Radiat Oncol Biol Phys* 1992; **23**:949–60.

28. Cardenas J, Ramirez T, Noriega J, De La Garza J, Gonzalez JP, Labastida S. Multidisciplinary therapy for locally advanced breast cancer: an update [abstract]. *Proc Am Soc Clin Oncol* 1987; **6**:67.

29. Calais G, Descamps P, Chapet S, et al. Primary chemotherapy and radiosurgical breast-conserving treatment for patients with locally advanced operable breast cancers. *Int J Radiat Oncol Biol Phys* 1993; **26**:37–42.

30. Perloff M, Lesnick GJ, Korzun A, et al. Combination chemotherapy with mastectomy or radiotherapy for stage III breast carcinoma: a Cancer and Leukemia Group B study. *J Clin Oncol* 1988; **6**:261–9.

31. Hobar PC, Jones RC, Schouten J, Leitch AM, Hendler F. Multimodality treatment of locally advanced breast carcinoma. *Arch Surg* 1988; **123**:951–5.

32. Conte PF, Alama A, Bertelli G, et al. Chemotherapy with estrogenic recruitment and surgery in locally advanced breast cancer: clinical and cytokinetic results. *Int J Cancer* 1987; **40**:490–4.

33. Aisner J, Morris D, Elias G, Wiernik PH. Mastectomy as an adjuvant to chemotherapy for locally advanced or metastatic breast cancer. *Arch Surg* 1982; **117**:882–7.

34. Boyages J, Langlands AO. The efficacy of combined chemotherapy and radiotherapy in advanced non-metastatic breast cancer. *Int J Radiat Oncol Biol Phys* 1987; **14**:71–8.

35. Hortobagyi GN. Local control for locally advanced breast cancer: many opinions, few facts [editorial comment]. *Int J Radiat Oncol Biol Phys* 1992; **23**:1085–6.

36. DeLena M, Varini M, Zucali R, et al. Multimodal treatment for locally advanced breast cancer. Results of chemotherapy–radiotherapy versus chemotherapy–surgery. *Cancer Clin Trials* 1981; **4**:229–36.

37. Lesnick G, Perloff M, Korzun A, et al. Neo-adjuvant chemotherapy for stage III breast cancer – 5-year report of CALGB 7784. In: *Neo-adjuvant Chemotherapy* (Jacquillat C, Weil M, Khayat D, eds). Paris: John Libbey, 1988:185–8.

38. Papaioannou AN. Preoperative chemotherapy: advantages and clinical application in stage III breast cancer. In: *Recent Results in Cancer Research.* Berlin: Springer-Verlag, 1985:65–90.

39. Spanos WJ, Montague ED, Fletcher FH. Late complications of radiation only for advanced breast cancer. *Int J Radiat Oncol Biol Phys* 1980; **6**:1473–6.

40. Booser DJ, Hortobagyi GN. Treatment of locally advanced breast cancer [review]. *Semin Oncol* 1992; **19**:278–85.

41. Singletary SE, McNeese MD, Hortobagyi GN. Feasibility of breast-conservation surgery after induction chemotherapy for locally advanced breast carcinoma. *Cancer* 1992; **69**:2849–52.

42. Singletary SE, Hortobagyi GN, Kroll SS, Bland KI (eds). Surgical and Medical Management of Local–Regional Treatment Failures in Advanced Primary Breast Cancer. *Surgical Oncology Clinics of North America*, Vol. 4, WB Saunders: Philadelphia. 1995:671–84.

43. Schwartz GF, Birchansky CA, Komarnicky LT, et al. Induction chemotherapy followed by breast conservation for locally advanced carcinoma of the breast. *Cancer* 1994; **73**:362–9.

44. Anonymous. Systemic treatment of early breast cancer by hormonal, cytotoxic, or immune therapy. 133 randomised trials involving 31,000 recurrences and 24,000 deaths among 75,000 women. Early Breast Cancer Trialists' Collaborative Group [see comments] [review]. *Lancet* 1992; **339**:1–15.

45. Anonymous. Systemic treatment of early breast cancer by hormonal, cytotoxic, or immune therapy. 133 randomised trials involving 31,000 recurrences and 24,000 deaths among 75,000 women. Early Breast Cancer Trialists' Collaborative Group [see comments] [review]. *Lancet* 1992; **339**:71–85.

46. Buzdar AU, Gutterman JU, Blumenschein GR, et al. Intensive postoperative chemoimmunotherapy for patients with stage II and stage III breast cancer. *Cancer* 1978; **41**:1064–75.

47. Grohn P, Heinonen E, Klefstrom P, Tarkkanen J. Adjuvant postoperative radiotherapy, chemotherapy, and immunotherapy in stage III breast cancer. *Cancer* 1984; **54**:670–4.

48. Saarto T, Blomqvist C, Tiusanen K, Grohn P, Rissanen P, Elomaa I. The prognosis of stage III breast cancer treated with postoperative radiotherapy and adriamycin-based chemotherapy with and without tamoxifen. Eight year follow-up results of a randomized trial. *Eur J Surg Oncol* 1995; **21**:146–50.

49. Caceres E, Zaharia M, Lingan M, Valdivia S, Moran M, Tejada F. Combined therapy of stage III adenocarcinoma of the breast [abstract]. *Proc Am Assoc Cancer Res* 1980; **21**:199.

50. Rubens RD, Bartelink H, Engelsman E, et al. Locally advanced breast cancer: the contribution of cytotoxic and endocrine treatment to radiotherapy. *Eur J Cancer* 1989; **25**:667–78.

51. Scholl SM, Fourquet A, Asselain B, et al. Neoadjuvant versus adjuvant chemotherapy in premenopausal patients with tumors considered too large for breast conserving surgery: preliminary results at a randomised trial:S6. *Eur J Cancer* 1994; **30A**:645–52.

52. Olson JE, Gray R, Sponzo R, Damsker J, Tormey D, Cummings F. Primary chemotherapy for non-resectable locally advanced breast cancer: 8 yr results of an ECOG trial [abstract]. *Breast Cancer Res Treat* 1990; **16**:148.

53. Semiglazov VF, Topuzov EE, Bavli JL, et al. Primary (neoadjuvant) chemotherapy and radiotherapy compared with primary radiotherapy alone in stage IIb–IIIa breast cancer. *Ann Oncol* 1994; **5**:591–5.

54. Schaake-Koning C, van der Linden EH, Hart G, Engelsman E. Adjuvant chemo- and hormonal therapy in locally advanced breast cancer: a randomized clinical study. *Int J Radiat Oncol Biol Phys* 1985; **11**:1759–63.

55. Gervasio H, De Oliveira CF, Albano J, et al. Neoadjuvant chemotherapy: a regimen (FNM) containing fluorouracil, mitoxantrone and methotrexate for the treatment of locally advanced breast cancer. A randomized trial comparing an initial chemotherapy versus a chemotherapy + radiotherapy combination [abstract]. *Progress and Abstracts of the 8th International Congress on Senology*, University of Texas, MD Anderson Cancer Center, Houston, TX 1994; **1**:263.

56. Ragaz J, Baird B, Rebbeck P, Goldie J, Coldman A, Basco V. Early results of the British Columbia breast cancer preoperative (Neo-Adjuvant) chemotherapy trial. In: *Neo-adjuvant Chemotherapy* (Banzet P, Holland J, Khayat D, Weil M, eds). Paris: Springer-Verlag, 1991:186–92.

57. Rubens RD, Sexton S, Tong D, Winter PJ, Knight RK, Hayward JL. Combined chemotherapy and radiotherapy for locally advanced breast cancer. *Eur J Cancer* 1980; **16**:351–6.

58. Pierga JY, Scholl S, Asselain B, et al. Neo-adjuvant versus adjuvant chemotherapy in operable breast cancer: a controlled trial [abstract]. In: *Proc Adjuvant Therapy of Primary Breast Cancer* 1992; 56.

59. De Oliveira CF, Gervasio H, Gordilho J, et al. Neoadjuvant (preoperative) chemotherapy for breast cancer. A randomized trial (Preliminary results) [abstract]. *Cancer Chemother Pharmacol* 1986; **18** (suppl 1):A22.

60. Scholl SM, Asselain B, Beuzeboc P, et al. Improved survival rates following first line chemotherapy in operable breast cancer. 4 year results of a randomized trial [abstract]. *Proceedings of the Fourth International Congress on Anti-cancer Chemotherapy*, Service d'Oncolgie Medicale Pitie Salpetriere, Paris, France 1993; 64.

61. Hortobagyi GN, Singletary SE, McNeese MD. Treatment of locally advanced and inflammatory breast cancer. In: *Diseases of the Breast* (Harris JR, Lippman ME, Morrow M, Hellman S, eds). Philadelphia: Lippincott-Raven, 1996:585–99.

62. McCready DR, Hortobagyi GN, Kau SW, Smith TL, Buzdar AU, Balch CM. The prognostic significance of lymph node metastases after preoperative chemotherapy for locally advanced breast cancer. *Arch Surg* 1989; **124**:21–5.

63. Abu-Farsakh N, Sneige N, Kemp B, Hortobagyi G. Clinical and pathologic findings of locally advanced breast carcinomas treated with preoperative chemotherapy [abstract]. *Modern Pathology* 1994; **7**:12A.

64. Quenel N, Wafflart J, Bonichon F, et al. The prognostic value of *c-erbB2* in primary breast carcinomas: a study on 942 cases. *Breast Cancer Res Treat* 1995; **35**:283–91.

65. Soubeyran I, Wafflart J, Bonichon F, et al. Immunohistochemical determination of pS2 in invasive breast carcinomas: a study on 942 cases. *Breast Cancer Res Treat* 1995; **34**:119–28.

66. Scholl SM, Pierga JY, Asselain B, et al. Breast

tumour response to primary chemotherapy predicts local and distant control as well as survival. *Eur J Cancer* 1995; **31A:**1969–75.

67. Frye D, Buzdar A, Hortobagyi G. Prognostic significance of axillary nodal involvement after preoperative chemotherapy in stage III breast cancer [abstract]. *Proc Am Soc Clin Oncol* 1995; **14:**95.

68. Vahdat L, Antman KH. Dose-intensive therapy in breast cancer. In: *High-Dose Cancer Therapy* (Armitage JO, Antman KH, eds). Baltimore: Williams & Wilkins, 1995:802–23.

69. Hortobagyi GN. Are the results of high-dose chemotherapy in breast cancer really better than standard treatment? *Bone Marrow Transplantation* 1995; **15:**S260–4.

70. Smith GA. Current status of vinorelbine for breast cancer. *Oncology* 1995; **9:**767–73.

71. Verweij J, Clavel M, Chevallier B. Paclitaxel (Taxol) and docetaxel (Taxotere): not simply two of a kind. *Ann Oncol* 1994; **5:**495–505.

72. Carmichael J, Possinger K, Phillip P, et al. Advanced breast cancer: a phase II trial with gemcitabine. *J Clin Oncol* 1995; **13:**2731–6.

73. Ten Bokkel Huinink W, Moore M, Smith I, et al. A phase II study of losoxantrone (DuP 941) in advanced breast cancer [abstract]. *Eur J Cancer* 1993; **29A:**S78.

74. Talbot DC, Smith IE, Mansi JL, Judson I, Calvert AH, Ashley SE. Anthrapyrazole CI 941: A highly active new agent in the treatment of advanced breast cancer. *J Clin Oncol* 1991; **9:**2141–7.

75. Goldhirsch A, Morgan R, Yau J, et al. A phase II study of DUP 937 in advanced breast cancer [abstract]. *Proc Am Soc Clin Oncol* 1992; **11:**76.

76. Hortobagyi GN, Buzdar AU. Present status of anthracyclines in the adjuvant treatment of breast cancer [review]. *Drugs* 1993; **45** (suppl 2):10–19.

77. A'Hern RP, Smith IE, Ebbs SR. Chemotherapy and survival in advanced breast cancer: the inclusion of doxorubicin in Cooper type regimens. *Br J Cancer* 1993; **67:**801–5.

78. Koyama H, Nishizawa Y, Wada T, Kabuto T, Shiba E, Iwanaga T. Intra-arterial infusion chemotherapy as an induction therapy in multidisciplinary treatment for locally advanced breast cancer. A long-term follow-up study. *Cancer* 1985; **56:**725–9.

79. Twelves CJ, Chaudary MA, Reidy J, Richards MA, Rubens RD. Toxicity of intra-arterial doxorubicin in locally advanced breast cancer. *Cancer Chemother Pharmacol* 1990; **25:**459–62.

80. de Dycker RP, Timmermann J, Schumacher T, Neumann RLA. Intra-arterial chemotherapy of advanced breast cancer. A phase II trial. *Breast Dis* 1991; **4:**181–91.

81. Lewis WG, Walker VA, Ali HH, Sainsbury JR. Intra-arterial chemotherapy in patients with breast cancer: a feasibility study. *Br J Cancer* 1995; **71:**605–9.

10

Routine management of disseminated disease (including anti-osteoclastic therapy)

Robert D Rubens

CONTENTS • **Principles of treatment** • **Clinical evaluation** • **Specific anti-tumour treatment** • **Specific complications** • **Conclusion**

Although, in developed countries, most patients with breast cancer present with localized disease, apparently resectable in its entirety, about half ultimately relapse with either recurrent or metastatic disease. Adjuvant systemic therapy has led to a significant decrease in relapse rate and improvement in survival, but some 15 000 women still die from breast cancer each year in the UK.

To emphasize the importance of disseminated breast cancer in oncological practice, it is instructive to compare the incidence and prevalence of this disease with those of other common cancers. The incidence of breast cancer in the UK is 25 000 new cases per annum, whereas its prevalence is estimated at 105 000. By contrast, the incidence of lung cancer is 40 000 per annum, but, with its high mortality, the prevalence is only 26 000. These figures reflect the prolonged clinical course of breast cancer in many patients resulting in a uniquely high prevalence, compared with other cancers, of more than four times the annual incidence.

Advanced breast cancer gives rise to a wide variety of clinical manifestations. Locoregional relapse in the breast, skin or lymph nodes may cause serious morbidity from fungation, ulceration or infection. Relapse in proximity to the brachial plexus can cause pain, sensory loss and motor disability, and is often associated with lymphoedema. Dissemination of the disease to distant sites is common. About 70% of patients with metastatic breast cancer develop clinically significant skeletal metastases which may give rise to pain, fractures, bone marrow suppression, hypercalcaemia or spinal cord compression. Serious morbidity may also result from pleural effusions or ascites, or metastases in the lungs, liver and brain.

There are therefore many potential approaches to treatment (Table 10.1). These include methods directed against the tumour itself, such as surgical resection, radiotherapy, endocrine treatment or cytotoxic chemotherapy, whereas certain complications may require specific interventions including paracentesis, orthopaedic surgical procedures or stenting of ducts, such as the ureters or bile duct, when obstructed by tumour.

This chapter concentrates principally on the use of specific systemic anti-tumour treatments (endocrine therapy and chemotherapy), but also covers the increasing importance of bisphosphonates for use in metastatic bone disease; attention is also given to the management of specific complications. The use of symptomatic and

Table 10.1 Treatments available for advanced breast cancer

Radiotherapy

Surgery

Endocrine therapy
  Ovarian ablation (surgical or irradiation)
  Gonadotrophin-releasing hormone agonists
    Goserelin
  Anti-oestrogens
    Tamoxifen
    Toremifene
  Aromatase inhibitors
    Aminoglutethimide
    Formestane, exemestane,
    Letrozole, fadrozole, vorozole,
    anastrozole
  Progestogens
    Medroxyprogesterone acetate
    Megoestrol acetate
    Norethisterone acetate

Cytotoxic chemotherapy
  Doxorubicin, epirubicin
  Cyclophosphamide
  Methotrexate
  5-Fluorouracil
  Mytomycin C
  Mitozantrone
  Paclitaxel, docetaxel
  Vinblastine
  Vinorelbine

Corticosteroids

Bisphosphonates
  Pamidronate
  Clodronate

Isotope therapy
  Strontium-89
  Samarium-153

Symptom control

supportive measures, for example, the use of analgesics, psychotropic drugs and antiemetics, is extremely important, but is not covered in this chapter. The role of the clinical nurse specialist and good communication among the patient, family and the medical team are of the utmost importance.

PRINCIPLES OF TREATMENT

Disseminated breast cancer is not curable, but with skilful use of available treatments the disease can often be controlled and valuable palliation provided, sometimes for many years. The principal objective of treatment is therefore to make patients' lives as active and symptom free for as long as possible with the fewest adverse effects from treatment. Whether or not treatment is capable of extending survival is controversial and this is not usually a primary objective of treatment. However, when the pattern of metastatic disease leads to rapidly progressive organ failure, such as metastatic liver disease with deranged hepatic function or pulmonary lymphangitis carcinomatosa, its reversal by treatment almost certainly prolongs life.

Although some oncologists prescribe systemic therapy at the first appearance of metastatic disease, it is the view of the author that the institution or change of treatment is normally indicated only in the presence of symptomatic progressive disease. Earlier treatment may confer side-effects without benefit and induce resistance of disease to the agent used, making it no longer available for palliative use. In an asymptomatic patient, an indication for treatment may, however, occasionally be to attempt to avoid or delay an anticipated imminent complication. For example, the progression of pulmonary metastases observed on sequential chest radiographs may lead to the expectation of respiratory symptoms and institution of treatment could be appropriate. The decision on whether or not to give treatment under these circumstances will depend upon previous observations of the pace of the disease and, sometimes, a patient's preference for treatment. Another example is the appearance of early symptoms and signs of a brachial plexopathy, when induction of tumour regression by systemic treatment may prevent irreversible neurological damage.

CLINICAL EVALUATION

Before new treatment is started for disseminated breast cancer, careful clinical evaluation and re-staging of patients are useful to provide a baseline reference against which to judge the response to treatment. However, the use of laboratory and radiological investigations that influence neither the management nor the outcome of patients is undesirable. Tests should always have a clear purpose, such as those needed to diagnose symptomatic problems, those necessary for giving cytotoxic chemotherapy safely and those appropriate for monitoring response to treatment. Blood counts are essential for the safe planning and monitoring of chemotherapy, and should be repeated before each course of treatment. Baseline biochemical screens for hepatic and renal function are appropriate, but regular repetition of tests is usually unnecessary. A chest radiograph before starting treatment is a simple and useful examination that gives information about pulmonary or pleural and sometimes skeletal disease. A baseline isotopic bone scan is appropriate to screen for skeletal lesions, but as it images function rather than structure, radiographs of abnormal regions are needed for full assessment.

Isotopic or ultrasonic scans of the liver are not needed routinely and should be confined to patients with clinically suspected liver disease or those with deranged hepatic biochemistry. Computed tomography of the brain is only needed if there is clinical suspicion of cerebral metastases and is not part of routine baseline staging. Magnetic resonance imaging is occasionally needed and is of particular use in the diagnosis of suspected spinal cord compression.

Assessing response to treatment can often be achieved simply by clinical examination supplemented by plain radiography of marker lesions. Sometimes ultrasonography and computed tomography may be useful. Biological markers for breast cancer in serum are not particularly specific, and a routine role for their measurement in monitoring treatment has not been established. The evaluation of metastatic bone disease is considered in more detail later.

SPECIFIC ANTI-TUMOUR TREATMENT

Selection of treatment

Selection of specific systemic treatment for disseminated breast cancer is based on the consideration of three important factors (Figure 10.1):

1. The extent, pattern and aggressiveness of the disease
2. Indices of likely hormone sensitivity such as steroid receptor status
3. Menopausal status.

For patients with rapidly progressive visceral lesions, such as lymphangitis carcinomatosa causing severe breathlessness or hepatic metastases with deranged liver biochemistry, death is likely to ensue rapidly unless disease progression can be reversed. This pattern of disease rarely responds to endocrine treatment, chemotherapy being needed if there is to be a chance of disease control. For patients with less aggressive disease, it is helpful to consider the oestrogen and progesterone receptor status of the tumour.[1] Patients with low tumour levels of these receptors are unlikely to respond to endocrine treatment and chemotherapy should be considered. If patients have steroid receptor-positive tumours, consideration of menstrual status can assist in the selection of endocrine treatment before chemotherapy needs to be used.

If information on steroid receptor levels is not available, other factors can be used to give an indication of the potential hormone sensitivity of a tumour. For example, patients who have had a disease-free interval of more than 2 years after primary treatment tend to have hormone-dependent tumours. There is also a correlation between steroid receptor status and the differentiation of ductal carcinomas, poorly

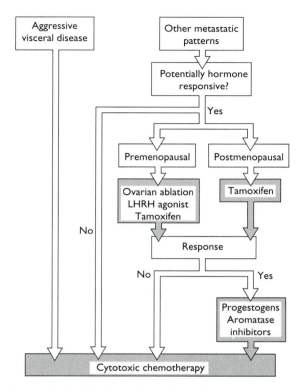

Figure 10.1 Selection of specific anti-tumour treatment in advanced breast cancer. LHRH, luteinizing hormone-releasing hormone.

differentiated ductal carcinomas usually being receptor negative; lobular tumours are generally steroid receptor positive.

Endocrine therapy

The rationale for endocrine therapy is to reduce the oestrogenic stimulus to breast cancer growth. This may be achieved by removal of sites of oestrogen production, removal of the source of, or inhibiting, gonadotrophins, blocking oestrogenic action, antagonizing oestrogens with either androgens or progestogens, or inhibition of oestrogen synthesis. Depending upon selection criteria, response rates to first-line endocrine treatment range from 30% to 50%, and to second line they are about 20%.

The established treatment for premenopausal patients with oestrogen receptor-positive tumours is ovarian ablation, either surgically or by pelvic irradiation. Tamoxifen 20 mg daily is the principal agent used to block binding of oestrogen to its receptor, and is the preferred first-line endocrine treatment in postmenopausal women. The use of gonadotrophin-releasing hormone analogues or tamoxifen is a reasonable alternative to ovarian ablation in premenopausal patients. Prednisolone is active against breast cancer and was shown in two successive trials to enhance the response of the disease to either ovarian ablation or tamoxifen.[2] Provided that there is no contraindication to the use of prednisolone, it is reasonable to combine this agent with these forms of endocrine treatment.

Patients who respond to first-line endocrine treatment for advanced disease and subsequently relapse may then be considered for other endocrine treatments, which may also be more suitable for women who have had adjuvant systemic therapy. With increasing use of adjuvant tamoxifen and the induction of permanent amenorrhoea by adjuvant chemotherapy, tamoxifen and ovarian ablation may not be appropriate treatment options for many patients relapsing after primary treatment.

The development of agents to inhibit oestrogen synthesis has been of particular interest in recent years. The first such agent, aminoglutethimide, was originally introduced to inhibit the desmolase enzyme responsible for the conversion of cholesterol to pregnenelone in the adrenal cortex, so interfering with the production of all adrenocortical hormones. It was regarded as a 'medical adrenalectomy'. However, it was subsequently recognized that the principal action of the drug is to inhibit the conversion of C19 androgens to C18 oestrogens by aromatase, a more specific effect achieved at drug concentrations that do not inhibit desmolase. Moreover, inhibition of aromatase also impairs the peripheral synthesis of oestrogens from androgens in adipose tissue, the liver and breast cancer itself. These findings have stimulated the search for more specific aromatase inhibitors, both steroidal (such as formestane, exemestane) and non-steroidal (such as voro-zole, fadrozole, letrozole and anastrozole). These agents are assuming increasing importance in the endocrine treatment of breast cancer.

Progestational agents, such as medroxyprogesterone acetate, norethisterone acetate and megoestrol acetate, are useful against breast cancer. They act both at the level of the tumour cell and by inhibiting gonadotrophins.

The endocrine treatments outlined above are simple to use and devoid of serious side effects. There is no clear evidence indicating the superior efficacy of any one approach over another, and the sequential use of treatments as indicated above is reasonable for routine practice. There is no evidence to support the combined use of hormone treatments other than the addition of prednisolone to either ovarian ablation or tamoxifen.

With the variety of endocrine agents now available, there is no longer a place for the use of either oestrogens or androgens in the treatment of this disease. Oestrogens may cause serious cardiovascular and gastrointestinal toxicity, whereas the virilizing effects of androgens can be extremely distressing to female patients. The major surgical endocrine ablation procedures of hypophysectomy and bilateral adrenalectomy have become obsolete.

Cytotoxic chemotherapy

Cytotoxic drugs that have an established place in the treatment of disseminated breast cancer include anthracyclines (particularly doxorubicin and epirubicin), cyclophosphamide, 5-fluorouracil, methotrexate, mitomycin C and mitozantrone. They are often used together in combinations, for examples CMF (cyclophosphamide, methotrexate and 5-fluorouracil), MMM (mitomycin C, methotrexate and mitozantrone) or FAC (5-fluorouracil, doxorubicin and cyclophosphamide). No combination has emerged as clearly superior to the others and it is uncertain whether any of them is significantly more effective than doxorubicin or epirubicin alone. Anthracyclines have been widely recognized as the most active single agents until the recent introduction of the taxoids. Ideally, the contribution of any drug in a combination should be confirmed by a clinical trial so that the available treatments are used optimally. This has rarely been done, but such trials have demonstrated that vincristine has no value in combinations.[3]

When selecting drugs, side effects that need to be avoided should be considered. For example, the existence of bone marrow disease or previous extensive skeletal radiotherapy may preclude drugs that are particularly toxic to bone marrow such as mitomycin C. In other patients, the avoidance of alopecia may be particularly important, precluding the use of anthracyclines. Considerable progress has been made in reducing the toxic effects of chemotherapy, particularly the use of more effective antiemetics such as the $5HT_3$ (5-hydroxytryptamine) inhibitors. There are no good predictors of response to chemotherapy, although crude measures of tumour bulk and performance status do give some guidance: a large tumour burden and poor performance status correlate with low response rates.

Dose–response relationships have been demonstrated for cytotoxic drugs, and testing of the concepts of dose intensification has been facilitated by the use of haemopoietic growth factors, autologous bone marrow transplantation or the use of peripheral blood stem cells. However, there is no evidence so far to suggest that this enhances either the palliation or curability of breast cancer.

Although the response rate of metastatic breast cancer to first-line treatment in patients selected for clinical trials is in the range 50–70%, in unselected patients receiving such treatment in routine practice the objective response rate is closer to 30%.[4] Placing too much reliance on clinical trials to provide pertinent information in planning treatment for individual patients gives rise to the problem that they invariably have highly restrictive entry criteria and so do not necessarily represent the generality of patients with advanced breast cancer. Hence, patients excluded from clinical trials may include elderly people and those with poor performance status, non-evaluable disease, haematological and biochemical parameters deviating from defined ranges, concomitant illnesses, or certain previous treatments, or those who have specific metastatic patterns such as brain metastases. Furthermore, there is a lowered response to chemotherapy in patients who have had previous adjuvant chemotherapy.[5]

The optimal duration of chemotherapy is not known. If, after 6 weeks, a response is observed or the disease has remained static, continuation of treatment is appropriate provided that it is acceptable to the patient. If the disease is progressing, the treatment in question should be stopped. In patients responding to treatment, there is no evidence to support long-term treatment and regimens lasting 4–6 months are appropriate.

Response to second-line treatment in unselected patients falls to 20%, but may be considered in patients with progressive disease. In patients who have responded to primary chemotherapy and have had a long time to relapse of, say, 6 months or more, it is reasonable to consider using the same regimen again, but in other groups of patients, alternative drugs will need to be chosen.

There is no evidence to support the combined use of endocrine treatment and chemotherapy, and the two approaches may be antagonistic.[6]

Evaluating treatment

Whether or not a patient judges treatment for advanced breast cancer to be worth while will depend on any benefits, such as symptom relief or reduction in disability, which outweigh any adverse effects including physical toxicity, psychosocial disturbance and domestic disruption. The balance between beneficial and harmful effects can be particularly fine when using cytotoxic chemotherapy for the palliative treatment of cancer. Judgements about cost-effectiveness are difficult to make because the relevant factors are not easily compared with each other and they are not readily amenable to quantitative measurement. Clinical trials have usually relied on strict criteria for objective response to determine the efficacy of treatment, but in recent years more weight has been given to the evaluation of symptom relief and quality of life in assessing the effectiveness of treatment. The use of such instruments has demonstrated a correlation between the achievement of objective response and effective palliation, but probably only 20–30% patients have net benefit from first-line chemotherapy.[7]

SPECIFIC COMPLICATIONS

Bone metastases

Breast cancer is the most frequent cause of malignant involvement of the skeleton. Seventy per cent of patients with advanced disease develop clinically significant metastatic bone disease which is responsible for much of the morbidity and disability caused by breast cancer.[8] Problems include pain, pathological fractures, hypercalcaemia, myelosuppression, spinal cord compression and nerve root lesions. In about 20% of patients with disseminated breast cancer, the skeleton is the only clinically detectable site of metastases. The illness in these patients can follow a prolonged clinical course with a medial survival from the diagnosis of bone metastases of 24 months, 20% of patients surviving more than 5 years.

Monitoring metastatic bone disease for response to treatment is difficult in comparison with disease in soft tissues. Response is usually judged by the recalcification of previously lytic disease seen on plain radiographs. However, this method does not assess tumour regression directly, but rather a delayed consequential recalcification. This results in reported response frequencies at sites of skeletal disease being low compared with those in soft tissues. This almost certainly reflects the insensitivity of assessment methods rather than a true difference in response rates. Although isotopic bone scanning is a useful and sensitive test to screen for the presence of bone metastases, it is of no value in monitoring efficacy of treatment.

As a result of the limitations of imaging

techniques, efforts have been made to identify other parameters of response in bone.[9] Biochemical factors include the bone isoenzyme of alkaline phosphatase (ALP-BI), the osteoblast product osteocalcin and urinary calcium excretion. The increased osteoblastic activity, associated ultimately with a radiological response, is characterized by an elevation of the serum osteocalcin and ALP-BI one month after starting treatment, and a concomitant drop in urinary calcium excretion. The combination of a rise in ALP-BI and osteocalcin and a fall in urinary calcium excretion gives a diagnostic efficiency of 89% for discriminating between response and progression. Preliminary observations on the urinary excretion of the cross-linking amino acids of collagen, pyridinoline and deoxypyridinoline have shown a significant decrease in patients with bone metastases 4 weeks after starting treatment with the osteoclast-inhibiting agent pamidronate. The importance of these tests lies in the aim of the treatment of bone metastases being palliative rather than curative. Early information at one month, indicative of either response or progressive disease, is particularly helpful in determining whether or not treatment should be continued. This cannot be achieved if reliance is placed solely upon imaging tests.

The skeletal damage caused by metastatic disease is mediated largely by osteoclastic bone resorption. Malignant cells secrete factors which stimulate, both directly and indirectly, osteoclastic activity.[10] They include prostaglandin E and a variety of cytokines and growth factors such as transforming growth factor α and β, epidermal growth factor, tumour necrosis factor and interleukin-1. In addition to local paracrine factors, osteoclastic activity can also be stimulated by humoral factors in malignant disease, particularly parathyroid hormone-related peptide (PTHrP). Ectopic production of this hormone is a cause of osteoclastic bone resorption and hypercalcaemia, even in the absence of bone metastases.

The dominant role of the osteoclast in tumour-induced osteolysis provides the basis for the use of inhibitors of osteoclastic activity in the treatment of bone metastases. In recent years, the possibilities for inhibiting osteolysis have increased considerably with the development of the bisphosphonates.[11] These compounds are pyrophosphate analogues containing a P–C–P backbone rather than the P–O–P bond of pyrophosphate. This chemical substitution renders the bisphosphonates resistant to phosphatase degradation. The bisphosphonates bind to bone mineral and, through effects on the surface charge on hydroxyapatite, exert a marked physicochemical effect on crystal physiology. The result is a reduction in osteoclast numbers by a direct toxic effect of ingested bisphosphonates and inhibition of the differentiation of precursor cells into mature osteoclasts.

The three bisphosphonates in current clinical use are etidronate, clodronate and pamidronate. The efficacy of bisphosphonates in metastatic bone disease was first demonstrated by the reversal of hypercalcaemia, a complication for which these agents are now the treatment of first choice. Several controlled and uncontrolled studies of the bisphosphonates have now demonstrated their ability to reverse osteolysis, even in the absence of other anti-tumour treatment, with substantial symptomatic benefits.[12] The studies have shown relief of pain in about half the patients, and a significant reduction in the subsequent incidence of hypercalcaemia and pathological fractures, and in the need for palliative radiotherapy.

Bisphosphonates now have an established role in the treatment of bone metastases from breast cancer, but their optimal use is still being defined. From work on tumour-induced hypercalcaemia it has become clear that a dose–response relationship exists. New, more potent, bisphosphonate analogues for oral use, such as alendronate and ibandronate, are being developed.[11] However, in spite of the apparent convenience of oral bisphosphonates, high-dose intermittent intravenous treatment may ultimately be confirmed as the method of choice because of the poor bioavailability of the oral form.

Another approach to the treatment of metastatic bone disease is the administration of bone-seeking isotopes.[13] Strontium-89 is a pure β emitter and, like calcium, is a bone-seeking element. Samarium-153 also has β emission for therapeutic use and additional γ emission enables imaging to be done; complexing with a tetrabisphosphonate targets the skeleton. These agents can be effective for relieving bone pain, particularly in the late stages of disease when high doses of opiate analgesics are required and when external beam radiotherapy is no longer practicable.

A scheme for an approach to treatment of metastatic bone disease is given in Figure 10.2.

Several complications give rise to the substantial morbidity resulting from bone metastases, including pain, impaired mobility, pathological fracture, spinal cord compression, cranial nerve palsies, nerve root lesions, hypercalcaemia and suppression of bone marrow function. Localized pain and peripheral nerve

dysfunction can often successfully be treated by radiotherapy and the general management of pain is dealt with in Chapter 14. Consideration will be given to specific management of other complications.

Pathological fractures are common in patients with metastatic bone disease and affect long bones (particularly the femora and humeri), ribs and vertebrae. Radiological assessment of long bones suggests that, when metastatic destruction involves over 50% of the cortical thickness, the risk of fracture is so high that prophylactic orthopaedic surgery, such as intramedullary nailing or prosthetic hip replacement, is indicated. Stabilization of the bone is more readily done and rehabilitation facilitated while the bone is still intact. The principles of the treatment of a fracture are the same as those of prophylactic surgery, and it is usual to follow surgical stabilization by radiotherapy. Pathological fracture does not necessarily indicate generalized disease progression and restaging with a bone scan is appropriate. Progression of disease elsewhere may necessitate a change in specific anti-tumour systemic treatment or possibly prophylactic orthopaedic surgery at other sites.

Compression of the spinal cord or cauda equina in patients with metastatic disease of the spine is a medical emergency necessitating prompt diagnosis and treatment. Its causes include pressure from an enlarging extradural mass, spinal angulation following vertebral collapse, vertebral dislocation following pathological fracture or, rarely, pressure from intradural metastases. The standard diagnostic test was myelography, but this has been replaced by magnetic resonance imaging in many centres. Multiple levels of compression may be demonstrated. Back pain is the most common initial symptom and may be either local spinal or radicular in character, both being experienced close to the lesion site. Motor weakness, sensory loss and autonomic dysfunction are all common features of spinal cord or cauda equina compression. Treatment with high-dose corticosteroids should be instituted immediately on suspicion of the diagnosis, because the reversal of associated oedema can effect a

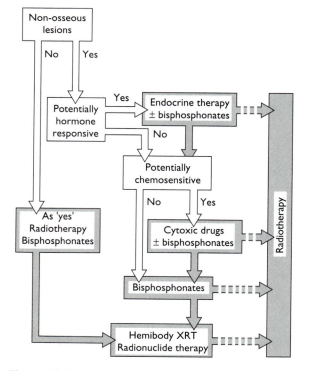

Figure 10.2 Management of metastatic bone disease. XRT, radiotherapy.

prompt reduction in neurological compression. This needs to be followed by definitive treatment, the choice being between surgical decompression and radiotherapy. Generally, radiotherapy is preferred and is the only option when there are multiple levels of compression. Surgery is more appropriately considered after radiotherapy for patients with residual spinal instability. Occasionally, spinal surgery can be valuable in patients with severe refractory radicular pain in the absence of cord compression.

Hypercalcaemia is another acute emergency associated with metastatic bone disease. Its clinical features include nausea, vomiting, dehydration and confusion. Although malignant hypercalcaemia is usually associated with demonstrable bone metastases, this is not always the case because it is occasionally caused by ectopic PTHrP production, leading to humorally mediated bone resorption. The immediate treatment is intravenous rehydration followed by an intravenous bisphosphonate. Etidronate, clodronate and pamidronate are all effective, but a randomized trial has demonstrated the superiority of pamidronate.[14] Normocalcaemia is achieved in almost all patients and, after a single infusion of pamidronate, it is maintained for about 3 weeks. Repeated administration prevents recurrence in many patients, although more prolonged control may be achieved by instituting more effective specific systemic anti-tumour treatment. The introduction of the bisphosphonates has replaced older treatments for hypercalcaemia which included corticosteroids, phosphate and mithramycin. In patients with hypercalcaemia caused by PTHrP, calcitonin is occasionally of value for inhibiting the high renal tubular reabsorption of calcium in these patients.

Extensive infiltration of the bone marrow by metastatic disease can cause leukoerythroblastic anaemia and pancytopenia predisposing to infection and haemorrhage. Radiotherapy, often needed for the treatment of bone metastases, can exacerbate this problem. Such patients are particularly sensitive to the myelotoxic effects of cytotoxic chemotherapy.

The incidence of breast cancer increases with increasing age and many older patients have coexisting osteoporosis. Certain treatments for breast cancer can exacerbate this problem, for example, ovarian ablation, ovarian failure induced by chemotherapy or the use of corticosteroids. Osteoporosis can also present diagnostic problems in elderly patients in whom it may be difficult to distinguish between osteoporotic and metastatic bone disease as a cause of vertebral collapse. Bisphosphonates are increasingly being used for the treatment of osteoporosis, and this is particularly compatible with the increasing indication for these agents in patients with breast cancer.

Serous effusions

Pleural effusions are common in patients with breast cancer.[15] They may occur as the sole evidence of metastatic disease or as part of more widespread dissemination. Diagnosis is based on physical signs and chest radiography. If symptomatic, immediate relief of breathlessness can be achieved by simple needle aspiration. If they are part of more widespread disease necessitating specific systemic treatment, further local treatment can be deferred until the response to systemic treatment is ascertained. For patients with isolated symptomatic pleural effusions, it is preferable to undertake a pleurodesis as more definitive treatment. Reliance on repeated pleural aspirations for the relief of symptoms can lead to pleural adhesion formation and loculation of fluid, making future drainage difficult and compromising the success of a formal pleurodesis. The most reliable method of pleurodesis is talc insufflation at thoracoscopy under general anaesthetic. For patients in whom this method is inappropriate, suitable agents for intrapleural instillation under local anaesthetic include mustine, tetracycline and bleomycin. Irrespective of the sclerosing agent used, complete drainage of pleural fluid is an important prerequisite before its instillation. Although talc can be insufflated throughout the thoracic cavity under direct vision, after instillation of other agents, it is important for the patient to be placed in several different positions to ensure uniform spread of the agent throughout the pleural cavity. After a few hours, the draining tube, which was left in place, can be unclamped to allow free drainage of further fluid and to ensure contact between and adherence of the two serosal layers. This may take several days, but is important to ensure adhesion of the parietal and visceral pleurae, effectively to obliterate the pleural cavity and so prevent further accumulation of effusions.

Pericardial effusion leading to cardiac tamponade is a relatively unusual complication of breast cancer. This medical emergency may be suspected in a patient with severe breathlessness of relatively short duration. The physical signs of increased venous pressure and pulsus paradoxus, together with cardiomegaly, on chest radiography indicate the diagnosis for which immediate relief can be achieved by percutaneous pericardiocentesis. After pericardial drainage, recurrent pericardial effusions are uncommon, possibly because the procedure results in an artificial pericardial window that allows subsequent drainage into the pleural cavity. Although instillation of sclerosant agents into the pericardial cavity has been used, this is unlikely to be effective because the incessant movement within the pericardium makes it improbable that adhesion of the two surfaces could be achieved.

Ascites is seen quite commonly in patients with breast cancer as a result of either peritoneal metastases or liver disease complicated by either portal hypertension or hypoalbuminaemia. Drainage of ascites is useful to relieve discomfort, but when secondary to hepatic failure and in the presence of low plasma albumin, it may precipitate hypovolaemic shock. Diuretics such as frusemide and spironolactone have limited value in controlling ascites, although prolonged infusions of frusemide have been reported to be useful. Transfer of ascites from the peritoneal cavity into the venous system is possible by means of a subcutaneous shunt connecting the peritoneal cavity to the subclavian or jugular vein, a one-way valve preventing retrograde flow. However, success with these shunts is variable because blockage is common. Usually, control of ascites will be dependent upon the sensitivity of the underlying disease to systemic treatment, with little place for the instillation of drugs intraperitoneally. Caution has to be exercised with systemically administered methotrexate because its slow diffusion back into the circulation after accumulation in ascitic fluid risks mucosal and bone marrow toxicity.

Liver metastases

About a quarter of patients who die from breast cancer have evidence of liver metastases before death. Their prognosis is poor in comparison to patients with disease confined to other sites, particularly when liver biochemistry deteriorates. Patients with symptomatic liver metastases and deranged biochemical tests often have tumours of oestrogen receptor-negative phenotype and response to endocrine treatment is unlikely. About a third have disease sensitive to chemotherapy and this is the preferred treatment for most patients with liver metastases. However, when asymptomatic liver metastases come to light as a result of staging in the context of more indolent disease, a trial of endocrine treatment may be appropriate. Chemotherapy is potentially compromised by impaired liver function, particularly the use of anthracyclines. Doxorubicin is largely excreted by the liver and, in the presence of impaired liver function, high blood levels persist, resulting in severe toxicity with mucositis and bone marrow suppression. Epirubicin, closely related to doxorubicin structurally, is particularly subject to glucuronidation and is metabolized more rapidly than doxorubicin. This feature may make epirubicin more appropriate for use in patients with liver metastases as the effective dose can be determined from the level of the aspartate aminotransferase.[16] In patients with markedly deranged liver function, it can sometimes be useful to give chemotherapy cautiously as low weekly doses rather than at higher doses at longer intervals. This approach has been found to be well tolerated and achieves about a 30% response rate.

Brain metastases

Brain metastases develop in a small proportion of patients with breast cancer. Focal neurological signs, deterioration of mental function or symptoms of raised intracranial pressure suggest the diagnosis which is usually readily confirmed by either computed tomography or magnetic resonance imaging. These metastases cause considerable morbidity and median survival from diagnosis is about 3 months. Temporary symptomatic relief can be achieved for many patients by the prescription of oral dexamethasone, which reduces cerebral oedema surrounding the lesions. For patients who are in the terminal stages of the disease, this may be all that is appropriate, but, for others, although prognosis is poor, cranial irradiation should be given in an attempt to reverse symptoms and disability, with a view to the patient retaining an independent functional state. In spite of the theoretical presence of the blood–brain barrier, chemotherapy as well as endocrine therapy may control cerebral disease in some patients.

Metastatic involvement of the meninges may mimic intracerebral metastases or result in impaired cranial or peripheral nerve function as a consequence of scattered nerve root involvement. Examination of the cerebrospinal fluid will often enable a cytological diagnosis to be made, associated with a high protein and low sugar level. Focal radiotherapy to control relevant symptoms is most useful, but occasionally intrathecal chemotherapy, administered either at lumbar puncture or intraventricularly through an Ommaya reservoir, can be considered.

CONCLUSION

Disseminated breast cancer is a complex illness with a wide spectrum of clinical manifestations and a variable clinical course. Many approaches to treatment are available which, used skilfully and selectively, can palliate the disease effectively for many patients, sometimes for prolonged periods of time.

REFERENCES

1. Roberts MM, Rubens RD, King RJB, et al. Oestrogen receptors and the response to endocrine therapy in advanced breast cancer. *Br J Cancer* 1978; **38**:431–6.
2. Rubens RD, Tinson CL, Coleman RE, et al. Prednisolone improves the response to primary endocrine treatment for advanced breast cancer. *Br J Cancer* 1988; **58**:626–30.
3. Steiner R, Stewart JF, Cantwell BMJ, Minton MJ, Knight RK, Rubens RD. Adriamycin alone or combined with vincristine in the treatment of advanced breast cancer. *Eur J Cancer Clin Oncol* 1983; **19**:1553–7.
4. Gregory WM, Smith P, Richards MA, Twelves CJ, Knight RK, Rubens RD. Chemotherapy of advanced breast cancer: outcome and prognostic factors. *Br J Cancer* 1993; **68**:988–95.
5. Rubens RD, Bajetta E, Bonneterre J, Klijn JGM, Lonning PE, Paridaens R. Treatment and relapse of breast cancer after adjuvant systemic therapy – review and guidelines for future research. *Eur J Cancer* 1994; **30A**:106–11.
6. Rubens RD, Begent RHJ, Knight RK, Sexton SA, Hayward JL. Combined cytotoxic and progestogen therapy for advanced breast cancer. *Cancer* 1978; **42**:1680–6.
7. Ramirez AJ, Towlson KE, Leaning MS, Richards MA, Rubens RD. Do patients with advanced breast cancer benefit from chemotherapy? *Br J Cancer* 1997; in press.
8. Coleman RE, Rubens RD. The clinical course of bone metastases from breast cancer. *Br J Cancer* 1987; **55**:61–6.
9. Coleman RE, Whitaker KW, Moss DW, Mashiter G, Fogelman I, Rubens RD. Biochemical prediction of response of bone metastases to treatment. *Br J Cancer* 1988; **58**:205–10.
10. Mundy GR. Hypercalcaemia of malignancy revisited. *J Clin Invest* 1988; **82**:1.
11. Bijvoet OLM, Fleisch HA, Canfield RE, Russell RGG (eds). *Bisphosphonate on Bones*. Amsterdam: Elsevier, 1995.
12. Coleman RE, Purohit OP. Osteoclast inhibition for the treatment of bone metastases. *Cancer Treat Rev* 1993; **19**:79–103.
13. Clarke SEM. Isotope therapy for bone metastases. In: *Bone Metastases: Diagnosis and Treatment* (Rubens RD, Fogelman I, eds). London: Springer Verlag, 1991:187–205.
14. Ralston SH, Gallacher SJ, Patel U, et al. Comparison of three intravenous bisphospho-

nates in cancer-associated hypercalcaemia. *Lancet* 1989; **ii:**1180.

15. Miles DW, Knight RK. Diagnosis and management of malignant pleural effusion. *Cancer Treat Rev* 1993; **19:**151.

16. Twelves CJ, Richards MA, Smith P, Rubens RD. Epirubicin in breast cancer patients with liver metastases and abnormal liver biochemistry: initial weekly treatment followed by rescheduling and intensification. *Ann Oncol* 1991; **2:**663–6.

11

Salvage therapy after adjuvant systemic therapy

Monica Castiglione-Gertsch, Pinuccia Valagussa

CONTENTS • **Diagnosis of recurrence** • **Special types of recurrence** • **Systemic treatment at relapse** • **Quality of life issues in recurrent breast cancer** • **Hormone replacement therapy** • **Comments and conclusions**

Breast cancer is the most frequently diagnosed malignancy in women in the West. More than 95% of cases are diagnosed at an operable stage, i.e. there is only the primary tumour in the breast tissue; in 30–50%, ipsilateral axillary lymph node metastases are also detected after an accurate work-up.

Despite radical local treatment, consisting mainly of surgery (mastectomy or breast-conserving procedures) and radiotherapy (generally to the conserved breast), most patients have recurrences and eventually die of overt metastatic disease. Independent of axillary nodal status, bone, either alone or with involvement of other sites, is the most frequently documented single lesion at the time of first disease relapse.[1–3] Other frequent sites of new disease are the liver, lung and pleura, as well as soft tissues, including the operated breast, the mastectomy scar, lymph nodes and skin metastases.[4] Despite new and possibly more effective treatment approaches, recurrent breast cancer is not curable and only a very limited number (4–5%) of patients are alive 18 years after disease relapse.[5] However, with appropriate treatment, valuable palliation can be provided, at times for many years.

Failure to achieve cure with a locoregional modality alone is currently attributed to occult micrometastases that are present at the time of diagnosis.[6] This hypothesis has received indirect support from results of clinical trials carried out over the last three decades. Available findings have confirmed that more aggressive locoregional treatments do not provide additional benefit, in terms of both disease-free and overall survival, compared with less radical surgery.[7–9] Overall, prospective randomized studies of adjuvant systemic treatments (chemotherapy, hormone manipulation or combinations of both) have shown that it is possible to change the natural history of resectable breast cancer, through a significant reduction in the annual odds of disease recurrence and death.[10] Whether adjuvant systemic therapy affects occurrence of new disease mainly in locoregional or distant sites, or in both is still controversial.[5,11] Similarly, in spite of the significant improvement in long-term survival, there is still concern that adjuvant therapies may compromise the possibility of effectively treating the disease after relapse.

DIAGNOSIS OF RECURRENCE

The extent and timing of postoperative follow-up programmes for patients with breast cancer are still debatable; intensive surveillance of asymptomatic patients does not have a convincing influence on outcome.[12] When the first trials of adjuvant systemic therapy were activated in the early 1970s, both extent and timing of follow-up examinations were planned with stringent requirements for the careful assessment of the side effects of adjuvant programmes and patterns of new disease; they were also important in the attempt to detect early recurrences and consequently institute appropriate salvage treatments while the tumour cell burden was still low. Findings from these evaluations indicated that the vast majority (ranging from 60% to 79% in different case series) of patients with recurrent disease presented with signs and/or symptoms of metastases, which were reported during physical examinations and then confirmed on radiological and laboratory investigations.[2,4] Among those women who were found to have asymptomatic recurrences at planned examinations, the lead time from diagnosis to symptoms has been estimated to be a median of about 8 months.

Recently published data on two randomized trials show that neither survival nor quality of life is improved with a more intensive follow-up programme.[13,14] In the first trial,[13] patients undergoing the intensive follow-up programme showed an excess of isolated bone (84 for the intensive follow-up versus 53 for the other group) and intrathoracic (lung and pleura) (28 for the intensive group versus 18 for the other patients, respectively) metastases. As expected, 5-year relapse-free survival was significantly lower for patients in the intensive follow-up programme, who showed an earlier diagnosis of relapse ($p = 0.01$). However, estimated mortality rate at 5 years (18.6% in the intensive follow-up group and 19.5% in the other group) and survival curves were comparable. In the second trial,[14] which included more than 1300 patients, no difference could be observed in survival for the patients followed in the two

programmes. It is of interest that metastases were detected in 31% and 21% of asymptomatic patients in the intensive follow-up group and the control group, respectively. In the control group, tests leading to detection of metastases in asymptomatic women were prompted by either anamnestic information or findings on physical examination. In this study, the mean time to detection of distant metastases was 53 and 54 months, respectively, showing no anticipation of diagnosis of recurrence for patients followed more intensively. Some aspects of quality of life were studied in this trial. The intensity of follow-up did not affect the examined dimensions of quality of life in the two surveillance groups.

Both trials support the view that, because breast cancer patients do not benefit from intensive follow-up programmes in terms of survival and quality of life, the allocation of high financial resources for this type of surveillance is not justified. In routine clinical practice, the frequent use of laboratory tests and radiological examinations should therefore be discouraged. Recommendations for clinical practice should endorse a follow-up strategy based on the appropriate clinical surveillance plus a yearly/2-yearly mammography, which should be bilateral after conservative surgery, to detect second primary breast cancers.

PATTERNS OF RELAPSE AFTER SYSTEMIC TREATMENT

As previously mentioned, whether the main effect of adjuvant systemic therapy consists of reduction in new disease manifestation in locoregional or distant sites, or in both, is still a matter of controversy. Description of the sites of first disease relapse has been summarized in many reports dealing with treatment outcome. However, there are still few evaluations with appropriate methods that show relapse site-specific incidence over time.

Investigators from the International (Ludwig) Breast Cancer Study Group (IBCSG) have reported their experience in 2830 node-positive breast cancer patients treated with either more effective or less effective systemic treatment.[11] The more effective treatment consisted of prolonged CMF (cyclophosphamide, methotrexate and fluorouracil) based regimens (1788 patients) or tamoxifen for 1 year (320 postmenopausal women), whereas treatment using one cycle of perioperative CMF (413 patients) or no adjuvant systemic treatment (309 postmenopausal women) was designated as less effective. Table 11.1 summarizes the

findings reported in the IBCSG analysis and compares them with the experience of the Milan Cancer Institute in the first CMF study.[5] In spite of the limitations of a between-study comparison, the difference between the two case series is striking. In the case series of the IBCSG, the CMF-based regimen apparently has no effect in bone and visceral dominant sites of disease recurrence; its efficacy seems to be limited to a dramatic reduction of soft tissue relapses (18% vs 36%). By contrast, in the Milan experience adjuvant CMF had a moderate effect on all sites of disease relapse. Of note, in the IBCSG control group, the cumulative incidence of soft tissue relapses at 5 and 10 years was twice (32% and 36%, respectively) that of the same type of relapses detected in the Milan Cancer Institute control group (15% and 18%, respectively). Another issue found in the IBCSG was the high incidence of bone metastases in patients treated with CMF plus low-dose prednisone, compared with patients in whom this latter drug was not administered.[15] Prednisone's mechanism of action may be partly responsible for the inefficacy of the more effective regimen in influencing bone metastases.

Relapse site-specific analyses are required to investigate issues relating to the consequences of recurrence, and are eagerly awaited from other research groups. They can be instrumental in the design of new and more effective adjuvant regimens.

SPECIAL TYPES OF RECURRENCE

Locoregional recurrence in general

Locoregional recurrence, defined as the reappearance of disease in the operated breast, chest wall or regional lymph nodes, affects up to 20–40% of women after surgery for breast cancer.[16] This incidence is influenced primarily by the type of local treatment and the number of initially positive axillary lymph nodes. However, several clinical trials,[7-9] and the recently published overview on local treatments, have shown that the extent of surgery

Table 11.1 Cumulative incidence of first sites of breast cancer relapse in two different case series

Case studies	Incidence	
	At 5 years (%)	At 10 years (%)
IBCSG[11]		
Soft tissue*		
More effective[†]	15	18
Less effective	31	36
Bone		
More effective	13	18
Less effective	14	17
Viscera		
More effective	13	17
Less effective	16	19
Milan Cancer Institute[5]		
Soft tissue*		
CMF	11	13
Control	15	18
Bone		
CMF	12	15
Control	18	22
Viscera		
CMF	19	22
Control	18	25

* Locoregional or distant.
† See text for explanation.

does not influence the overall survival of patients[17] and that even the rates of isolated local recurrences are not significantly different with different surgical procedures. At the time of locoregional recurrence, about one-third of all patients have overt distant metastases.[17–19]

Breast recurrence after breast-conserving surgery

Breast-conserving surgical procedures have become standard in many centres, so recurrence in the breast is therefore becoming a common event. The prognosis of this type of recurrence is considered to be excellent, but there are few data available on patients with adequate follow-up time. Caution appears to be necessary when dealing with breast recurrence after breast-conserving treatments, which could also have included radiotherapy.

Diagnosis of breast recurrence is generally done by either clinical examination or follow-up mammography. The long-lasting breast changes after surgery and radiotherapy may, however, considerably reduce the accuracy of mammography in these patients,[20] leading to the recommendation that, for suspicious cases, additional tests such as magnetic resonance imaging (MRI) and cytology may be necessary. The question of whether the anticipation of breast recurrence diagnosis with intensive surveillance will improve outcome remains open. Treatment of breast recurrence, regardless of whether adjuvant chemotherapy was administered, has generally consisted of surgical excision. No consistent data are available on the value of additional systemic therapies in this setting.

Local recurrence after mastectomy

Retrospective analyses, after local recurrence in mastectomized patients, show a 5-year disease-free survival (DFS) rate of 13–37% and an overall 5-year survival rate of 21–50%, the 10-year values being 7–12% and 22–26%, respectively. Occasionally, patients have enjoyed a disease-free interval of more than 15 years, but relapses later than that have also been described.[18,21] Treatment of these lesions depends on the type of local recurrence. Nodular recurrences can, in general, be surgically removed. Inflammatory and lymphangitic spread, however, often require a systemic approach, similar to the treatment of metastatic disease. Radiotherapy is usually recommended for locoregional recurrences[22] but treatment failure with the reappearance of locoregional disease is common (up to 25%), even after appropriate radiotherapy doses.[23,24] Moreover, a large percentage of these patients will eventually develop distant metastases.

Systemic treatment after local therapy (surgery and radiation) for chest wall recurrence has been studied in only one randomized trial, conducted by the Swiss Group for Clinical Cancer Research, which examined the possible benefit of secondary adjuvant manipulations.[25] In the 'good risk' group (defined as patients with oestrogen receptor-positive tumours or long disease-free interval), randomized to no systemic treatment or tamoxifen, the median disease-free survival after local recurrence was 26 months for the observation arm and 82 months for patients treated with the antioestrogen ($p = 0.007$). The 5-year DFS rate was 36% and 59%, respectively. The 5-year cumulative incidence for local disease manifestations was 28% and 10%, in the control arm and tamoxifen arm, respectively ($p < 0.001$), whereas distant metastases (25% for treated as well as for observed patients), mixed manifestations (5%/2%), death and second cancers (6%/4%) were not significantly affected by treatment. No survival difference could be demonstrated between observation and tamoxifen ($p = 0.77$). The 5-year survival rate was 76% for the observation and 74% for the tamoxifen arm.

These data suggest a possible benefit of systemic therapy for some patient populations. Although this approach cannot generally be recommended, systemic therapy, namely chemotherapy, can be considered for poor prognosis (e.g. oestrogen receptor-negative tumours, high proliferative activity).

Contralateral breast cancer as an isolated manifestation of disease recurrence

Women with a prior diagnosis of breast cancer have a threefold increased risk of developing a new tumour in the contralateral breast, compared with women with no previous breast cancer diagnosis.[26] Adequate local management of contralateral tumours follows the usual guidelines. Resectable breast cancers first undergo locoregional treatment modality (breast-saving procedures for small cancers, modified mastectomy for larger lesions) and administration of systemic treatment is dictated by the presence of unfavourable factors (nodal involvement, negative steroid receptors, undifferentiated malignancy, high proliferative rate) found at the time of diagnosis of the second primary. Locally advanced breast cancers are usually treated with primary chemotherapy, the type and sequence of successive locoregional treatments depending on the extent of tumour shrinkage as well as the presence or absence of inflammatory signs. Additional systemic therapy (chemotherapy and/or endocrine therapy) is generally planned to prolong the DFS.

It is worth mentioning that the vast majority of individual trials,[27] as well as the international overview,[10] have reported a statistically significant reduction in the odds (39%; $p < 0.00001$) of developing a contralateral breast cancer in women treated with adjuvant tamoxifen compared with patients not given this antioestrogen. This was observed despite the fact that the mean duration of recurrence-free survival was longer in tamoxifen-allocated than in control patients, thereby giving treated women more time during which contralateral disease could develop. No protective effect for contralateral breast cancer has been reported after adjuvant chemotherapy.

SYSTEMIC TREATMENT AT RELAPSE

The proper management of patients developing new disease manifestations after adjuvant systemic therapy can represent a therapeutic problem. The length of the disease-free interval, sites and extent of recurrence, performance status and steroid receptors are all parameters that are important in selecting the appropriate treatment for patients with previously untreated metastatic breast cancer. In addition, the modality of the adjuvant therapy, as well as the treatment duration and intensity of the drugs to which these patients were previously exposed, deserve careful consideration.

In 1981, Chlebowski and co-workers[28] suggested that adjuvant systemic chemotherapy might be associated with a poor response to treatment on relapse. In the same year, however, investigators from the MD Anderson Cancer Institute in Houston[29] confuted this hypothesis and reported that patients presenting with disease recurrence after adjuvant FAC (fluorouracil, doxorubicin [Adriamycin] and cyclophosphamide) could indeed achieve consistent tumour shrinkage after either endocrine therapy or chemotherapy, with a remission rate of 39–40% for a median duration of 16 months. Subsequently, other reports on limited case series appeared in the medical literature and, overall, the conclusions about the efficacy of salvage therapy after adjuvant treatment have been contradictory.

Findings from randomized studies of adjuvant chemotherapy

In 1986, the Milan Cancer Institute reported, for the first time, data on the effectiveness of salvage therapy by grouping together findings from two trials of adjuvant CMF, one comparing 12-monthly cycles of CMF versus no adjuvant therapy and the second comparing 12 versus 6 cycles of CMF. The findings were updated a few years later on a larger case series.[30] The essential results for patients given systemic treatment at disease relapse are summarized in Table 11.2. A total of 67 premenopausal women, 55 of whom were previously treated with adjuvant CMF, were subjected to therapeutic castration. In patients with measurable disease, there was no difference in the rate of objective (complete plus partial) remission between patients previously given CMF and those relapsing after loco-regional treatment alone. It is of note that drug-induced amenorrhoea did not influence treatment outcome. A total of 139 CMF-treated patients and 17 control patients received additive endocrine therapy, mainly tamoxifen. Both the rate of objective remissions and the remission duration favoured control patients. It is, however, worth stressing that about half the patients in the control group presented with dominant recurrence in soft tissues, compared with only one-third of the patients given adjuvant CMF. This different pattern of disease presentation may, at least in part, be responsible for the different treatment outcome.

The most important findings are those obtained in women given chemotherapy at the time of diagnosis of disease recurrence. More than 40% presented with visceral involvement, regardless of previous treatment modality. Overall, the rate of objective remissions and their duration were similar between control and CMF-treated patients (Table 11.2). However, in the adjuvant CMF failures, treatment response to salvage chemotherapy was influenced by the length of the DFS interval from the end of adjuvant therapy. In fact, when DFS was less than 12 months, none of the eight patients re-treated with CMF achieved a remission, which was attained in 9 of 29 women given salvage doxorubicin-containing regimens. In contrast, when DFS lasted more than one year, outcome was similar after CMF re-treatment (48%) and doxorubicin-containing regimens (45%). Regardless of the treatment modality used as salvage therapy, median overall survival was similar between control and CMF patients, both when measured from the date of first disease relapse (35 vs 31 months) and when measured from the date of diagnosis and surgical treatment of the primary tumour (60 vs 60 months).

Different findings were reported by investigators from Guy's Hospital in London[31] who analysed the impact of salvage treatment in patients entered into their randomized study of adjuvant CMF versus control. A total of 176 women (CMF 65, control 111) were evaluated; endocrine treatment was given to 123 patients at some time after first relapse, whereas 94

Table 11.2 Efficacy of systemic treatment in patients failing after adjuvant chemotherapy for node-positive breast cancer

	Control	CMF
Therapeutic castration		
Total patients	12	55
Objective remission* (%)	12	20
With amenorrhoea (%)		21
No amenorrhoea (%)		19
Duration, median (months)	12	20
Additive endocrine therapy		
Total patients	17	139
Soft tissue lesions[†] (%)	47	33
Objective remission (%)	59	37
Duration, median (months)	32	25
Chemotherapy		
Total patients	42	93
Visceral disease[†] (%)	42	46
Objective remission		
Total (%)	38	38
To CMF (%)	38	37
DFS[‡] < 12 months (%)		0
DFS > 12 months (%)		48
To ADM regimens (%)		38
DFS < 12 months (%)		31
DFS > 12 months (%)		45
Duration, median (months)	20	21

Data from two successive studies carried out at the Milan Cancer Institute.[28]
* In patients with measurable disease.
† Dominant site of disease.
‡ From end of adjuvant CMF.
ADM regimens: doxorubicin [Adriamycin]-containing regimens.

women received chemotherapy after relapse. Overall, patients previously treated with adjuvant CMF achieved a significantly lower response rate and showed a shorter time to progression than women in the control group, independent of treatment modality (chemotherapy or endocrine treatment) that was first applied for the metastatic stage. However, survival after relapse was similar in the two groups of patients, lasting for a median of 16 months regardless of prior exposure to adjuvant chemotherapy.

A comparison between the findings reported by the Milan Cancer Institute[30] and those from Guy's Hospital[31] is hampered by differences in the two case series and the lack of important details. Salvage therapies described in the Italian experience were, indeed, the first treatment applied at the diagnosis of first disease relapse, whereas in the British series patients received systemic treatment on development of distant metastases, locoregional recurrences being normally treated by excision and/or radiotherapy. Plausible, therefore, at least one-third of the patients in the Guy's Hospital series were given systemic treatment upon further

disease progression. In addition, a description of the dominant sites of disease presentation when systemic treatment was delivered was not reported by the British investigators.

Findings from chemotherapy trials on advanced disease

Results from three representative reports, evaluating the impact of previous adjuvant chemotherapy on patients entered into prospective studies of chemotherapy for advanced disease, are summarized in Table 11.3.

In 1980, the Cancer and Leukaemia Group B (CALGB) activated a randomized study to assess whether the addition of tamoxifen could

Table 11.3 Selected studies in advanced breast cancer evaluating response to chemotherapy after relapse in patients with or without adjuvant chemotherapy

Research group	Regimens* for advanced disease	No. of patients with/without adjuvant chemotherapy	Comments
CALGB[32]	CAF ± TAM	46/379	Prior adjuvant chemotherapy as a stratification variable No effects on treatment outcome
ECOG[33]	DAVTH	145/356	Multivariate analysis Detrimental effect of prior chemotherapy However, previously treated patient had a better treatment outcome when DFS was >24 months from first diagnosis
FESG[34]	FAC FEC Epirubicin	137/340	Multivariate analysis Detrimental effect of prior chemotherapy in terms of response rate and time to treatment failure but not on overall survival from initial diagnosis

*See text for acronyms.

enhance response rate and response duration of CAF (cyclophosphamide, doxorubicin and fluorouracil) chemotherapy. Patients failing prior adjuvant chemotherapy were eligible if their adjuvant programme had been completed at least 6 months previously; more importantly, prior adjuvant treatment was a stratification variable next to dominant site of metastatic disease. A total of 425 evaluable patients was entered into this study, 46 of whom had received prior adjuvant chemotherapy.[32] There was no difference in response rate (59% vs 50%), response duration (12 vs 10.7 months), time to treatment failure (10.6 vs 9.4 months) or survival (19.6 vs 17.5 months) between patients previously untreated with chemotherapy and those previously exposed to cytotoxic drugs. Interestingly, only 29% of women with a DFS of 12 months or less from the end of prior adjuvant chemotherapy achieved objective remission, compared with 51% of those with a longer interval. The authors concluded that women who relapsed 6 months or more after completion of adjuvant chemotherapy do not have inherently drug-resistant tumours.

The Eastern Co-operative Oncology Group (ECOG) has evaluated factors predicting for treatment outcome using a treatment consisting of DAVTH (mitolactol, doxorubicin, vincristine, tamoxifen and fluoximesterone) for metastatic breast cancer.[33] Overall, exposure to prior adjuvant chemotherapy did not affect treatment response to salvage treatment, but median time to treatment failure and overall survival were influenced negatively. However, when the duration of DFS, plausibly from first breast cancer diagnosis, was considered, prior adjuvant chemotherapy influenced treatment outcome negatively in those with a DFS between 1 and 24 months, but not when the DFS was longer than 24 months (objective remission 26% vs 46%, median time to treatment failure 3.4 vs 9.5 months, median survival 8.3 vs 21.8 months).

A similar type of analysis was performed by the French Epirubicin Study Group (FESG) which examined the effect of prior exposure to CMF-type adjuvant regimens in two successive studies for advanced breast cancer.[34] In their report only patients without metastases at the time of initial diagnosis were included. Regimens for advanced disease were either FAC, FEC with epirubicin at two different doses substituting for doxorubicin, or epirubicin alone. The clinical characteristics of the patients showed important and statistically significant differences between patients previously given adjuvant chemotherapy and those who were not. The most important imbalances included prior adjuvant endocrine therapy, prior treatment with radiation and duration of DFS. In this series, multivariate analysis revealed that prior exposure to adjuvant CMF-type chemotherapy had a negative effect on response rate (31% vs 48%, $p = 0.03$), median time to treatment failure (182 days vs 268 days, $p = 0.007$) and median survival from starting salvage chemotherapy (410 days vs 560 days, $p = 0.008$). However, median overall survival from initial diagnosis was similar in all patients with or without adjuvant chemotherapy. It is interesting that, in the large subgroup of node-positive breast cancer patients, survival from salvage chemotherapy was not affected by prior exposure to CMF-type adjuvant regimens.

Salvage chemotherapy after relapse from a doxorubicin-containing adjuvant regimen

Most of the findings available concern treatment outcome of patients relapsing after CMF or CMF-like combinations. In many of these patients salvage chemotherapy, when delivered, consisted of an anthracycline-containing regimen. Today, more patients receive an anthracycline-containing regimen in the adjuvant programme. Therefore there is additional concern about the choice of cytotoxic salvage treatment, especially when considering the potential myocardial toxicity of anthracyclines, with administration of cumulative doses of 450–500 mg/m^2 for doxorubicin and 1000 mg/m^2 for epirubicin, or when there is irradiation to the chest wall or thoracic area.

For this reason, attempts at designing different drug combinations have been carried out in the past. Unfortunately, the vast majority of these reports were in an abstract form, lacking important details about patients previously treated with adjuvant chemotherapy. In more recent years, new drugs have been found to be effective in advanced breast cancer, namely taxanes (paclitaxel and docetaxel) and vinorelbine.

Among these three drugs, paclitaxel is probably the most frequently tested single agent in patients classified as resistant to anthracyclines.[35] Overall, objective responses varied from 29% to 50% when paclitaxel was administered at the dose of 175 mg/m^2 or more in this subset of patients. Besides the usual methodological problems inherent to interstudy comparisons, the definition of resistance to doxorubicin or epirubicin varied greatly among the different trials, and included both absence of response in metastatic disease and relapse within 12 months from the end of adjuvant chemotherapy. In the experience of the Milan Cancer Institute,[36] 46% of 24 women who failed within 12 months of primary or adjuvant doxorubicin-containing chemotherapy achieved an objective remission on paclitaxel, compared with 31% of 26 patients previously given doxorubicin-containing regimens for metastatic disease.

Although detailed data are not as yet available, treatment outcome following docetaxel[37] and vinorelbine[38] confirm that both drugs are also effective in patients previously treated with adjuvant chemotherapy; these compounds warrant further studies in this patient subset.

Salvage treatments after relapse from adjuvant tamoxifen

In spite of the large number of patients treated with adjuvant tamoxifen in prospective controlled studies, there is little information about outcome of salvage treatments in patients who failed this adjuvant modality. The Stockholm Breast Cancer Study Group reported the effect of tamoxifen alone or associated with fluoximesterone, in 54 postmenopausal women with recurrent disease diagnosed at least 2 years after the end of the adjuvant programme.[39] A total of 28 women had received adjuvant tamoxifen and 26 no endocrine adjuvant treatment. Notably, 12 of the 28 patients also received adjuvant CMF chemotherapy, as did 11 of the 26 women in the control group. The objective response to salvage endocrine therapy was significantly lower in patients from the tamoxifen group (14%), compared with the controls (54%, $p < 0.01$). The median time to disease progression was also significantly shorter (4 vs 15 months, $p < 0.05$) for women exposed to adjuvant tamoxifen. The authors reported that differences between the two groups with regard to prognostic factors could not explain the difference in treatment outcome.

Rubens[40] recently summarized the effect of salvage treatment in 142 patients relapsing either while receiving adjuvant tamoxifen or after completing 2 years of treatment. Salvage endocrine therapy was able to achieve objective remission in 11% of patients, whereas the response rate after salvage chemotherapy was 30%. No information on duration of response and survival was reported.

QUALITY OF LIFE ISSUES IN RECURRENT BREAST CANCER

The goal of treatment in most breast cancer relapses is palliation, because no cure can be achieved with the currently available tools. Palliation means not only the relief of pain, but also the improvement of all disease-related symptoms (gastrointestinal disturbances such as lack of appetite and nausea, weight loss, psychological distress, etc.), as well as the possible prevention of disease-related complications (hypercalcaemia, bone fracture, cord compression, etc.). Palliation means conserving the patient's quality of life for as long as possible.

Can we define quality of life?

There have been several attempts to define quality of life: Freud is supposed to have said that quality of life consists of work and love, others have defined it as the difference between expectations and achievements. The quality of life is a complex multidimensional concept which includes physical, biological, psychological, emotional, cognitive, social and economic aspects.[41] A patient's quality of life is influenced by different factors, which are weighted differently by each individual. It is easy for each one of us to describe our own needs for quality of life; however, it is very difficult to develop collective norms from the subjective reality of a single patient.

Can quality of life be measured?

In the past decade quality of life has become one of the most important endpoints in cancer treatment. Different methods and instruments for the valid and reliable measurement of quality of life during palliative treatments have been validated in past years. Two main approaches can be used for the assessment of quality of life during treatment: qualitative and quantitative. The qualitative approach, generally more psychoanalytically oriented, is applicable especially for the assessment of quality of life of a single patient; the quantitative measurements with different instruments, such as the LASA or Linear Analogue Self-Assessment (Figure 11.1), allow for the comparison between quality of life outcomes within different treatment and patient populations.

Mood:
Happy _____ Miserable
Well-being:
Good _____ Lousy

Figure 11.1 Examples of LASA scales (Linear Analogue Self-Assessment)

Can we improve the quality of life of patients with metastatic breast cancer?

Medical treatment in general is not always followed by clinical improvement and does not invariably mean patient benefit, especially when using cytotoxic agents for metastatic disease.[41,42] The most important task, while treating a woman with metastatic breast cancer, is to maintain the balance between therapy-induced improvement of symptoms and therapy-induced unfavourable side effects. A study carried out by the Australian Group has shown that, against the expectation of the investigators, continuous chemotherapy yielded better quality of life and better survival than the intermittent application of the same chemotherapy, in spite of increased toxicity (mainly nausea and vomiting) reported by the patients treated continuously.[43]

Psychosocial treatment of patients with metastatic breast cancer

Psychosocial treatment for patients with metastatic breast cancer should be considered for each patient, especially when considering the frequency of psychological morbidity, including anxiety, fear, depression and therapy or disease-induced sexual dysfunctions. Psychosocial interventions have been shown not only to improve the well-being and quality of life of the patients, and to reduce anxiety, depression and pain significantly, but also to prolong their survival.[44–46] A possible explanation for this rather surprising finding is that psychologically supported patients may adhere better to aggressive treatment options; however, this hypothesis requires further investigation. The question of whether all patients should be offered psychological intervention is scientifically still open, and the decision depends not only on additional knowledge but also on the allocation of medical resources.

The selection of psychosocial support should be an inter-/multidisciplinary task involving not only the patient, her family and the treating physician, but also several others, such as nursing personnel, social workers, psychologists, psychiatrists, etc.

HORMONE REPLACEMENT THERAPY

Breast cancer patients often have important sexual dysfunctions and menopausal symptoms resulting mainly from treatment (amenorrhoea following chemotherapy, hot flashes with anti-oestrogens, oestrogen-depletion symptoms from aromatase inhibitors, etc.). The use of hormone replacement therapy after breast cancer is still controversial, and for patients with metastatic disease there is some concern that such treatment may stimulate disease progression.[47] In fact, oestrogen can promote proliferation of certain breast cancer cell lines in vitro and our knowledge about the proliferative activity of progesterone is minimal.

Long-term oestrogen depletion symptoms such as osteoporosis and cardiovascular disorders obviously are irrelevant in the presence of metastatic breast cancer.

Short-term oestrogen-depletion symptoms such as hot flashes may severely impair patients' quality of life but, in general, they can be fairly well controlled with clonidine or belladonna alkaloids combined with ergotamine tartrate and phenobarbitone (Bellergal). Vaginal dryness can show an improvement through use of local oestrogen, and the availability of preparations with low systemic absorption makes its use safer.

Some patients, however, will not improve with these treatments and will require systemic hormone replacement therapy. For those patients, the benefit of hormones in terms of quality of life may largely outweigh the concerns about safety. However, because of the lack of firmly reassuring data, caution and increased surveillance of the patients are required.[48,49]

COMMENTS AND CONCLUSIONS

There is no doubt that the recently published data on the decrease in mortality rates from breast cancer are of historical importance. This goal is likely to have been achieved through new developments in diagnostic tools, as well as through a more widespread use of systemic adjuvant treatment modalities in high-risk patients. In fact, the international overview[10] has confirmed that, overall, effective adjuvant systemic therapies can alter the natural history of operable breast cancer. Nevertheless, a consistent fraction of treated patients is at risk of developing new tumour manifestations and these patients eventually die of overt metastatic disease.

Many clinical trials have required testing of patients at frequent intervals in order to detect recurrence as early as possible: a low tumour burden is more amenable to therapeutic intervention as a result of a decreased probability of cell resistance to therapy. Unfortunately, there is no evidence that intensive surveillance, allowing earlier detection of recurrence, has a favourable effect on overall survival.[13,14] This may be because the current treatment for metastatic disease is still palliative rather than curative.

A great concern in women failing after adjuvant systemic therapy is that adjuvant programmes may compromise the potential for effective treatment of the disease at relapse. Findings reported so far in the medical literature remain somewhat contradictory. It is common experience that, in advanced breast cancer, second-line chemotherapy regimens are unable to achieve response rates and response durations similar to those obtained with first-line combinations. Does this also hold true after adjuvant chemotherapy? Does adjuvant chemotherapy induce resistance to subsequent drug treatments? Despite decades of adjuvant trials, no definitive answer is available.

In the absence of adequate experimental data, considerations of the putative mechanisms of an impaired response after previous adjuvant chemotherapy rely on theoretical speculations. One possibility is that previous adjuvant chemotherapy could induce acquired resistance and therefore counteract the effects of later treatments. Findings from Guy's Hospital,[31] as well as those from the ECOG[33] and the FESG,[34] would indeed support this hypothesis. Alternatively, resistance may be transient, reversible and relative, and this second hypothesis is mainly supported by findings from the vast experience of the Milan Cancer Institute[30] and by results from the CALGB study.[32] Patients failing during or fairly shortly after the end of adjuvant chemotherapy have a very low response rate to salvage chemotherapy, one plausible explanation being that these women have a relatively highly resistant cell population. Patients who show new disease manifestations after a longer DFS can obtain response rates and response durations that are no different from those achievable in patients who have never received chemotherapy.[30] These patients have either a less extensive drug-resistant cell population or resistance was transient and reversible.

The balance of evidence indicates that prior adjuvant systemic treatment may compromise the response of the disease to systemic therapy after relapse. However, an important observation from almost all the previously mentioned studies is that no survival differences were detected between previously treated and previously untreated patients, from both date of relapse and date of first diagnosis. This held true after prolonged follow-up as exemplified by the 20-year experience[5] of the Milan Cancer Institute (Figure 11.2). Thus, the reported significant decrease in the annual odds of death can be attributed to the early administration of adjuvant treatment.

Most of the patients will not achieve a long-lasting remission with salvage treatment. Nevertheless, physicians should be encouraged always to administer adequate systemic treatments at the time of first relapse, regardless of prior exposure to cytotoxic drugs or hormonal manipulations, to yield the greatest palliation and the best quality of life for the patients.

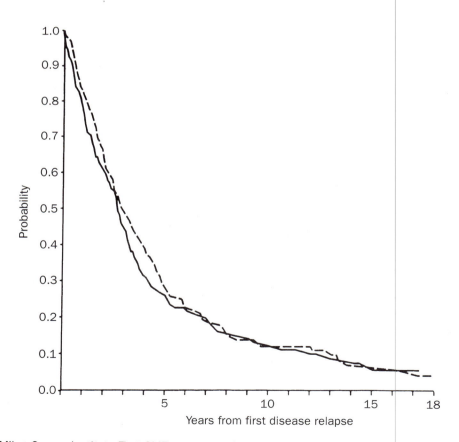

Figure 11.2 Milan Cancer Institute First CMF programme in node-positive breast cancer. Survival from first disease-relapse in the control group (———) compared with CMF-treated patients (- - -).

REFERENCES

1. Goldhirsch A, Gelber RD. Treatment of overt metastatic breast cancer. In: *Baillière's Clinical Oncology. International Practice and Research. Breast Cancer* (Veronesi U, ed.). 1988; **2**:215–29.

2. Valagussa P, Tesoro Tess JD, Rossi A, et al. Adjuvant CMF effect on site of first recurrence, and appropriate follow-up intervals, in operable breast cancer with positive axillary nodes. *Breast Cancer Res Treat* 1982; **1**:349–56.

3. Primary Therapy of Breast Cancer Study Group (PTBCSG). Identification of breast cancer patients with high risk of early recurrence after radical mastectomy. II: Clinical and pathological correlations. *Cancer* 1978; **42**:2809–26.

4. Hayes DF, Kaplan WD. Evaluation of patients following primary therapy. In: *Breast Diseases* 2nd edn (Harris JR, Hellman S, Henderson IC, Kinne DW, eds). Philadelphia: JB Lippincott Co., 1991:505–25.

5. Bonadonna G, Valagussa P, Moliterni A, et al. Adjuvant cyclophosphamide, methotrexate, and fluorouracil in node-positive breast cancer. The results of 20 years of follow-up. *N Engl J Med* 1995; **332**:901–6.

6. Henderson IC, Canellos GP. Cancer of the breast: A past decade. *N Engl J Med* 1980; **302**:17–30, 78–90.

7. Veronesi U, Valagussa P. Inefficacy of internal mammary node dissection in breast cancer surgery. *Cancer* 1981; **47**:170–5.

8. Veronesi U, Banfi A, Salvadori B, et al. Breast conservation is the treatment of choice in small breast cancer: long-term results of a randomized trial. *Eur J Cancer* 1990; **26**:668–70.

9. Fisher B, Redmond C, Poisson R, et al. Eight-year results of a randomized clinical trial comparing total mastectomy and lumpectomy with or without irradiation in the treatment of breast cancer. *N Engl J Med* 1989; **320**:822–8.

10. Early Breast Cancer Trialists' Collaborative Group. Systemic treatment of early breast cancer by hormonal, cytotoxic or immune therapy: 133 randomised trials involving 31000 recurrences and 24000 deaths among 75000 women. *Lancet* 1992; **339**:1–15, 71–85.

11. Goldhirsch A, Gelber RD, Price KN, et al. Effect of systemic adjuvant treatment on first sites of breast cancer relapse. *Lancet* 1994; **343**:377–81.

12. Tomiak E, Piccart M. Routine follow-up after primary therapy for early breast cancer: Changing concepts and challenges for the future. *Ann Oncol* 1993; **4**:199–204.

13. The GIVIO Investigators. Impact of follow-up testing on survival and quality of life in breast cancer patients: A multicenter randomized controlled trial. *JAMA* 1994; **271**:1587–92.

14. Rosselli del Turco M, Palli D, Cariddi D, et al. Intensive diagnostic follow-up after treatment of primary breast cancer: A randomized trial. *JAMA* 1994; **271**:1593–7.

15. Marini G, Murray S, Goldhirsch A, et al. The effect of adjuvant prednisone combined with CMF on patterns of relapse and occurrence of second malignancies in patients with breast cancer. *Ann Oncol* 1996; **7**:245–50.

16. Recht A, Hayes DF. Specific sites and emergencies: Local recurrence. In: *Breast Diseases* (Harris JR, Hellman S, Henderson IC, Kinne DW, eds). Philadelphia: JB Lippincott Co., 1987:508–24.

17. Early Breast Cancer Trialists' Collaborative Group. Effects of radiotherapy and surgery in early breast cancer. An overview of the randomized trials. *N Engl J Med* 1995; **33**:1444–55.

18. Andry G, Suciu S, Vico P, Faverly D, Mattheiem W. Locoregional recurrences after 649 modified radical mastectomies: incidence and significance. *Eur J Surg Oncol* 1989; **15**:476–85.

19. Beck TM, Hart NE, Woodard DA, Smith CE. Local or regionally recurrent carcinoma of the breast: Results of therapy in 121 patients. *J Clin Oncol* 1983; **1**:400–5.

20. Bedwinek JM, Fineberg B, Lee J, Ocwieza M. Analysis of failures following local treatment of isolated local-regional recurrence of breast cancer. *Int J Radiat Oncol Biol Phys* 1981; **7**:581–5.

21. Ciatto S. Detection of breast cancer local recurrences. *Ann Oncol* 1995; **6** (suppl 2):23–6.

22. Magno L, Bignardi M, Micheletti E, Bardelli D, Plebani F. Analysis of prognostic factors in patients with isolated chest wall recurrence of breast cancer. *Cancer* 1987; **60**:240–4.

23. Aberizk WJ, Silver B, Henderson IC, Cady B, Harris JR. The use of radiotherapy for treatment of isolated locoregional recurrence of breast carcinoma after mastectomy. *Cancer* 1986; **58**:1214–18.

24. Halverson KJ, Perez CA, Kuske RR, et al. Isolated local-regional recurrence of breast following mastectomy: radiotherapeutic management. *Int J Radiat Oncol Biol Phys* 1990; **19**:851.

25. Borner M, Bacchi M, Goldhirsch A, et al., for the Swiss Group for Clinical Cancer Research. First isolated locoregional recurrence following mastectomy for breast cancer: results of a phase III

multicenter study comparing systemic treatment with observation after excision and radiation. *J Clin Oncol* 1994; **12**:2071–7.

26. Prior P, Waterhouse JA. Incidence of bilateral tumours in a population-based series of breast cancer patients. I. Two approaches to an epidemiological analysis. *Br J Cancer* 1978; **37**:620–34.

27. Nayfield SG, Karp JE, Ford LG, et al. Potential role of tamoxifen in prevention of breast cancer. *J Natl Cancer Inst* 1991; **83**:1450–9.

28. Chlebowski RT, Weiner JM, Luce J, et al. Significance of relapse after adjuvant treatment with combination chemotherapy or 5-fluorouracil alone in high risk breast cancer. *Cancer Res* 1981; **41**:4399–403.

29. Buzdar AU, Legha SS, Hortobagyi GN, et al. Management of breast cancer patients failing adjuvant chemotherapy with adriamycin-containing regimens. *Cancer* 1981; **47**:2798–802.

30. Valagussa P, Brambilla C, Zambetti M, Bonadonna G. Salvage treatments in relapsing resectable breast cancer. *Recent Res Cancer Res* 1989; **115**:69–76.

31. Houston SJ, Richards MA, Bentley AE, et al. The influence of adjuvant chemotherapy on outcome after relapse for patients with breast cancer. *Eur J Cancer* 1993; **29A**:1513–18.

32. Kardinal CG, Perry MC, Korzun AH, et al. Responses to chemotherapy or chemohormonal therapy in advanced breast cancer patients treated previously with adjuvant chemotherapy. A subset analysis of CALGB study 8081. *Cancer* 1988; **61**:415–19.

33. Falkson G, Gelman G, Falkson CI, et al. Factors predicting for response, time to treatment failure, and survival in women with metastatic breast cancer treated with DAVTH: a prospective Eastern Cooperative Oncology Group study. *J Clin Oncol* 1991; **9**:2153–61.

34. Bonneterre J, Mercier M, for the French Epirubicin Study Group. Response to chemotherapy after relapse in patients with or without previous adjuvant chemotherapy for breast cancer. *Cancer Treat Rev* 1993; **19** (suppl B):21–30.

35. Rowinsky EK, Eisenhauer EA, Chaudhry U, et al. Paclitaxel (Taxol) Investigators' Workshop. *Semin Oncol* 1993; **20** (suppl 3):1–60.

36. Gianni L, Munzone E, Capri G, et al. Paclitaxel in metastatic breast cancer: a trial of two doses by 3-hr infusion in patients with clinical resistance to anthracyclines. *J Natl Cancer Inst* 1995; **87**:1169–75.

37. Aapro MS, Lavelle F, Bissery MC, et al. The impact of docetaxel (Taxotere) on current treatment. *Semin Oncol* 1995; **22** (suppl 4):1–33.

38. Abeloff MD, Hayes DF, Henderson IC, et al. The current status of vinorelbine (Navelbine) in breast cancer. *Semin Oncol* 1995; **22** (suppl 5):1–87.

39. Fornander T, Rutqvist LE, Glas U. Response to tamoxifen and fluoxymesterone in a group of breast cancer patients with disease recurrence after cessation of adjuvant tamoxifen. *Cancer Treat Rep* 1987; **71**:685–8.

40. Rubens RD. Effect of adjuvant systemic therapy on response to treatment after relapse. *Cancer Treat Rev* 1993; **19** (suppl B):3–10.

41. Osoba D. Lessons learned from measuring health-related quality of life in oncology. *J Clin Oncol* 1994; **12**:608–16.

42. Pickering WG. Does medical treatment mean patient benefit? *Lancet* 1996; **347**:379–80.

43. Coates A, Val Gebski M, Bishop JF, et al. Improving the quality of life during chemotherapy for advanced breast cancer. A comparison of intermittent and continuous treatment strategies. *N Engl J Med* 1987; **317**:1490–5.

44. Spiegel D, Bloom JR, Kraemer HC, Gottheil E. Effect of psychosocial treatment on survival of patients with metastatic breast cancer. *Lancet* 1989; **i**:888–91.

45. Mulder CL, van der Pompe G, Spiegel D, Antoni MH, De Vries MJ. Do psychosocial factors influence the course of breast cancer? A review of recent literature, methodological problems and future directions. *Psycho-Oncology* 1992; **1**:155–67.

46. Bloch S, Kissane DW. Psychosocial care and breast cancer. *Lancet* 1995; **346**:1114–15.

47. Powles TJ, Hickish T, Casey S, O'Brien M. Hormone replacement after breast cancer. *Lancet* 1993; **342**:60–1.

48. Marchand DJ. Estrogen-replacement therapy after breast cancer. Risks versus benefits. *Cancer* 1993; **71**:2169–76.

49. Di Saia PJ. Hormone-replacement therapy in patients with breast cancer. A reappraisal. *Cancer* 1993; **71**:1490–500.

12

Radiotherapy plus chemotherapy: concomitant or sequential delivery

Beryl McCormick

Conventional treatment of the woman with breast cancer involves the use of both systemic therapy and locoregional radiation after surgery in most patients who opt for breast-conserving surgery. The 'sequence' or order of these two therapies has become a topic of interest among both medical and radiation oncologists.

In 1988, the US National Cancer Institute issued a clinical alert to all physicians, recommending the consideration of systemic therapy for women with pathologically node-negative breast cancer. Before this alert, women with node-negative breast cancer, who made up a significant subset of all women opting for breast-conservation surgery, were infrequently treated with systemic therapy. Thus, the need to identify a correct treatment sequence did not exist. In addition, before the computation of worldwide treatment results for the Oxford Overviews,[1] chemotherapy was rarely recommended for postmenopausal women with breast cancer, with the anti-estrogen tamoxifen substituting for chemotherapy in those post-menopausal women requiring systemic as well as local treatment.

In 1991, Recht and colleagues[2] observed and published some striking results related to the order of radiotherapy and chemotherapy after breast-conserving surgery. In their retrospective study, the actuarial rate of local failure in the breast at the 5-year point was 4% in patients who received radiotherapy followed by chemotherapy, but rose to 41% in patients who had the reversed order of treatments. Recht and colleagues called for a randomized trial to confirm their results, and encouraged caution in clinical utilization of this information.[2]

A number of similar retrospective studies analyzing the effect of sequencing radiotherapy and chemotherapy after breast-conserving surgery appeared in the literature over the next few years. Conclusions, as discussed later, were mixed. In autumn 1995, the Joint Center for Radiation Therapy (JCRT) first presented results of their randomized sequencing trial, and results have recently been published. The increased risk for local, in-breast failures was again noted in the subset of patients randomized to receive all chemotherapy followed by radiation. This same group was, however, also observed to have a benefit in terms of distant disease-free survival and survival with this sequence. The reverse was seen in patients who received radiotherapy immediately after surgery, followed by systemic chemotherapy.[3]

Concomitant radiotherapy and chemotherapy would appear to be the solution to the sequencing controversy from the point of view of cancer control, but this option carries with it an increased risk of enhanced radiation side effects, less than optimal cosmetic outcome, and the hypothetical problem of prolonged bone marrow recovery and delay in the timing of the chemotherapy. These issues arise from observations at single institutions which have explored concomitant treatments, and are discussed below.

MODELING AND SEQUENCING

Modeling a clinical problem can often help the reader to visualize the possible solutions. The Norton model[4] of breast cancer cell or growth curves is illustrated in Figure 12.1 which follows the gompertzian mathematical curve. Some cancer cells grow faster and some grow slower, and to illustrate this the median gompertzian growth curve has been selected. In Figure 12.2 the three areas of potential growth in women diagnosed with operable breast cancer at an early stage are shown, along with the possible interventions.

The model for a patient after a wide local excision with negative margins is shown in

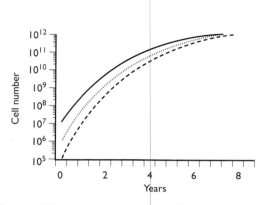

Figure 12.2 Gomperztian model of breast cancer, with no surgery, radiotherapy or chemotherapy. (—) Growth of the cells and the index primary in the breast; this is treated by the surgical intervention of lumpectomy. (– – –) Potential growth of cells beyond the lumpectomy cavity elsewhere in the treated breast; for this there is intervention by external beam radiation to the whole breast. (· · ·) Potential for growth elsewhere in the patient, beyond the locoregional area (metastatic spread); this is treated by the use of adjuvant systemic therapy.

Figure 12.3, where it can be seen that the surgeon has effectively removed the index lesion. The clinician now has several choices in terms of administering any further required therapy. Radiation can be given first, with a delay to the start of chemotherapy. This solution addresses the potential for growth in the breast, but delays the administration of systemic therapy. A second possible solution is to initiate chemotherapy first, delaying the start of the radiation. It could be hypothesized that, if the tumor cells are sensitive to the systemic treatment selected, while the main effect of the chemotherapy is systemic, the chemotherapy may also inhibit the growth of the cells locally within the breast. A third possible solution is to give both the radiotherapy and chemotherapy together, simultaneously addressing both potential areas for growth. However, this solution raises the question of whether or not the radiation may interfere with the recovery of the blood counts between cycles of chemotherapy and whether the chemotherapy may exaggerate anticipated radiation side effects.

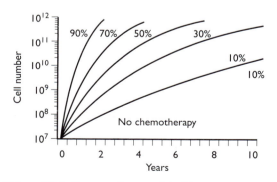

Figure 12.1 Gomperztian model of breast cancer: the Norton model.

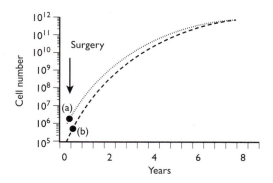

Figure 12.3 Gomperztian model of breast cancer, after a wide local excision with negative margins. (· · ·) and (– – –) as in Figure 12.2. (a) Tumor bulk if radiotherapy given first; (b) tumor bulk if chemotherapy started before radiotherapy.

Sequencing: other possible variables on outcome

The impact of sequencing of chemotherapy and radiotherapy after breast-conserving surgery must be considered in the context of other variables, which are also known to influence both local control and distant disease-free survival. Starting with the patient herself, young age, independent of other factors, is now widely recognized as influential in the outcome of breast cancer.[5–16] The extent of the surgical procedure must also be considered: a wide excision, such as a quadrantectomy, is associated with a lower local recurrence rate, all else being equal, than a smaller biopsy which may leave behind tumor cells in and around the biopsy cavity. A related variable is the status and size of the final 'margins'.

The complete pathology evaluation, which addresses the margins and other factors, is known to exert an influence on recurrence rates in the conserved breast. Pathological factors evaluated in several retrospective and prospective studies, and their impact on local recurrence rates, are given in Table 12.1.[17] The lack of consensus reflects different centers analyzing different potential predictors for failure, and the need to look at each in the context of other variables, such as the type of surgery.

The overall prognosis for the patient, as calculated from the complete pathology report and including tumor size, grade and number of positive lymph nodes, is likely to be related to the risk of local failure as well as to the risk of distant failure. Although most radiation studies to date have not identified nodal status as a risk factor for local failure, Bartelink, speaking for the EORTC (European Organization for Research and Treatment of Cancer) study group, noted that a high node count 'appeared to be a prognostic factor for local regional control',[18] in the context of breast-preserving surgery. As indications for breast-conserving surgery are extended to women with larger lesions, it is likely that more patients will have high lymph node counts in the future, yielding larger numbers of high-risk patients for analysis of this question.

The type and dosage of chemotherapy also influence local control, as well as distant disease-free survival, and must be considered

Table 12.1 Pathological predictors of local failure	
Predictor	**Institution**
Extensive intraductal component	Joint Center for Radiation Therapy
	Netherlands Cancer Institute
	Marseilles (premenopausal patients only)
MCR	Marseilles (premenopausal patients only)
High grade	Marseilles (premenopausal patients only)
	Gustave-Roussy
Intralymphatic extensions	NSABP-B6
	Institut Curie

Note: not all predictors were evaluated by all institutions. Surgery and radiation varied significantly between institutions.

when discussing the sequencing question. The National Surgical Adjuvant Breast Project B0-6 Study, comparing women randomized to be treated with segmental mastectomy and radiation, or the same breast-conserving surgery without radiation, or mastectomy, supports this hypothesis in part. It has been noted that patients who are node positive and receive both radiotherapy and chemotherapy have the highest local control rates, when compared with patients who are node negative, and receive the same surgery and radiation but no chemotherapy, as shown in Figure 12.4.[19] Finally, although radiation doses are quite standard throughout the Western World, the time elapsing from the date of final surgery to the initiation of radiation, labelled the surgery–radiation interval by the JCRT,[20] must be considered as well. Initially, the first report on this subject from the JCRT defined 16 weeks as the interval: it was noted that the highest local failure rates occurred in patients whose radiation was delayed more than 16 weeks from the final breast-conservation procedure, presumably for the delivery of some or all of the chemotherapy.[2] A subsequent report looked not only at the timing issue, but also at patients' characteristics and pathological factors. This report compared patients with intervals for surgery to radiation in 4-week gradients, up to 12 weeks in total. All three groups were balanced with regard to patient characteristics, and no adverse impact of delay was noted.[21] It is interesting that the volume of tissue removed around the index lesion was largest in the subset of patients delayed 9–12 weeks.

The importance of sequencing is apparent, but related co-variables must be analyzed, as in any clinical dilemma, in order to have better understanding of outcomes and to improve them for women with breast cancer.

Clinical trials: chemotherapy–radiotherapy interactions on normal tissues

Women who opt for breast-conserving surgery are by definition interested in preserving their breasts. What has been labelled a 'cosmetic outcome', and what actually represents the physical findings of the treated breast over time, must be considered, as well as the impact of radiotherapy and chemotherapy on rib fractures, lung fibrosis, and cardiac and brachial plexus complications.

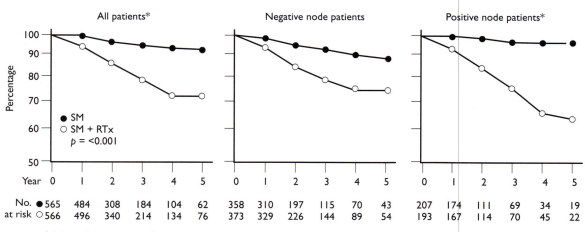

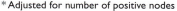

*Adjusted for number of positive nodes

Figure 12.4 Life-table analysis showing the percentage of patients remaining free of breast tumor after segmental mastectomy (SM) or segmental mastectomy with breast irradiation (SM + RTx).

Cosmesis

Although two previous cancer centers analyzed their data, looking for a possible impact of adjuvant chemotherapy on cosmetic outcome in the treated breast,[22,23] Danoff and colleagues[24] first established this link in 1983, when 27 patients receiving concurrent or sequential breast radiotherapy and adjuvant chemotherapy (cyclophosphamide, methotrexate and 5-fluorouracil [CMF] or CMF with prednisone [CMF-P]) were compared with 19 patients treated only with radiation, with a median follow-up of 2 years. Of the adjuvant chemotherapy group 19% scored in the fair–poor cosmesis range, compared with 11% in the radiation-only group. Arm edema was observed in 22% of the adjuvant chemotherapy group, but none in the radiation group.

In a related study, Beadle reached a similar conclusion, observing that the adverse cosmetic impact of adjuvant chemotherapy was primarily on retraction upwards of the treated breast, when compared with women receiving radiation only at the JCRT.[25] Various chemotherapy regimens were used (CMF, MF, doxorubicin [Adriamycin] and cyclophosphamide [AC]), sometimes given concurrently, although more often sequentially. Gore et al,[27] also reporting for the JCRT, first analyzed the sequence of radiotherapy and chemotherapy. He noted no differences in local control or relapse-free survival, and the paper focused on cosmetic outcomes. Forty-one patients received concurrent CMF and radiation, and another 41 received radiation followed by CMF chemotherapy. Using the cosmetic grading system of Harris,[26] 52% of the sequentially treated patients and only 12% of the concurrent patients achieved an excellent cosmetic outcome at the 2-year follow-up mark. Fair–poor results were noted in 30% of the concurrently treated patients, but only 10% (all rated 'fair') of the sequential patients.[27] Later reports from the same institutions with longer follow-up and larger patient numbers continued to document the adverse impact of adjuvant chemotherapy on cosmesis.[28,29]

Taylor analyzed multiple factors influencing cosmesis including the use of concurrent or sequential chemotherapy with radiation after breast-conserving surgery. Her results document that concurrent delivery resulted in a significant decrease in excellent cosmetic outcome, when compared with sequential delivery, or no chemotherapy. Some patients in her study, who received a concurrent regimen of CMF, had the methotrexate omitted during the 6-week course of radiotherapy. She noted a trend towards better cosmesis in those patients, compared with methotrexate-inclusive CMF, but numbers were small in these subsets and no statistical significance was attached to the observation.[30]

Wazer also reported on chemotherapy as one of many factors influencing cosmetic outcome; in this study, CMF or CAF (doxorubicin instead of methotrexate) chemotherapy was given either sequentially or concurrently, with methotrexate or doxorubicin omitted as in the Taylor study, over the period during which the patient received radiotherapy. Using this regimen, no adverse impact of chemotherapy was noted on breast cosmesis.[31]

Borger related the development of breast fibrosis to adjuvant chemotherapy, using the linear–quadratic model. Seven independent factors were identified which related to severity of breast fibrosis; adjuvant chemotherapy was one, associated with a twofold risk for fibrosis. The chemotherapy in that study was CMF, but details of the timing of its delivery with the breast radiation were not given.[32]

Other normal tissue complications

When considering combining postoperative radiotherapy and chemotherapy, an important tissue to evaluate for toxicity is the bone marrow. Lippman, using data from the National Cancer Institute trial randomizing women with stage I and II breast cancer to either mastectomy or breast-conserving surgery and radiation, focused on this issue.[33] He reported on node-positive women in that study, who received identical chemotherapy using an AC regimen. The women assigned to both groups received the first cycle of chemotherapy postoperatively. Chemotherapy was then discontinued during the 7 weeks of radiotherapy, and for an equivalent time period in the mastectomy group. The chemotherapy was then restarted in both groups for a total of 11 cycles. In examining both chemotherapy cycles and individual patients, dose reduction was required more commonly in the radiation group. However, in comparing ability to re-escalate dose, and absolute drug received in both groups, no statistical significance was observed in the two subsets. The authors concluded that by using a tangential radiation technique to the breast, and absolute granulocyte counts, rather than total white blood cell counts, their data suggested that 'it was possible to administer aggressive combination chemotherapy to patients concurrently receiving radiation to the breast and regional lymph nodes'.[33]

Yet 5 years later, Bentzen noted that: 'increasing use of combined radiotherapy and adjuvant systemic therapy in the treatment of breast cancer has stressed the need for more clinical data on normal tissue injury from combined treatment. While fairly comprehensive experimental studies have been conducted, clinical data are sparse and rarely analyzed in a manner allowing direct quantification of the observed effects.[34]' He then continued into his data presentation, documenting an increased probability of developing subcutaneous fibrosis after mastectomy and chest wall radiation in patients receiving CMF chemotherapy, compared with the same treatment and cyclophosphamide only.[34]

In the course of arriving at the correct sequencing of radiotherapy and chemotherapy after breast-conserving surgery, the issue of bone marrow tolerance remains a central one. Related to this is the relationship of differences in dose intensity and dose density of chemotherapy to long-term disease outcomes.

Glick and colleagues[35] initiated a trial for women with breast-conserving surgery, employing immediate radiotherapy and CMF chemotherapy postoperatively. Over the weeks of radiation, methotrexate was withheld during the chemotherapy treatments. When the patient completed radiotherapy, methotrexate was added for the additional six cycles of conventional CMF chemotherapy. The mean CF dose was 95% in the first two cycles and the mean CMF dose was 89% for the following six cycles. The authors concluded that this was an effective and safe way of combining both modalities.[35] In a follow-up report at 10 years, the authors noted a 70% overall survival for node-positive patients. Local failure in the treated breast was 5% at 5 years and 13% at 10 years.[36]

Denham reported on a retrospective study for the Trans-Tasman Radiation Oncology Group.[37] He compared 138 patients requiring radiotherapy and chemotherapy after a mastectomy or breast-conserving surgery, with patients receiving chemotherapy only during this same time period; CMF chemotherapy was used. Using the absolute lymphocyte count, median counts for cycles 2–6 were statistically significantly lower in the chemotherapy/radiotherapy group than for those patients receiving chemotherapy only. Focusing on absolute neutrophil counts, the median counts for cycles 2–6 were significantly decreased only in patients receiving radiotherapy in addition to intravenous CMF chemotherapy, in contrast to oral CMF chemotherapy.[37]

This same study had a second retrospective comparison to evaluate other normal tissue complications. In that study design, patients treated with concurrent radiotherapy and chemotherapy were compared with those receiving only radiotherapy. No significant differences were noted in the acute radiation reactions, including skin edema, esophagitis and pneumonitis. As a result of differences in surgical procedures between the two study groups, the authors also could not demonstrate any differences in late treatment effects, with the exception of more telangiectasia and pigmentation noticed in the subset receiving both chemotherapy and radiotherapy.[37] In two companion papers, the JCRT also addressed the incidence of late tissue complications and chemotherapy. Lingos studied factors related to the development of radiation pneumonitis.[38] Two factors, the use of adjuvant chemotherapy and the use of a supraclavicular field in addition to the two tangent fields, correlated, on both univariant and multivariant analysis, with this complication. It was of note that women with supraclavicular fields and sequential chemotherapy had a 1.3% incidence of pneumonitis, compared with a 8.8% incidence in those given concurrent chemotherapy and supraclavicular radiotherapy.[38] Pierce analyzed the development of brachial plexopathy, rib fractures and pericarditis, in women receiving radiotherapy to the whole breast. Chemotherapy was a contributing factor to the development of both rib fractures and brachial plexopathy.[39] Olsen also analyzed the development of brachial plexopathy, in patients in the Danish Breast Cancer Group Trials receiving CMF chemotherapy alone, or CMF plus radiation, or CMF plus tamoxifen plus radiotherapy in premenopausal patients.[40] Postmenopausal patients were similarly randomized to receive radiotherapy plus tamoxifen, tamoxifen alone or tamoxifen plus CMF. There was a statistically significant increase in patients developing brachial plexopathy, when chemotherapy was used with radiotherapy.[40]

IS TIMING CRITICAL FOR THE INITIATION OF CHEMOTHERAPY?

Although it is beyond the scope of this chapter to discuss the impact of timing and dosing of adjuvant chemotherapy on long-term breast cancer outcomes, the fact that administration of chemotherapy is optimal when it is timely, and that it delivers the dose intended, is now general knowledge. Most of our knowledge regarding the delay of chemotherapy comes from retrospective analysis of chemotherapy protocols where reasons other than the intent of the protocol designers are responsible for the delay in the chemotherapy. Nevertheless, some useful information can be extrapolated from studies designed for reasons other than analyzing the impact of sequencing in early staged breast cancer.

Lara Jimenez reported, in abstract form, from Granada, Spain, on 248 node-positive breast cancer patients who were randomized to

receive radiotherapy followed by chemotherapy, chemotherapy followed by radiotherapy, or 'sandwich' treatment, consisting of CMF chemotherapy for three cycles, then radiotherapy, and then CMF for three more cycles. The surgical procedure, however, was mastectomy, not lumpectomy. The 'sandwich' group achieved highest local control and disease-free survival, when compared with the other two groups at 10 years, with statistically significant results.[41]

Scholl recently reported on a randomized trial for patients with tumor sizes measuring between 3 and 7 cm, and nodes that were either not clinically palpable or freely mobile on clinical examination. After a diagnosis by drill biopsy, patients were randomized to receive 5-fluorouracil, doxorubicin and cyclophosphamide (FAC) chemotherapy, followed by radiotherapy and then surgery for persistent tumor, or full-dose radiotherapy, followed by surgery if persistent, and finally by four cycles of the same chemotherapy. Breast-conservation rates were similar in both arms of the study, but more interesting was the statistical difference in survival at 5 years, with a median follow-up time of 54 months, favoring the patients with chemotherapy delivered first.[42]

Sertoli recently reported an Italian study randomizing women with T1–T3, N0 and N1 breast cancer to a single cycle of perioperative chemotherapy.[43] After surgery, node-negative patients received no further treatment, but node-positive patients went on to receive additional CEF chemotherapy (epirubicin replacing methotrexate), alternating with CMF chemotherapy, for a total of 12 cycles in each randomization arm. All lymph node-positive patients also received 5 years of tamoxifen therapy. With a median study time of 5.5 years, differences in relapse-free survival approach statistical significance favoring perioperative chemotherapy. Focusing only on the estrogen receptor-negative subset of patients, a survival advantage ($p = 0.003$) was noted, again favoring the perioperative chemotherapy.[43]

More relevant are the chemotherapy delay data from the recent JCRT randomized study, where patients received radiotherapy first,

Table 12.2 Sequencing radiation and chemotherapy

Reference/Study	Breast-conserved patients	Analyzed by specific time interval?	Interval	'Delay' increased local failure?	Multi-variant analysis used?	Significant predictors for LR in multi-variant analysis	Comments
Hartsell et al[44]	84	Yes	120 days	Yes	Yes	Margins	All patients had some chemotherapy before RT; 'early' patients had TAM + concomitant RT
Antoniades et al[45]	137	No		No	No		
Heimann et al[46]	233	No		No	No		82% negative margins
Leonard et al[47]	262	Yes	1, 3, 4, 6 months	No	Yes	T size, age < 50 (NS)	71% negative margins
Buzdar et al[48]	85	No		No	No		
Slotman et al[49]	508	Yes	50 days	Yes	Yes	T size, margins, time interval	Only 30% had chemotherapy/hormone treatment
McCormick et al[50]	471	No		No	No		Early group had no chemotherapy
Recht et al[2]	295	Yes	16 weeks	Yes	No		Retrospective JCRT
Recht et al[3]	244	No	No	Yes	No		Prospective Delayed RT increased local failure only in cases of close/involved margins

RT, radiotherapy; TAM, tamoxifen; NS, not significant.

followed by methotrexate, folinic acid, 5-fluorouracil, cyclophosphamide, prednisone and doxorubicin, or the reverse sequence. In the radiotherapy-first group, the median interval from first breast surgery to start of chemotherapy was 119 days, compared with 52 days in the chemotherapy-first group. All patients had stage I or II breast cancer, and were treated with breast-conserving surgery. The rate of distant metastases was 36% in the radiotherapy-first group, compared with 25% in the chemotherapy-first group; this was a significant difference.[3]

CLINICAL STUDIES: OUTCOMES WITH SEQUENCING

As noted in the introduction, a number of authors have looked into their breast databases, in an attempt to provide answers on what is the optimal sequencing of chemotherapy and radiotherapy after breast-conserving surgery. Table 12.2 lists the studies that have been reported or published, by author and stage of disease. It is notable that, in spite of the early interest in defining an optimal surgical/radiation interval,[20] only four of the studies analyzed their patients by specific time intervals, and each used a different interval. In addition to the JCRT studies, the two studies supporting a negative impact on local control of 'delay' in radiotherapy, Hartsell[44] and Slotman,[49] are notable for the inclusion of a multivariant analysis including interval from surgery to initial radiotherapy, and other factors as well. In Hartsell's multivariant analysis, the time interval fell out as a predictor for local recurrence, and only the involved margins remained statistically significant. In Slotman's study,[49] tumor size, margins and time interval achieved significance. In that study, it is notable that only 30% of the patients received any endocrine or chemotherapy, and the remaining 70% had a delay in radiotherapy for other reasons. Thus, unlike most of these studies, 70% of patients in that study had no therapy from the time of surgery to the time of radiotherapy.

In the studies where there was no impact on the delay of radiotherapy, several other observations are in order. In the reports of both Heimann[46] and Leonard,[47] almost all the patients in all treatment arms had negative margins going into adjuvant chemo–radiotherapy. Antoniades' retrospective study[45] is remarkable because all patients started some systemic therapy immediately after surgery, although the chemotherapy group had delayed sequential radiation. Tamoxifen was started concomitantly in all 'early' irradiated patients. In the author's experience at Memorial Hospital, although margins were unknown in a large proportion of the patients treated in the early 1980s, it has been the practice to ask for a rim of 1–2 cm of normal tissue around the tumor, or in the later part of the decade to review all 'close' or 'involved' margins and ensure that there is no invasive cancer or extensive intraductal cancer at any margin in any patient before accepting the patient for treatment.

In Recht's randomized study,[2,3] the local failure rate for the radiotherapy-first group was 5%, compared with 14% for the chemotherapy-first group. Using a polychotomous logistic model, negative tumor margins were associated with 'little difference' in the risks of recurrence regardless of sequence. Using the same model for patients with either negative nodes or four or more involved nodes, a higher local recurrence rate was seen in the chemotherapy-first group, and a higher distant failure rate in the radiotherapy-first group.

One question frequently asked is the incidence of local failures within the treated breast during the delivery of all chemotherapy first, before the radiotherapy starts. In the experience of the author's query, as well as that of several other authors (Table 12.2), this is a rare event, usually accompanied by rapid systemic failure as well.

CONCLUSIONS

The optimal sequencing of chemotherapy and radiotherapy after breast-conserving surgery is a clinical question which must be answered by looking at several important outcomes. Although local control is an important goal in the intent of breast-conserving treatment, the optimal therapy to ensure distance disease-free survival rates and overall survival rates must drive our treatment decisions. In the 5 years that have elapsed since the initial report from the JCRT, linking the impact of sequencing to local failure rates in the breast, much progress has been made. In two of the three multivariant analysis from the retrospective studies in Table 12.2, margin involvement emerged as a significant predictor for local failure. In two of the other studies, most patients had pathologically negative margins. Returning to the modeling of the gompertzian curves, clinical experience to date supports a delay in the start of radiotherapy, to deliver chemotherapy when the surgical procedure has achieved negative margins. When margins are involved, from the experience of the prospective JCRT study in which local control was decreased by delay in radiotherapy, but disease-free survival was decreased by delay in chemotherapy, it would appear that it is in the patient's best interest to return to the operating room with the intent of re-excising and establishing negative margins, if clinically possible.

The use of concomitant chemo–radiotherapy has apparent advantages. Starting both therapies immediately must be balanced with the clinical documentation that normal tissue complications and poor cosmetic outcomes are probably higher with this choice of therapy. The University of Pennsylvania[35] abstract did not address this important endpoint; although it might be advantageous for the patient to complete all therapy in a shorter time course, there has been no demonstration that the local control rate is higher than with a sequencing program using chemotherapy first in patients with negative margins, followed by radiotherapy. The impact of leaving out the methotrexate in the first two cycles, compared with its inclusion, has not been addressed in a randomized way in terms of impact on survival and disease-free survival.

Optimal surgery, from the point of view of both cosmetic outcome and local control, involves removing the index primary mass with negative margins. At this time, this gives clinicians the latitude needed for delivery of chemotherapy, followed by breast radiotherapy. Although concomitant delivery of both is intriguing, this option has not yet been evaluated in a prospective randomized trial.

REFERENCES

1. Early Breast Cancer Trialists' Collaborative Group. Systemic treatment of early breast cancer by hormonal, cytotoxic or immune therapy. *Lancet* 1992; **339**:1–15, 71–85.
2. Recht A, Come SE, Gelman RS, et al. Integration of conservative surgery, radiotherapy, and chemotherapy for the treatment of early-stage, node-positive breast cancer: Sequencing, timing, and outcome. *J Clin Oncol* 1991; **9**:1662–7.
3. Recht A, Come SE, Gelman RS, et al. The sequencing of chemotherapy and radiation therapy after conservative surgery for early-stage breast cancer. *N Engl J Med* 1997; in press.
4. Norton L. A Gompertzian model of human breast cancer growth. *Cancer Res* 1988; **48**:7067–71.
5. Nemoto T, Vana J, Bedwani RN, et al. Management and survival of female breast cancer: Results of a national survey by the American College of Surgeons. *Cancer* 1980; **45**:2917–24.
6. Ribeiro GG, Swindell R. The prognosis of breast cancer in women aged less than 40 years. *Clin Radiol* 1981; **32**:231–6.
7. Ries G, Pollack ES, Young JL Jr. Cancer survival: Surveillance, epidemiology, and end results program, 1973–79. *J Natl Cancer Inst* 1983; **70**:693–707.
8. Adami HO, Malker B, Meirik O, et al. Age as a prognostic factor in breast cancer. *Cancer* 1985; **56**:898–902.
9. Host H, Lund E. Age as a prognostic factor in breast cancer. *Cancer* 1986; **57**:2217–21.
10. Kurtz J, Spitalier J-M, Amalric R, et al. Mammary recurrences in women younger than forty. *Int J Radiat Oncol Biol Phys* 1988; **15**:271–6.
11. Matthews RH, McNeese MD, Montague ED, et al. Prognostic implications of age in breast cancer patients treated with tumorectomy and irradiation or with mastectomy. *Int J Radiat Oncol Biol Phys* 1988; **14**:659–63.
12. Lees AW, Jenkins HJ, May CL, et al. Risk factors

and 10-year breast cancer survival in Northern Alberta. *Breast Cancer Research and Treatment* 1989; **13**:143–51.

13. Lee CJ, McCormick B, Mazumdar M, et al. Infiltrating breast carcinoma in patients age 30 years and younger: long term outcome for life, relapse, and second primary tumors. *Int J Radiat Oncol Biol Phys* 1992; **23**:9969–75.

14. Fowble BL, Schultz DJ, Overmoyer B, et al. The influence of young age on outcome in early stage breast cancer. *Int J Radiat Oncol Biol Phys* 1994; **30**:23–33.

15. de la Rochefordiere A, Asselain B, Campana F, et al. Age as prognostic factor in premenopausal breast carcinoma. *Lancet* 1993; **341**:1039–43.

16. Nixon AJ, Neuberg D, Hayes DF, et al. Relationship of patients' age to pathological features of the tumor and prognosis for patients with stage I or II breast cancer. *J Clin Oncol* 1994; **12**:888–94.

17. McCormick B. Invasive breast carcinoma: Patient selection for conservative management. *Semin Radiat Oncol* 1992; **2**:74–81.

18. Bartelink H, van Tienhoven G, van Dongen JA, et al. Locoregional recurrence after mastectomy or breast conserving therapy; analysis of clinical prognostic factors and results of salvage therapy in a randomized EORTC trial. *Int J Radiat Oncol Biol Phys* 1992; **24**:220.

19. Fisher B, Bauer M, Margolese R, et al. Five-year results of a randomized clinical trial comparing total mastectomy and segmental mastectomy with or without radiation in the treatment of breast cancer. *N Engl J Med* 1985; **312**:665–73.

20. Recht A, Harris JR, Come SE. Sequencing of irradiation and chemotherapy for early breast cancer. *Oncology* 1994; **8**:19–37.

21. Nixon AJ, Recht A, Neuberg D, et al. The relation between the surgery-radiotherapy interval and treatment outcome in patients treated with breast-conserving surgery and radiation therapy without systemic therapy. *Int J Radiat Oncol Biol Phys* 1994; **30**:17–21.

22. Botnick L, Gomes S, Rose C, et al. Primary breast irradiation and concomitant chemotherapy (CMF). In: *Alternates to Mastectomy* (Harris J, Hellman S, Silber W, eds). Philadelphia: JB Lippincott Co., 1982.

23. Lichter A. The National Cancer Institute experience – primary radiotherapy and adjuvant chemotherapy. In: *Alternates to Mastectomy* (Harris J, Hellman S, Silber W, eds). Philadelphia: JB Lippincott Co., 1982.

24. Danoff B, Goodman R, Glick J, Haller D, Pajak T. The effect of adjuvant chemotherapy on cosmesis and complications in patients with breast cancer treated by definitive irradiation. *Int J Radiat Oncol Biol Phys* 1983; **9**:1625–30.

25. Beadle GF, Come S, Henderson C, et al. The effect of adjuvant chemotherapy on the cosmetic results after primary radiation treatment for early stage breast cancer. *Int J Radiat Oncol Biol Phys* 1984; **10**:2131–7.

26. Harris J, Levene M, Svensson G, Hellman S. Analysis of cosmetic results following primary radiation therapy for stages I and II carcinoma of the breast. *Int J Radiat Oncol Biol Phys* 1979; **5**:257–61.

27. Gore SM, Come SE, Griem K, et al. Influence of the sequencing of chemotherapy and radiation therapy in node-negative breast cancer patients treated by conservative surgery and radiation therapy. In: *Adjuvant Therapy of Cancer V* (Salmon SE, ed.). Orlando, FL: Grune & Stratton, 1987:365–73.

28. Abner AL, Recht A, Vicini FA, et al. Cosmetic results after surgery, chemotherapy, and radiation therapy for early breast cancer. *Int J Radiat Oncol Biol Phys* 1991; **21**:331–8.

29. de la Rochefordiere A, Abner AL, Silver B, et al. Are cosmetic results following conservative surgery and radiation therapy for early breast cancer dependent on technique? *Int J Radiat Oncol Biol Phys* 1992; **23**:925–31.

30. Taylor ME, Perez CA, Halverson KJ, et al. Factors influencing cosmetic results after conservation therapy for breast cancer. *Int J Radiat Oncol Biol Phys* 1995; **31**:753–64.

31. Wazer DE, DiPetrillo T, Schmidt-Ullrich R, et al. Factors influencing cosmetic outcome and complication risk after conservative surgery and radiotherapy for early-stage breast carcinoma. *J Clin Oncol* 1992; **10**:356–63.

32. Borger JH, Kemperman H, Sillevis Smitt H, et al. Dose and volume effects on fibrosis after breast conservation therapy. *Int J Radiat Oncol Biol Phys* 1994; **30**:1073–81.

33. Lippman ME, Lichter AS, Edwards BK, et al. The impact of primary irradiation treatment of localized breast cancer on the ability to administer systemic adjuvant chemotherapy. *J Clin Oncol* 1984; **2**:21–7.

34. Bentzen SM, Overgaard M, Thames HD, et al. Early and late normal-tissue injury after postmastectomy radiotherapy alone or combined with chemotherapy. *Int J Radiat Biol* 1989; **56**:711–15.

35. Glick JH, Fowble BL, Haller DG, et al. Integration of full-dose adjuvant chemotherapy with definitive radiotherapy for primary breast cancer: Four year update. *NCI Monograph* 1988; **6**:297–301.

36. Markiewicz D, Fox K, Schultz D, et al. Concurrent chemotherapy and radiation for breast conservation therapy of early stage breast cancer [abstract]. *Proc of ASCO* 1996; **15**:97.

37. Denham JW, Hamilton CS, Christie D, et al. Simultaneous adjuvant radiation therapy and chemotherapy in high-risk breast cancer – toxicity and dose modification: A Transtasman Radiation Oncology Group Multi-Institution Study. *Int J Radiat Oncol Biol Phys* 1995; **31**: 305–13.

38. Lingos TI, Recht A, Vicini F, et al. Radiation pneumonitis in breast cancer patients treated with conservative surgery and radiation therapy. *Int J Radiat Oncol Biol Phys* 1991; **21**:355–60.

39. Pierce M, Recht A, Lingos TI, et al. Long-term radiation complications following conservative surgery (CS) and radiation therapy (RT) in patients with early stage breast cancer. *Int J Radiat Oncol Biol Phys* 1992; **23**:915–23.

40. Olsen NK, Pfeiffer P, Johannsen L, et al. Radiation-induced brachial plexopathy: neurological follow-up in 161 recurrence-free breast cancer patients. *Int J Radiat Oncol Biol Phys* 1993; **26**:43–9.

41. Jimenez LP, Garcia PJ, Pedruza V. Adjuvant combined modality treatment in high risk breast cancer patients: 5th EORTC Breast Cancer Working Conference [abstract]. *Oncology* 1991; **8**:A293.

42. Scholl SM, Fourquet A, Asselain B, et al. Neoadjuvant versus adjuvant chemotherapy in premenopausal patients with tumours considered too large for breast conserving surgery: Preliminary results of a randomized trial: S6. *Eur J Cancer* 1994; **30A**:645–52.

43. Sertoli MR, Bruzzi P, Pronzato P, et al. Randomized cooperative study of perioperative chemotherapy in breast cancer. *J Clin Oncol* 1995; **13**:2712–21.

44. Hartsell WF, Recine DC, Griem KL, Murthy AK. Delaying the initiation of intact breast irradiation for patients with lymph node positive breast cancer increases the risk of local recurrence. *Cancer* 1995; **76**:2497–503.

45. Antoniades J, Chen C, Gabuzda TG, et al. Stage II carcinoma of the breast treated in sequence by surgery, chemotherapy and irradiation [abstract]. *Proc ASCO* 1993; **12**:132.

46. Heimann R, Powers C, Fleming G, et al. Does the sequencing of radiotherapy and chemotherapy affect the outcome in early-stage breast cancer: A continuing question [abstract]. *Proceedings of the 36th Annual ASTRO Meeting* 1994; **30**:243.

47. Leonard CE, Wood ME, Zhen B, et al. Does administration of chemotherapy before radiotherapy in breast cancer patients treated with conservative surgery negatively impact local control? *J Clin Oncol* 1995; **13**:2906–15.

48. Buzdar AU, Kau SW, Smith TL, et al. The order of administration of chemotherapy and radiation and its effect on the local control of operable breast cancer. *Cancer* 1993; **71**:3680–4.

49. Slotman BJ, Meyer OWM, Njo KH, Karim ABMF. Importance of timing of radiotherapy in breast conserving treatment for early stage breast cancer. *Radiother Oncol* 1994; **30**:206–12.

50. McCormick B, Norton L, Yao TJ, et al. The impact of the sequence of radiation and chemotherapy on local control after breast-conserving surgery. *Cancer J Sci Am* 1996; **2**: 39–45.

13

Long-term side effects from systemic drug therapy

Lígia Bruno da Costa, Jean Pierre Armand

CONTENTS • **Cardiotoxicity of chemotherapeutic drugs** • **Secondary malignancies after chemotherapy** • **Acute leukaemia or myelodysplastic syndrome** • **Tamoxifen**

One of the major indisputable advances of the past 20 years in breast cancer is the use of adjuvant systemic treatment with chemotherapy and hormone therapy. Long-term toxicities resulting from adjuvant chemotherapy have since then become an important issue because they may be a limiting factor, especially in patients for whom cure is expected or who have long survival rates. The concept of cost-effectiveness is of major importance in such cases; it raises the question: 'Are the potential benefits worth the cost (i.e. cost of morbidity and mortality)?' Although most side effects seen in adjuvant breast cancer chemotherapy are transient and relatively well tolerated (i.e. alopecia, myelosuppression, gastrointestinal disturbances), long-term side effects, such as cardiac toxicity, as well as secondary malignancies and death, may occur as a result of treatment. If the benefit obtained in terms of survival is obvious, the cost, in terms of morbidity, is of major concern to decide how to optimize the cost–benefit risk: is it better to modify systemic treatment or use prophylactic agents, or to ensure that a better selection of patients receives adjuvant treatment? Breast cancer is a privileged model for the study of the long-term side effects, not only because patient populations are large, but also because these populations have been studied in randomized studies and followed up over decades. However, even if the current guidelines recognize a survival benefit in a selected group of patients with cancer of the breast and negative lymph nodes when given adjuvant chemotherapy, a secondary malignancy must be considered an eventuality that must be clearly explained to the patient. It is important to followup breast cancer patients over time because of the risk of secondary cancers, although this risk is much lower than it is after treatment of Hodgkin's disease. Breast cancer is undoubtedly a more common tumour, and even if there is a substantial decrease in the risk of secondary cancers compared with patients with Hodgkin's disease, large numbers of patients are likely to be affected.

CARDIOTOXICITY OF CHEMOTHERAPEUTIC DRUGS

The drugs used in cancer chemotherapy can affect many organ systems; anthracycline antibiotics used in breast cancer adjuvant therapy, in particular, affect mainly the heart, sometimes causing arrhythmias.

Anthracycline compounds

Anthracyclines are a class of red pigmented antibiotics that are isolated from the actinomycete *Streptomyces* sp. Their anti-tumour effect results mainly from intercalation into the DNA of actively cycling cells, with subsequent blockage of DNA synthesis and cell death; their major limiting toxicity is cardiac.

Anthracyclines are perhaps among the most important drugs in the adjuvant treatment of breast cancer. Their late cardiotoxicity is primarily related to cumulative doses, although they can also cause acute cardiac dysfunction. Information concerning anthracycline-induced cardiomyopathy is mostly derived from studies with doxorubicin and to a lesser extent those with daunorubicin. Classically, doxorubicin cardiotoxicity can present in three different ways: acute, subacute and late (chronic) effects. For the purpose of this chapter we will discuss only the late effects. In children, generally the effects occur months or years after doxorubicin administration and may cause cumulative dose-related myocardial cell damage which can ultimately culminate in clinical congestive heart failure (CHF).

This late-onset clinical cardiac toxicity has undergone limited evaluation in adult breast cancer patients, in whom the frequency of anthracycline late cardiac toxicity is not precisely known, but is most probably very low according to published data. The major problem with anthracycline cardiac toxicity in adults is the subacute effects.

The data published up until now about late-onset clinical cardiac toxicity is mostly derived from paediatric patients. According to Von Hoff, for patients receiving full doses of doxorubicin at the standard dose interval of every 3 weeks, the risk of clinical CHF remains very low until a total dose of 400–500 mg/m^2 (Figure 13.1) has been reached. After a total dose of 550 mg/m^2 the risk of CHF rises rapidly. The risk of developing clinical CHF in unselected patients receiving more than 400–500 mg/m^2 of doxorubicin ranges from 7% to 15%, whereas for patients receiving more than 550 mg/m^2 the risk rises in a more or less linear fashion; patients receiving a total dose of 1000 mg/m^2 have practically a 50% probability of developing clinical CHF; this mainly concerns patients treated during childhood.

The actual incidence of clinical CHF may be higher in this paediatric group of patients than previously reported in retrospective trials. Prospective clinical trials performed with strict monitoring of these young patients seem to show an incidence of early signs of clinical CHF of about 25% or more with a cumulative dose of 450 mg/m^2 or greater.

Pathophysiology

Anthracycline-induced cardiomyopathy seems to result from a series of repeated chemical injuries to the myocardium (some of which are resolved), which gradually obstruct cellular defences producing cell damage with decreased contractility and eventual cell death. These facts are consistent with its gradual onset, the variability of its course, risk factors for increased susceptibility, and laboratory and pathological findings. The common mechanism for anthracycline-induced cardiomyopathy appears to be free radical damage, which culminates in the formation of a Fe^{3+}–doxorubicin complex which increases free radical generation considerably. Anthracycline-induced free radical damage is now, however, confined to the myocardium. It can also play a role in tumour cell killing (FE^{3+}–doxorubicin–DNA complex), although this is thought to be related primarily to other mechanisms (e.g. DNA intercalation, inhibition of topoisomerase II).

Diagnosis

The late onset of anthracycline cardiomyopathy in children generally occurs 5 or more years after completion of anthracycline therapy,[1–6] but

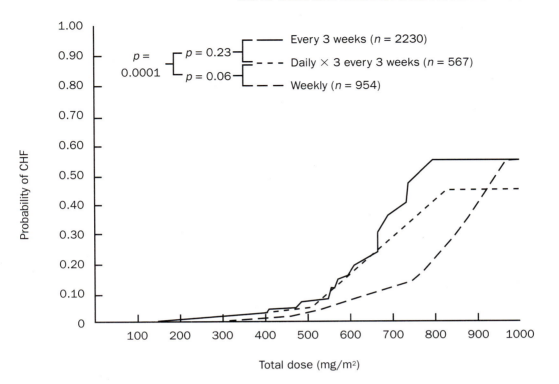

Figure 13.1 Incidence of clinical congestive heart failure, according to cumulative dose of doxorubicin by schedule. (Reproduced from Von Hoff et al[3], with permission.)

there is little or no evidence of this late cardiotoxicity in adult breast cancer patients.

In breast cancer patients, clinical evidence of CHF may be observed only in the overwhelming majority of cases within weeks or a few months of the last dose of anthracycline (acute or subacute cardiotoxicity).

Generally, an increased incidence of late cardiotoxicity in children (cardiomyopathy) correlates with increasing cumulative doses of anthracyclines, and left chest wall irradiation is an additive risk factor.[2,3,6] In some of the published paediatric cases, a selective right heart dysfunction has been noted in right ventricular radionuclide cardiac scans. Such findings may precede left ventricular dysfunction, and have led to speculation that monitoring of right heart function may serve as an early warning signal for impending left heart dysfunction.

A system for staging anthracycline-induced haemodynamic changes in humans was developed by Bristow et al[1] (Table 13.1).

Steinhertz and colleagues reported[2,3] the sudden death from late cardiomyopathy, up to 15 years after anthracycline therapy, of several young patients treated for paediatric tumours. Pathological findings on biopsy specimens and *post mortem* showed predominantly fibrosis and hypertrophy of the remaining myocytes, with little residual vacuolization.[2,3] Thus, even asymptomatic patients who have been treated in childhood with anthracyclines for paediatric tumours need long-term cardiac surveillance, and new symptoms suggestive of arrhythmia or syncope require vigorous investigation. Cardiac status at non-invasive testing during the year after completion of therapy in children is predictive of the likelihood of late abnormalities

---

Table 13.1 Clinical staging of doxorubicin cardiac toxicity

Grade	Abnormality
0	Within normal limits
1	Mild abnormality any of the following:
	(a) Resting haemodynamics: RVEDP >8 to <12 mmHg or mean RAP ≥7 to <10 mmHg, LEVDP ≥12 to <15 mmHg or mean PCW pressure >10 to <15 mmHg, CI ≥2.2 and <2.5 l/min per m, arteriovenous O_2 difference >5 vol%
	(b) Exercise haemodynamics: RVEDP > 5 to <9 mmHg above resting pressure; PCW >5 to <11 mmHg above resting pressure, exercise factor (change in cardiac output/change in oxygen consumption) ≥4–6
2	Moderate abnormality, any of the following:
	(a) Two or more of the above
	(b) Pressure at rest: PCW or LVEDP ≥15 to <20 mmHg, RVEDP ≥12 to <17 mmHg or RA >10 to ≤15, CI <2.2 to ≤1.8 with arteriovenous O_2 difference >5 vol%
	(c) Exercise haemodynamics: RVEDP ≥9 mmHg above resting pressure, PCW ≥10 mmHg above resting pressure at rest, exercise factor <4
3	Severe abnormality, any of the following:
	(a) Two or more moderate abnormalities
	(b) Haemodynamics at rest: PCW or LVEDP ≥20 mmHg, REVDP ≥18 or ≥16 mmHg, CI <1.8 l/min per m with arteriovenous difference >5 vol%

Adapted from Bristow et al[1] with permission.
CI, cardiac index; LVEDP, left ventricular end-diastolic pressure; RVEDP, right ventricular end-diastolic pressure; PCW, pulmonary capillary wedge; RAP, right arterial pressure.

and serves as a yardstick for the frequency of follow-up.

Radionuclide cardiac angiography to determine left ventricular ejection fraction (LVEF) is one of the methods most frequently used to assess chronic anthracycline cardiac toxicity. At least one multiple image acquisition scan should be performed at baseline, in the middle of treatment and/or when the dose of 300 mg/m² has been reached, then at the dose of 450 mg/m², and patients should undergo strict monitoring (at least every 100 mg/m² of dose increase) thereafter. Patients at increased risk (>70 years, previous anthracycline therapy, left chest wall irradiation and pre-existing car-diac disease) may be monitored more frequently. Decrements in LVEF that remain within the 'normal' range but fall 0.2 below the baseline range, as well as decreases in LVEF to a value that is clearly abnormal (<0.45), may indicate anthracycline damage and withdrawal of anthracycline therapy may be advisable in such cases.

For some experienced centres, endomyocardial biopsy is a mandatory confirmatory procedure, because it is highly specific for the interpretation of anthracycline-induced myocardial damage. In these centres, anthracycline therapy is withheld when the Billingham biopsy (Table 13.2) score is 2 or more. Biopsy is

Table 13.2 Histopathological scale of doxorubicin cardiomyopathy	
Grade	**Description**
0	Within normal limits
1	Minimal numbers of cells (<5% of total number of cells in block) with early change (early myofibrillar loss and/or distended sarcoplasmic reticulum)
1.5	Small group of cells involved (5–15% of total number, some showing definite change (marked myofibrillar loss and/or cytoplasmic vacuolization)
2	Groups of cells (16–25% of total number), some showing definite change (marked myofibrillar loss and/or cytoplasmic vacuolization)
2.5	Groups of cells (26–35%), some showing change (marked myofibrillar loss and/or cytoplasmic vacuolization)
3	Diffuse cell damage (>35% of total number of cells with marked change total loss of contractile elements, loss of organelles, mitochondrial and nuclear degeneration)

Adapted from Billingham et al[45] with permission

also considered for young patients with a cumulative dose of $450 \, mg/m^2$ or more in the case of doxorubicin.

Doppler echocardiography is a very useful tool, in experienced hands, for pre-treatment evaluation of the heart (assessment of valvular and pericardial status, as well as myocardial systolic and diastolic function), and also for clinical follow-up during and after the end of anthracycline treatment.

Myoscintigraphic scans are a more recent investigational technique using monoclonal antibodies directed to myosin, labelled with indium-111 (^{111}In) or iodine-131 (^{131}I) which may complement the results of radionuclide cardiac scans. It may also provide more direct evidence of myocardial damage and circumvent inadequate specificity.

More recent non-invasive techniques are under investigation which may render nuclear quantification modalities obsolete in patients whose hearts can be imaged ultrasonically. These techniques include computer-assisted echocardiographic technologies, which can be broken down into automated border detection-derived quantification of cardiac volumes and LVEF.

How to decrease anthracycline toxicity
Dose schedule changes
Factors other than the cumulative dose may modify the risk of doxorubicin-induced cardiomyopathy. These include the schedule of administration, mediastinal or left thoracic wall irradiation, pre-existing cardiac disease, age over 70 years, nutritional status and perhaps their combination with other cytotoxic drugs.

An interrelationship of the dose schedule, the cumulative dose and cardiotoxicity has been clearly established for anthracyclines. This shows that toxicity is related primarily to peak drug concentration and the anti-tumour effect of these agents is related to drug exposure. Legha et al[2] demonstrated that prolonged continuous infusions (up to 96 hours) resulted in lower peak plasma levels.

Comparison of endomyocardial biopsy scores in patients receiving doxorubicin showed that those who received their dose in a 48- or 96-hour infusion had significantly lower biopsy scores, and therefore less cardiomyopathy, than patients who received the bolus dose. In addition, patients who received 96-hour infusions had lower biopsy scores than those who received 24-hour infusions. Another study by Shapira and colleagues[7] using radionuclide cardiac angiography to evaluate cardiotoxicity demonstrated a decline of only 6% in LEVF after a total cumulative dose of 400 mg/m² administered in a 6-hour continuous infusion, compared with a drop of 21% in patients who received the same range of total doxorubicin bolus doses. These results have been confirmed, in a prospective study by Casper and colleagues[8], using a 72-hour continuous infusion in 82 patients with soft tissue sarcoma.

Bristow and colleagues[1] also demonstrated that dividing the planned monthly doxorubicin dose into smaller weekly doses also decreased clinical cardiotoxicity, as measured by clinical examination, radionuclide ejection fraction or endomyocardial biopsy, without apparent loss of anti-tumour activity, compared with shorter (24-hour) or bolus infusions, and allowed the administration of higher cumulative doses. Although continuous infusion or weekly schedules reduced cardiotoxicity, they did not totally prevent it.

Thoracic and mediastinal irradiation have been shown in most, but not all, analyses to increase the risk of doxorubicin cardiotoxicity significantly. Bristow et al[1] calculated that previous mediastinal irradiation increased the risk of doxorubicin-associated heart failure by a factor of 1.6, but only if more than 6 grays (Gy) were delivered to the cardiac apex. Unfortunately, this interaction has received meagre attention, and the interrelationship of dose fractionation, the timing of radiotherapy and the potentiation of cardiotoxicity is unknown. Pre-existing cardiac risk factors, including active CHF, a history of myocardial infarction within one year, hypertension or diabetes mellitus and previous exposure to anthracyclines, appear to have a deleterious effect on cardiac tolerance of doxorubicin, although this

effect is not well characterized. In practically all studies, a history of CHF has precluded administration of doxorubicin.

Age has been found to influence cardiac tolerance of doxorubicin. Young children and elderly people (>70 years) are more likely to experience CHF at lower cumulative doses of doxorubicin.

Multidrug regimens, especially those containing alkylating agents such as cyclophosphamide, etoposide, actinomycin D, mitomycin D, melphalan, vincristine and bleomycin, have been implicated as potentiators of doxorubicin cardiotoxicity.

Analogues

Epirubicin is similar to doxorubicin in terms of anti-tumour activity, but has less associated nausea and vomiting. In preclinical animal models it appears to be less cardiotoxic than doxorubicin. However, in clinical trials it has not yet provided a major reduction in cardiotoxicity when administered at equivalent myelotoxic (equimyelotoxic) doses to doxorubicin. The cumulative dose at which the risk of clinical cardiotoxicity starts to rise significantly is between 900 and 1000 mg/m², especially for epirubicin.

Related compounds

Mitozantrone is an anthraquinone that is structurally similar to the anthracyclines. In both animal and human studies, it appears to be less cardiotoxic than doxorubicin. Some studies performed with cardioprotectors (ICRF-187) seem to suggest the possible existence of another mechanism of cardiotoxicity related to the anthraquinones, because ICRF-187 inhibits doxorubicin cardiotoxic effects but not those of mitozantrone. Data collected from selected single agent and two randomized studies indicated that, for equimyelotoxic doses of mitozantrone, there is a lower incidence of CHF than for doxorubicin. As with doxorubicin, the important risk factors for mitozantrone cardiotoxicity are previous mediastinal irradiation, cardiovascular disease and anthracycline (doxorubicin) exposure, of which the last is the most important. In patients previously unexposed to anthracyclines, the risk of cardiotoxicity does not begin to rise significantly (5% with <2% clinical CHF) until a dose of about 160 mg/m^2 has been reached. This represents the equimyelotoxic dose, which is equivalent to about 800 mg/m^2 of doxorubicin. For patients who have received doxorubicin previously (in a median cumulative dose of 239 mg/m^2), the risk starts to rise when the cumulative mitozantrone doses reaches about 100 mg/m^2. Mitozantrone should not, however, be considered to be as active as the anthracyclines.

Cardioprotection

ICRF-187 (ADR 529) is a bisdioxopiperazine compound which is hydrolysed intracellularly to form a chelating agent that binds intracellular iron and prevents free radical production. This compound was used in randomized trials and markedly reduced the incidence and sever-

ity of cardiomyopathy induced by anthracyclines in breast cancer patients. The limiting toxicity of ICRF-187 is myelosuppression, but that did not add significant toxicity to the anthracycline regimens.

SECONDARY MALIGNANCIES AFTER CHEMOTHERAPY

Secondary malignancies have been widely documented in Hodgkin's disease, the first cancer to be cured by chemotherapy. In breast cancer, a longer follow-up is needed to evaluate the risk of secondary malignant neoplasm (MN) after adjuvant therapy (Tables 13.3 and 13.4). Numerous other factors may also have an impact on this risk, including the total dose of drug administered, the number of patients evaluated, the types of therapy administered,

Table 13.3 Type of secondary malignancies documented within 15 years of surgery

	Number of cases		Median months from surgery (range)	Median age (years) at surgery
	Total	With adjuvant chemotherapy		
Acute myeloid leukaemia	3	3	38 (8–121)	51
Chronic lymphocytic leukaemia	4	4	68 (34–139)	47
Thyroid carcinoma	3	3	48 (43–61)	45
Lung carcinoma	5	5	98 (22–143)	52
Gastrointestinal carcinoma	22*	21*	97 (17–168)	54
Gynaecological tumours	22	18	68 (2–138)	51
Pancreatic carcinoma	4	4	71 (27–108)	52
Renal carcinoma	2	1	148–151	39–52
Bladder carcinoma	6	5	49 (21–160)	51
Soft tissue sarcoma	5	4	48 (20–107)	44
Cutaneous	3	2	95 (20–140)	62
Other malignancies	8*	8*	56 (15–158)	49

*One patient with concomitant gastrointestinal cancer and multiple myeloma.

Table 13.4 Absolute risk of secondary malignancies after CMF-based adjuvant chemotherapy (2241 patients; 19 382 person-years at risk)

	No. observed	No. expected	Absolute risk*
Acute myeloid leukaemia	3	1.3	0.9
Lung carcinoma	5	3.4	0.8
Gastrointestinal carcinoma	21	22.4	–
Gynaecological tumours	18	17.8	–
Pancreatic carcinoma	4	2.0	1.0
Bladder carcinoma	5	2.1	1.5
Soft tissue sarcoma	4	1.3	1.4

*Absolute risk was calculated by subtracting the expected number of cases from the number observed, dividing the difference by the person-years of observation and multiplying the quotient by 10^4 to estimate the excess number of cases per 10 000 person-years.

the pre-existent individual risk of developing a malignancy and other causes of death.[9] Some secondary malignancies developed in patients as a result of genetic and iatrogenic factors and their interaction.

Genetic factors (Li–Fraumeni syndrome)

The Li–Fraumeni syndrome consists of the association of multiple cancers (sarcoma, breast cancer and soft tissue sarcoma) diagnosed generally before the age of 45 years within the same family. The genetic abnormality present in some families with Li–Fraumeni syndrome is characterized by a mutation in the *p53* gene.

Factors associated with type of adjuvant treatment

Surgery

In the early years of adjuvant treatment of breast cancer, the most common secondary malignancy ascribed to surgery was an angiosarcoma in an oedematous arm (Stewart–Treves syndrome), a complication occasionally described after a radical mastectomy. A recent publication by Edeiken and col-

leagues[10] also reported some cases of angiosarcoma that developed in radiotherapy fields, after a lumpectomy on breast irradiation. They suggest that there is a very low risk of developing a secondary angiosarcoma associated with the current conventional adjuvant treatment of breast cancer.

Radiotherapy

No specific type of cancer has been observed after therapeutic irradiation. Radiation-induced leukaemias frequently occur around 5 years after irradiation. Solid tumours typically occur more than 10 years after treatment, but may occur earlier in particularly susceptible people. Carcinomas of the skin are a known consequence of skin irradiation. Basal cell carcinomas are particularly common after relatively low radiation doses. After evaluation, the risk of secondary solid tumours rose as the radiation dose to the site increased and as time after treatment increased to as long as 20 years. Even in the studies in which actual doses to the site were not estimated, the risk was usually highest in the field, lower at the periphery of the field, and much lower at a distance from the radiation field. An excess risk is seen after both external-beam irradiation and interstitial radiotherapy.

The risk of contralateral breast cancer

Interest and concern have accumulated regarding the risk of cancer in the contralateral breast after adjuvant radiotherapy, because the radiation doses received by the other breast are in the range known to be carcinogenic, especially in young women. In a review of a case-control study including more than 40 000 women with breast cancer in Connecticut, Boice et al[11] reported that women with breast cancer have a threefold increased risk of developing another cancer of the other breast. A small increase in risk was found to be associated with an average dose of about 3 Gy to the contralateral breast. Although treatment has varied substantially in recent practice, the total dose was within the range of that delivered to the contralateral breast with current techniques. Fewer than 3% of all second breast cancers in the study could be attributed to previous radiotherapy. Consistent with the studies discussed previously is the increase in the relative risk (RR) observed in irradiated women surviving 10 or more years, but only in those who were treated when aged less than 45 years (RR = 1.85). The risk in this sample increased with additional radiation doses, with the range analysed extending from 1.99 Gy or less to 4 Gy or more, and the relative risks varying from 1.54 to 2.35, respectively ($p = 0.003$).

Levitt and Mandel[12] have pointed out the difficulties inherent in studies of radiation oncogenesis in the opposite breast, and emphasized that the risk–benefit factors entailed should be weighed carefully. Although the issue remains highly controversial, it would seem prudent to conclude from these data that the dose to the contralateral breast, in breast cancer patients aged under 45 years, should be reduced to a minimum, using radiotherapy techniques such as those described by Frass and associates[13].

Lung cancer risk and radiotherapy

Only a few studies have quantified how ionizing radiation can cause lung cancer after adjuvant radiotherapy for initial breast cancer, and its risk in relation to the radiation dose. The long-term risk for lung cancer was evaluated in a recent retrospective study by Inskip and associates[14], including 8976 women treated with radiation for breast cancer and who survived for up to at least 10 years. Sixty-one evaluable cases of lung cancer (out of 72) were identified in this group of patients. The information about current and past smoking habits in this female population was sparse and thus not mentioned in the study. For these 10-year survivors of breast cancer, the results showed that the overall relative risk of lung cancer associated with initial radiotherapy for breast cancer was 1.8 (95% confidence interval, 95%CI = 0.8–3.8), and the overall relative risk increased with time after treatment, so that the overall relative risk for periods of 15 years or more after radiotherapy was 2.8 (95%CI = 1.0–8.2). The mean dose was 15.2 Gy to the ipsilateral lung, 4.6 Gy to the contralateral lung and 9.8 Gy for both lungs combined. The excess overall relative risk was 0.08/Gy, based on the average dose to both lungs and 0.20/Gy to the affected lung. The authors concluded that the breast cancer radiotherapy regimens used before the 1970s (mainly cobalt) were associated with an elevated risk of lung cancer many years after treatment. About nine cases of radiotherapy-induced lung cancer per year would be expected to occur among 10 000 women who received an average lung dose of 10 Gy and survived for at least 10 years. Radiotherapy techniques and machines (linear accelerators) used nowadays for adjuvant treatment of breast cancer avoid extensive exposure of the lungs to radiation, compared with treatments employed in the past, so that the actuarial risk of secondary lung cancer does not play a major role in clinical decisions regarding treatment for breast cancer. Nevertheless efforts to reduce unnecessary exposure of the lungs and heart should strive to reduce possible adverse radiation effects further.

ACUTE LEUKAEMIA OR MYELODYSPLASTIC SYNDROME

The evaluation of several adjuvant studies in breast cancer has yielded some data on the risk of developing secondary malignancies. The possibility of *de novo* acute leukaemia occurring coincidentally, and not being related to the alkylating agent, is plausible as a result of the high prevalence of breast cancer among women. Most of the secondary malignant neoplasms reported after chemotherapy have been acute myeloid leukaemias or acute non-lymphocytic leukaemias (AMLs) or non-Hodgkin's lymphoma. Alkylating agents were the first agent, and continue to be the aetiological agents most frequently implicated. In the early 1970s the first cases of secondary AMLs were reported in breast cancer patients treated with melphalan; these patients were expected to have a prolonged survival: among the 11 patients with AML and a history of breast cancer, six had a family case history of dysmyelopoiesis consisting of erythroid hyperplasia, megaloblastoid changes, ringed sideroblasts, vacuolated myeloblasts, erythroblasts and abnormal megakaryocytes. Both the myelodysplastic syndrome (MDS) and acute leukaemia have been associated with melphalan (alkylating agent). The myelodysplastic syndrome, usually characterized by refractory cytopenias, occurs in at least half the patients before acute leukaemia develops. The latent period (median time to overt leukaemia) is 2–5 years and the risk of secondary leukaemia is amplified as cumulative doses of alkylating agents increase.

The relative leukaemogenicity of various drugs has not been fully established, but the risk appears to differ according to the drug. Although all alkylating agents have been implicated, melphalan is probably the most potent leukaemogenic agent. The leukaemias that occur after chemotherapy with alkylating agents or nitrosourea have very distinctive characteristics. The AMLs are generally of cell types FAB (French–American–British classification) M1 or M2 and erythroleukaemia, and they occur typically between 2 and 10 years after therapy, with the peak interval at around 5 years. There is usually a clinical history of pancytopenia, and the leukaemia may occur as part of the spectrum of myelodysplastic syndromes. Treatment of this type of acute leukaemia is disappointing and median survival is measured in months, even if there have been some reports of short-term success. Cytogenetic abnormalities occur in more than 90% of patients. Chromosomes 5 and 7 are involved in almost 90% of those with cytogenetic abnormalities. Le Beau et al[15] described characteristic abnormalities (deletions) of all or parts of the long arm of chromosomes 5 and 7 [del(5q) and 7 del(7q)], which give strong support to the diagnosis of chemotherapy-associated acute leukaemia rather than *de novo* leukaemia. This had led researchers to speculate on the involvement of genes in these chromosomes in the pathogenesis of the alkylating agent-induced leukaemias. Variations in host susceptibility in developing these leukaemias have not been evaluated adequately, but may be related to interindividual variations in drug metabolism.

More recently the epipodophyllotoxins and other inhibitors of topoisomerase II (anthracyclines, mitozantrone and dactinomycin) were thought to be associated with AMLs. These common forms of secondary AMLs related to topoisomerase II inhibitors differ from those appearing after treatment with alkylating agents, because they occur earlier, namely 15 months after therapy, there is no period of pancytopenia, they are of the FAB M4 or M5 morphological type, the most frequent genetic abnormality involves a translocation in chromosomes 11q23 and 21q22, and they are generally found in patients with solid tumours. However, only 40–80% of cases have a chromosome 11q defect in bone marrow cells. Also, it is not clear whether the translocations, thought to be associated with leukaemia after treatment with topoisomerase II inhibitors, are caused by such exposure, because translocations involving chromosome 11q23 – specifically, t(4;11)(q21;q23) – are common in acute lymphocytic leukaemia (ALL) and translocation t(9;11)(p21;q23) is relatively specific for M5 leukaemia of whatever cause. Several potential candidate genes have been identified in this region, including the proto-oncogene *ETSI*, THY1 surface antigen, the CD3 surface antigen of T lymphocytes, NCAM and a gene for ataxia–telangiectasia. Rowley et al[16] and Detourmignies et al[17] implicated inhibitors of topoisomerase II in their report on therapy-associated acute promyelocytic leukaemia.

They pointed out that the same translocation, t(15;17), could be identified in both *de novo* and treatment-related acute promyelocytic leukaemias which develop after therapy with this class of drugs. In addition, t(8;21), t(9;11) and inv(16) were found in therapy-associated acute promyelocytic leukaemias and other therapy-associated AMLs.

Several other studies have also documented the development of leukaemia after adjuvant therapy with drugs, such as platinum salts alone or in combination with anthracyclines and/or their derivatives for breast cancer. Pedersen-Bjergaard et al[18] reported one of the most controversial studies about anthracycline-related leukaemias (4-epidoxorubicin), in pre-treated advanced breast cancer patients. They concluded that single agent 4-epidoxorubicin may be slightly leukaemogenic or non-leukaemogenic at cumulative doses up to 1000 mg/m^2, but that it is leukaemogenic when used in combination with alkylating agents or *cis*-platinum and the leukaemia presents the same characteristics (M5 and M6 type, translocation in 11q123, short latency period) as those related to topoisomerase II inhibitors. Furthermore, these results suggested a synergistic effect with 4-epidoxorubicin and *cis*-platinum in the combination regimens, or, in some cases, even with the alkylating agents administered previously. The authors concluded that an increased risk of secondary AML may exist after treatment with 4-epidoxorubicin, at least if it is combined with cisplatin or an alkylating agent.

Colombat et al (*Proceedings XVe Forum de Cancérologie*, Paris, 1995; 240: 419) reported five cases of therapy-related AML in breast cancer patients that were attributed to mitozantrone (Novantrone) in a combination regimen with fluorouracil, cyclophosphamide and, in two cases, vindesine. This presumption resulted from the fact that these five cases did not present any of the features characteristic (cytogenetic, cytopenias and later onset) of alkylating agent-related leukaemia, but on the contrary, they shared many characteristics of the topoisomerase II inhibitor-related leukaemia.

A true evaluation of the late effects of adjuvant chemotherapy for breast cancer, and the interrelationship of the type and duration of chemotherapy, radiotherapy and their interaction were described in a large study by Fisher and associates.[19] It represents one of the first large case-control studies, including 8483 women with data collected from the National Surgical Adjuvant Breast and Bowel Project (NSABP) clinical trials. The authors reported 43 evaluable (out of 53) cases of secondary leukaemia, including seven cases of myelodysplasia. Most patients in this study were aged over 50 years when the breast cancer was diagnosed. Of the 8430 women, 2068 had surgery alone (three cases of secondary leukaemia), 1116 surgery + radiotherapy (six cases of secondary leukaemia) and 5299 chemotherapy (27 cases of secondary leukaemia + 7 of MDS). Of the 5299 patients who received adjuvant regimens containing L-phenylalanine mustard (alkylating agent), 27 cases of secondary leukaemia (0.5%) and seven cases of the myeloproliferative syndrome (0.1%) were observed. None of the patients treated with surgery or radiotherapy alone was reported to have a myeloproliferative syndrome. The mean interval from the diagnosis of breast cancer to the development of leukaemia was 5 years. No cases of secondary leukaemia were reported before the second and after the seventh year. The results showed a cumulative risk of acute leukaemia (for patients free of metastases and of a second primary tumour) of $1.29 \pm 0.28\%$ at 10 years for all patients, of $0.06 \pm 0.05\%$ at 10 years for patients undergoing surgery alone, $1.39 \pm 0.49\%$ for those receiving postoperative regional radiotherapy and $1.54 \pm 0.36\%$ (including the myeloproliferative syndrome) for those receiving melphalan. This risk was not significantly greater than that observed following radiation ($p = 0.58$ and 0.29). In this study a statistically significant increased risk of acute myelogenous leukaemia occurred after adjuvant chemotherapy ($p < 0.001$) with melphalan, and to a lesser extent after postoperative regional radiation ($p < 0.01$). The risk of secondary leukaemia was higher in patients aged under 50 years, compared with those over 50. These data confirmed the leukaemogenicity of

L-phenylalanine mustard. The authors concluded that the risk of secondary leukaemia, including the myeloproliferative syndrome, is lower than that reported after chemotherapy for other solid tumours and haematological malignancies, and that the benefit (survival rates and cost-effectiveness) from adjuvant chemotherapy for breast cancer (in node-positive patients) largely exceeded the risk of secondary leukaemia.

Other analyses have, however, failed to demonstrate an increased incidence of acute leukaemia, probably as a result of the different chemotherapeutic agents used in the adjuvant treatment of breast cancer. For example, Valagussa and colleagues reported only three cases of acute leukaemia in 2241 women treated in randomized studies,[20] with an adjuvant cyclophosphamide–methotrexate–fluorouracil (CMF)-based regimen. Of a total of 2465 women, 224 received no adjuvant chemotherapy after locoregional therapy for breast cancer and they were used as controls; the remaining 2241 were treated with chemotherapy (1359 with CMF for 6–12 months and an additional 882 patients with CMF + doxorubicin for 8–12 months). No adjuvant endocrine manipulation was included. Fifteen years after surgery, the probability of survival was 47.3% for the entire series, 34.7% for women with no adjuvant chemotherapy and 48.8% for patients treated with CMF-based adjuvant therapy. After the CMF-based regimen 77 secondary cancers (see Table 13.4) were observed with a cumulative risk of 6.5 ± 0.8%. No apparent difference was observed with administration of doxorubicin (with 5.1 ± 1.0%, without 6.4 ± 0.9%). Of the 77 cases of second malignancies only three were AML with a cumulative risk of 0.23 ± 0.15% at 15 years and a relative risk of 2.3 (see Table 13.2). The maximum planned dose of cyclophosphamide was 7200 mg/m² when given intravenously and 16 800 mg/m² when given orally. The authors concluded that the dose of alkylating agent (cyclophosphamide) used in their CMF-based regimen is probably linked to a barely detectable increased incidence of AML and breast irradiation did not enhance this low risk.

These findings were further extended and documented by Curtis et al[21] in a study of 82 700 women treated for breast cancer. The risk for leukaemia after regional radiation alone was increased twofold, with an average dose of 7.5 Gy to active bone marrow. The risk associated with treatment with alkylating agents, without radiation, was increased tenfold; with both radiation and alkylating agents, this increase rose to 17-fold. These radiation and chemotherapy doses are much higher than doses used for adjuvant treatment or primary radiotherapy after lumpectomy. Women receiving melphalan were ten times more likely to develop leukaemia than those receiving cyclophosphamide (relative risk 31.4 vs 3.1). All the leukaemias that developed after cyclophosphamide occurred in women who had received a dose larger than 20 000 mg. The difference in the total dose of cyclophosphamide may explain the variability in the risk of leukaemia in these populations. Based on the risks found in their study, Curtis et al[21] estimated that only about five in 10 000 patients treated for 6 months with a cyclophosphamide-based adjuvant regimen would be expected to develop treatment-induced leukaemia within 10 years of breast cancer diagnosis.

In conclusion, the risk of leukaemia after breast cancer therapy is mainly the result of treatment with alkylating agents, particularly melphalan. The risk is also related to the total dose of the drugs used; it is low in the cyclophosphamide dose range currently used in the adjuvant setting. The risk of leukaemia after regional radiotherapy (chest wall and nodes), using the older techniques, also appears to be minimally increased but is unknown after breast-conserving radiotherapy. Chemotherapy should be used with special care in premenopausal node-negative patients with breast cancer because of the likelihood of long survival rate (two or three decades). However, in patients with histologically positive lymph nodes, the risk of a secondary malignancy seems to be lower than that of dying of breast cancer. These findings reinforced the fact that the magnitude of benefit in survival achieved with adjuvant chemotherapy, in most cases, considerably exceeds the risk of secondary malignancies. Nevertheless, the non-selective and unnecessarily prolonged use of potentially toxic regimens must be avoided, especially in patients who have a very low risk of relapse (patients with negative axillary lymph nodes).

TAMOXIFEN

Tamoxifen is a non-steroidal agent that competes with oestrogen for oestrogen binding sites; it has either agonistic or antagonistic effects, depending upon the species, end-organ and endpoint measured. Cole et al[22], in 1971, were the first group to report the clinical efficacy of tamoxifen for advanced metastatic breast cancer. Furthermore, pharmacological and clinical evaluation were successfully performed and tamoxifen was approved, at the end of the 1970s, for the treatment of metastatic breast cancer in postmenopausal women. Once proven clearly efficient in patients with hormone receptor-positive metastatic breast cancer (rate of objective response of 60–70%), tamoxifen was subsequently approved as the initial endocrine therapy for oestrogen receptor (ER)- positive metastatic breast cancer in premenopausal women. Also used as adjuvant hormonal therapy for the management of primary operable breast cancer, tamoxifen provided a substantial improvement in overall survival,[23] and reduced the risk of cancer in the contralateral breast;[23–25] it thus became an important form of systemic adjuvant therapy for early breast cancer. Tamoxifen is currently the most widely used hormonal manipulation in the treatment of breast cancer, and has recently been approved for the treatment of metastatic breast cancer in men. More than three million breast cancer patients have received tamoxifen every year out of over 5.8 million patients.

Long-term toxic effects

Thromboembolic disease has been reported to occur occasionally with long-term tamoxifen treatment,[24] although a causal relationship has not been definitively established. Some studies have suggested a decrease in functional activity of antithrombin III levels with tamoxifen, whereas other reports have failed to note such a phenomenon. The analysis of NSABP B-14[24] does indeed suggest that tamoxifen is associated with an increased risk of vascular thrombosis: 1.5% of patients in the tamoxifen group versus 0.2% in the placebo group experienced a thrombotic event, and this included two (0.14%) deaths in the tamoxifen group as a result of pulmonary emboli. For this reason, women with a personal history of thrombosis were excluded from the NSABP B-14 study. Data currently available from other adjuvant trials also indicate a possible increase (with a low overall incidence) in thromboembolic disorders (1–3%) with tamoxifen.[24,26]

Leukopenia may occur transiently and usually resolves without the need to interrupt tamoxifen therapy. There are, nevertheless, at least three published reports about the association between leukopenia and long-term tamoxifen treatment. The last reported case of Miké et al[27] concerned a fatal neutropenia in postmenopausal women aged over 70 years and was directly associated with long-term (>7 years) tamoxifen treatment.

Secondary tumours
Endometrial cancer
It is well known that tamoxifen exerts oestrogenic effects on the endometrium of some postmenopausal women. The strongest evidence regarding the growth-promoting ability of tamoxifen in pre-existing endometrial disease, rather than a truly carcinogenic potential, was provided by clinical trials in which tamoxifen was evaluated for its usefulness in preventing breast cancer recurrences in women.

Breast cancer prevention trials
Some preliminary data from a British study that investigated the use of tamoxifen in the prevention of invasive breast carcinoma in women (at high risk) were published in 1994 by Kedar et

al[28], concerning the effect of tamoxifen on the uterus and ovaries of postmenopausal women. The authors recruited a cohort of 111 postmenopausal women aged between 46 and 71 years who were randomly (double-blind) assigned to receive either tamoxifen ($n = 61$) or a placebo ($n = 50$) with a mean follow-up of 2 years. Evidence of an abnormal endometrium ($p < 0.001$) was observed in 39% of women in the tamoxifen group compared with 10% of controls. The mean value ($\pm$ the standard deviation) for endometrial thickness among women in the tamoxifen group was 9.1 $\pm$ 4.3 mm, compared with 4.8 $\pm$ 2.8 mm in the control group ($p < 0.001$). Atypical hyperplasia was observed in 16% and polyps in 5% of the women in the tamoxifen group versus 0% hyperplasia and 2% polyps in the placebo group. A statistically significant negative correlation was noted between the duration of tamoxifen treatment and the mean uterine arterial peak systolic velocity ($p < 0.05$). No endometrial cancers were observed in this trial.

Adjuvant tamoxifen trials (Table 13.5)

Fisher and colleagues published a recent update[24] from the ongoing NSABP B-14 trial, the largest prospective, randomized (double-blind), controlled trial of adjuvant tamoxifen alone versus a placebo in a cohort of women with breast cancer and a favourable prognosis. The design, patient selection and the extensive detailed report of this trial provide a rich source for the assessment of some of the toxic effects of tamoxifen.

The NSABP B-14 trial enrolled 2843 women with primary operable ER-positive breast cancers who were randomly assigned to receive a placebo or tamoxifen 20 mg/day. An additional 1220 women on tamoxifen for breast cancer were registered for inclusion, at a later date, in a randomized trial designed to assess the efficacy of tamoxifen therapy given for 5 versus 10 years. After an average of 8 years for the randomized group and 5 years for the non-randomized registered group of patients on tamoxifen, two of the 1424 placebo recipients

(who subsequently developed recurrent breast cancer and colon cancer respectively, and were treated with tamoxifen), 15 of the 1419 randomized to receive tamoxifen for 5 years and eight of the 1220 registered patients on tamoxifen developed endometrial cancer. Of the 15 randomized patients, treated with tamoxifen, who developed secondary endometrial carcinoma, 14 (93%) were over 50 years of age, six (40%) had prior hormone replacement therapy, 10 had tumour known to be of a good or moderate grade and three died of the disease (including one patient who had never taken tamoxifen). The authors reported that the endometrial cancers occurring after tamoxifen therapy did not appear to be of a histological type with a poorer prognosis than cancers occurring in women who did not receive tamoxifen.

The relative risk of developing endometrial cancer among women treated with tamoxifen compared with the placebo group was 7.5 (95%CI = 1.7–32.7), as determined by the proportional hazards model. Among women in the randomized tamoxifen arm, the average annual hazard rate of endometrial cancer for women aged over 50 years was about sixfold that of women aged under 50 years (2.3/1000 versus 0.4/1000 patients per year). The authors noticed that the placebo group had an abnormally low number of cases of endometrial cancer (lower than expected). Using results from the 1984–88 Surveillance Epidemiology and End Results (SEER) study as baseline rates, they reanalysed their data and calculated an estimate of the relative risk of developing endometrial cancer of 2.2.

They reported an absolute risk of tamoxifen-induced endometrial cancer of one to two cases annually per 1000 women treated and a relative risk that is two to three times greater than that seen in women with breast cancer not treated with tamoxifen.

The first large trial to report the increased incidence of secondary endometrial cancer was the Stockholm Trial.[29] This study included 1846 postmenopausal women below 71 years of age with early breast cancer who were randomized after primary surgery to receive tamoxifen 40 mg/day for 2 or 5 years versus no hormonal

Table 13.5 Tamoxifen adjuvant trials

Reference	No. of patients on tamoxifen	No. of controls	Tamoxifen Dose (mg/day)	Duration (years)	Median follow-up time (years)	Menopausal (M) status	ER+	No. of endometrial cancer T	C	Risk (RR) of endometrial cancer (95%CI)
Fornander et al[29] 1989 (Sweden)	931	915	40	2–5	4.5	Post-M < 71 years	–	13	2	6.4 (1.4–28)
Andersson et al[30] 1991 (Denmark)	864	846	30	4	8	Post-M (N+)	–	–	–	3.3 (0.6–3.0)
Fisher et al[24] 1994 (USA/NSABP)	1419 +1220 (NR)	1424	20	5–8	8 / 5	Post-M + / Pre-M	ER+	15 / 8	2	7.5 (1.7–32.7) with SEER data (RR = 2.2)
Rutqvist et al[25] 1995 (Sweden)	2995	1919	40	2–5	5–8	Post-M	–	34	8	5.6 (1.9–16.2)
Castiglione et al[31] 1990 (Switzerland)	167	153	20 + p	1	8	Post-M (66–80 years)	–	4	2	Not available
Boccardo et al[32] 1992 (Italy)	168+ 171 + CT	165 CT	30	5	8	Pre-M + Post-M < 65 years	–	1	0	Not available
Stewart et al[23] 1992 (Scotland)	374	373	20	5	5	Pre-M + Post-M < 79 years	–	2	2	Not available
Ribeiro and Swindel[26] 1992 (New York, USA)	199 282	174 306	20	1	10	Pre-M + Post-M	–	1	1	Not available

M, menopausal; ER+, oestrogen receptor positive; NR, non-randomized; P, prednisone; CT, control + tamoxifen.

therapy. At a median follow-up of 4.5 years, the risk of second primary breast cancer was substantially reduced by tamoxifen (RR = 0.55; 95%CI = 0.31–0.98; p = 0.05) compared with that of controls. However, a small increase in the risk of secondary uterine cancer (corpus) was noticed in those patients treated with tamoxifen (RR = 6.4; 95%CI = 1.4–28; p < 0.01). Two patients in the tamoxifen group also developed liver cancer.

In the most recent update of the trial,[29] which included a total of 2729 women and a median follow-up of 9 years, 23 endometrial cancers were observed in the group treated with tamoxifen versus four in the control arm. The results of this analysis validated those found in the first report and confirmed a decrease in the incidence of second breast cancers in patients treated with tamoxifen (RR = 0.6; 95%CI = 0.4–0.9; p = 0.008), but showed that endometrial carcinomas are more frequent among women treated with tamoxifen (RR = 5.6; 95%CI = 1.9–16.2; p < 0.001).

A combined analysis performed by Rutqvist et al,[25] including 4914 women from the Stockholm, Danish[30] and South Swedish trials, reported 34 endometrial cancers in women treated with tamoxifen compared with eight in the control group. These three studies were specifically combined because the Stockholm data showed an increased incidence of endometrial cancer and the Danish and South Swedish data showed an increased incidence in gastrointestinal cancer. Therefore, a considerable nonrandom selection bias exists in the three studies combined.

Evidence arising from those randomized clinical trials[24,25,30] indicates that women treated with tamoxifen for breast cancer seem to be at increased risk of developing endometrial cancer. These trials were large studies mostly restricted to postmenopausal women,[25,30] with follow-up durations of at least 4.5 years. On the other hand, several smaller trials of adjuvant tamoxifen therapy failed to show an increased risk of endometrial cancers. One example is the study published by Castiglione et al[31] which included 320 postmenopausal women with node-positive breast cancer, randomly assigned

to receive either tamoxifen (n = 167) or no further treatment (n = 153). Four secondary malignancies occurred among patients treated with tamoxifen versus two in the control group. None of these secondary carcinomas was uterine. Boccardo et al[22] also reported the results of another randomized study of women with node-positive, ER-positive breast cancer who were randomized to receive chemotherapy (n = 165), 30 mg tamoxifen per day (n = 168), or combined tamoxifen and chemotherapy (n = 171). At a median follow-up of 5 years, no excess endometrial carcinoma or hyperplasia was observed among women treated with either tamoxifen or combined tamoxifen and chemotherapy, compared with those who received chemotherapy alone. Only one case of endometrial cancer occurred in a woman who received both tamoxifen and chemotherapy.

Stewart,[23] from the Scottish trials, reported no increased risk of endometrial cancer among women taking tamoxifen in 747 women with node-negative breast cancer randomized to receive either 20 mg/day adjuvant tamoxifen for 5 years (n = 373), or tamoxifen only in the event of recurrent breast cancer (n = 373). Two cases of endometrial cancer were reported, one in each treatment group. Ribeiro and Swindell[26] published a study of 961 women with operable breast cancer who were randomly assigned (according to their menopausal status) to receive either tamoxifen 20 mg/day for one year or to undergo radiotherapeutic castration (in premenopausal women, n = 373; postmenopausal women, n = 588) and either tamoxifen 20 mg/day or no further treatment (control group). At a median follow-up of 10 years, no increased risk of endometrial cancer was detected among women treated with tamoxifen.

The small sample size may partly explain why the smaller studies have failed to detect an increased risk of endometrial cancer among women treated with tamoxifen. Other differences in the study design, such as the variation in the dose and duration of tamoxifen therapy among treated women, could also account for this failure. Another relevant difference between studies was the criteria used for patient selection: two[29,30] of the three largest studies, which demonstrated an increased risk of endometrial cancer, were restricted to postmenopausal women. The remainder, namely the NSABP trial and three[23,26,32] of the four smaller studies, included both pre- and postmenopausal women. It is possible that the risk of endometrial cancer with tamoxifen therapy may be different for pre- and postmenopausal women. DeMuylder et al[33] found that the risk of endometrial cancer increased with age, and the differences in age distribution among patients in these trials may have contributed to the discrepancies in the final results.

In addition to the evidence from clinical trials, case-control and other cross-sectional studies (Table 13.6) support the conclusion that tamoxifen may be a promoter of endometrial

Table 13.6 Tamoxifen results of case-control studies

Reference	No. of patients with endometrial cancer	No. of controls	Dose tamoxifen (mg/day)	Relative risk of endometrial cancer	Conclusions
Van Leeuwen et al 1994[35]	98	285	40	T1 = 1.3 (0.7–2.4) $p = 0.049$ T1 = 2.3 (0.9–5.9) $p = 0.046$ T2 = 3.0 (0.6–15.8)	Risk of endometrial cancer increases with tamoxifen treatment duration
Sasco et al 1996[36]	43	177	20	T1 = 1.5 (0.44–4.9) T = 1.5 (0.42–5.6) T2 = 3.5 (0.94–12.7) >5 years	The risk of endometrial cancer increases with duration of tamoxifen therapy Radiotherapeutic castration increases the risk for endometrial cancer more than tamoxifen OR: 7.7 (1.8–32.8)
Lê et al 1996 (un-published)	34	102	20	T = 2.0 (0.5–7.8) T2 = 3.0 (0.2–51.5)	The risk of endometrial cancer increases with duration of tamoxifen therapy When controlling for other risk factors of endometrial cancer (obesity++, pelvic irradiation and parity): RR = T2; OR = 1.3 (0.05–33.7)

T = tamoxifen use > 2 years < 5 years; T1 = tamoxifen use > 1 years–2 years; T2 = tamoxifen use > 5 years; OR = odds ratio.

cancer in women.[34] Data from a recent case-control study, by van Leeuwen et al,[35] reported a relative risk of developing endometrial cancer of 1.3 (95%CI = 0.7–2.4) for women who received tamoxifen, compared with women who had not received this drug. The risk of endometrial cancer was increased 2.3-fold (95%CI = 0.9–5.9) and three-fold (95%CI = 0.6–15.8), for a duration of tamoxifen use of more than 2 years and 5 years, respectively, compared with women never treated with tamoxifen. Similarly, Sasco et al[36] reported a case-control study assessing the effect of tamoxifen combined with other treatments for breast cancer on the development of endometrial carcinoma. The authors identified 43 cases of endometrial carcinoma (at least one year after breast cancer). The relative risk of endometrial cancer increased with the duration of tamoxifen therapy as shown in previous reports,[34,35] and was equal to 1.5 (95%CI = 0.44–4.9) for less than 2 years of tamoxifen use, 1.5 (95%CI = 0.42–5.6) for 2–5 years and 3.5 (95%CI = 0.94–12.7) for more than 5 years. However, the most important finding in this study was that radiotherapeutic castration increased the risk of endometrial cancer more than tamoxifen (overall risk, OR = 7.7, 95%CI = 1.8–32.8). Similar results were found by Ewertz et al[37] and Hardell.[38,39] The most recent report was a case-control study conducted by Lê et al (unpublished) which analysed 34 cases of secondary endometrial cancers (at least one year after breast cancer) and 102 controls from a cohort of 7712 breast cancer patients treated at the Institut Gustave-Roussy, Villejuif, France. When compared with never-users of tamoxifen, the unadjusted relative risk of endometrial carcinoma for women with 2–5 years of tamoxifen therapy was very similar to that observed in the above studies. When other risk factors for endometrial cancer were taken into account, in particular obesity and to a lesser extent pelvic irradiation, and parity, the relative risk of endometrial carcinoma associated with over 5 years of tamoxifen therapy falls to 1.3 (95%CI = 0.05–33.7).

Evidence provided by the case-control studies mentioned above allows us to conclude that tamoxifen therapy of long duration (>5 years), alone or associated with other breast cancer treatments (not taking into account other risk factors of endometrial cancer), may be associated with an increased relative risk for endometrial cancer.

Other reports, such as that of Magriples et al,[40] suggested that women taking tamoxifen for breast cancer may be at an increased risk of developing endometrial carcinoma of a more aggressive histological type compared with women not on tamoxifen. The study of Fornander et al[41] found, somewhat surprisingly, that among women with endometrial cancer, women on tamoxifen did not have endometrial cancer with histological grades of a poor prognosis, yet they were more likely to die of the disease. Andersson et al[30] noticed that women on tamoxifen with endometrial cancer had a short duration of survival after diagnosis of the disease (2.2 years in the group on tamoxifen vs 4.2 years in the control). These findings support some concern that the prognosis for endometrial cancer may be poorer among women treated with tamoxifen for breast cancer than for women not exposed to the drug.

There is also evidence in numerous reports of endometrial and other gynaecological abnormalities associated with tamoxifen treatment. Gusberg and Runowicz have implicated adenomatous endometrial hyperplasia as a precursor of endometrial carcinoma. Similarly, tamoxifen has also been associated with an increased frequency of vaginal discharge and it is possible that some ascertainment bias may exist as a result of more frequent visits to physicians for gynaecological complaints. Lahti et al[42] studied the action of tamoxifen on the endometrium, through assessment of its mean width by ultrasonography. The results showed a width of 10.4 mm in patients treated with tamoxifen versus 4.2 mm in controls. Among the women treated with tamoxifen, 28% had atrophy of the endometrium compared with 87% in the control group. According to the recent observation of Barakat,[43] in 75 postmenopausal breast cancer patients on tamoxifen who underwent evaluation by dilatation and curettage, 15% of the symptomatic patients had polyps, 2% had hyperplasia and 11% had endometrial carcinoma, whereas only 9% of the asymptomatic patients had polyps and no other histological abnormalities.

To the question 'Does routine pelvic and/or endovaginal sonography and annual endometrial sampling reduce the morbidity and/or mortality from tamoxifen-induced endometrial cancers?' Cohen et al[44] demonstrated that vaginal ultrasonography and endometrial sampling in asymptomatic postmenopausal breast cancer patients treated with tamoxifen showed more frequent positive histological findings, such as hyperplasia, proliferation, polyps and cancers, than in a similar untreated group.

Whether the increased incidence of endometrial carcinoma in tamoxifen-treated patients is real or results from lead-time bias (increased detection of lesions that would otherwise have remained silent) in patients who take tamoxifen is not totally clear. Physicians should nevertheless be aware of the apparent increase in the rate of endometrial carcinoma during and/or after tamoxifen therapy, and patients should be informed of these risks.

The cumulative incidence of endometrical cancers in all women treated with tamoxifen in the major adjuvant trials is 0.9%, compared with 0.2% in the control groups, i.e. an extra seven women per 1000 who took adjuvant tamoxifen developed endometrial carcinoma.

Conclusion

Among women treated with adjuvant tamoxifen for breast cancer, despite the methodological differences and low statistical power of many of the existing epidemiological studies, there is modest but definitive evidence of an increased risk for endometrial cancer. It is possible that tamoxifen will act as a growth promoter of pre-existing disease in the endometrium in these women.

However, the proven clinical benefits of tamoxifen in controlling breast cancer seem to far outweigh the risk of endometrial carcinoma and, therefore, tamoxifen should not be withheld for the management of breast cancer in women.

Meanwhile, all women who receive tamoxifen therapy should have at least once yearly gynaecological examinations and should be advised to report to their physicians any abnormal vaginal bleeding or change in vaginal discharge and/or pelvic pain or pressure in order to have further evaluation.

In addition, many issues still need to be addressed in the design of future clinical trials. These issues include the way in which tamoxifen exerts its action, as well as the biological effects it has on other organs and tissues. These studies also need to identify accurately the patients at greatest risk of developing endometrial carcinoma from tamoxifen therapy, and the most efficient, simple and cost-effective means of screening these patients in search of endometrial cancers. In addition, the question of whether tamoxifen-induced carcinomas have a different prognosis from naturally occurring tumours needs to be answered adequately in larger studies. Ideally, we need to find a way to minimize or totally eradicate the endometrial effects of tamoxifen without altering its therapeutic value.

REFERENCES

1. Bristow, MR, Mason JW, Billingham ME, Daniels JR. Dose–effect and structure–function relationship in doxorubicin cardiomyopathy. *Am Heart J* 1981; **102**:709–18.

2. Legha SS, Benjamin RS, Mackay B, et al. Reduction of doxorubicin cardiotoxicity by prolonged continuous intravenous infusion. *Ann Intern Med* 1982; **96**:133–9.

3. Von Hoff DD, Layard MW, Basa P, et al. Dose–effect risk factors for doxorubicin-induced congestive heart failure. *Ann Intern Med* 1979; **91**:710–17.

4. Brambilla C, Rossi A, Bonfante V, et al. Phase II study of doxorubicin versus epirubicin in advanced breast cancer. *Cancer Treat Rep* 1986; **70**:261–6.

5. Ewer MS, Ali MK, Mackay B, et al. A comparison of cardiac biopsy grades and ejection fraction estimations in patients receiving Adriamycin. *J Clin Oncol* 1984; **2**:112–17.

6. Hurteloup P, Ganzina F. Clinical studies with new anthracyclines: epirubicin, idarubicin, esorubicin. *Drugs Exp Clin Res* 1986; **12**:233–46.

7. Shapira J, Gottfried M, Lishner M, Ravid M. Reduced cardiotoxicity of doxorubicin by a 6-hour infusion regimen. *Cancer* 1990; **65**:870–3.

8. Casper ES, Gaynor JJ, Hadju SI, et al. A prospective randomized trial of adjuvant chemotherapy with bolus versus continuous infusion of doxorubicin in patients with high-grade extremity soft tissue sarcoma and an analysis of prognostic factors. *Cancer* 1991; **68**:1221–9.

9. Early Breast Cancer Trialists' Collaborative Group. Systemic treatment of early breast cancer by hormonal, cytotoxic, or immune therapy. 133 randomized trials involving 31,000 recurrence and 24,000 deaths among 75,000 women. *Lancet* 1992; **339**:1–15, 71–85.

10. Edeiken S, Russo DP, Knecht J. Angiosarcoma after tylectomy and radiation therapy for carcinoma of the breast. *Cancer* 1992; **70**:644.

11. Boice JD Jr, Harvey EB, Blettner M, et al. Cancer in the contralateral breast after radiotherapy for breast cancer. *N Engl J Med* 1992; **326**:781–5.

12. Levitt SH, Mandel JS. Breast carcinogenisis: risk of radiation (Editorial). *Int J Radiat Oncol Biol Phys* 1985; **11**:1421.

13. Frass BA, Robertson PL, Lichter AS. Dose to the contralateral breast due to primary breast irradiation. *Int J Radiat Oncol Biol Phys* 1985; **11**:485.

14. Inskip PD, Stovall M, Flannery JT. Lung cancer risk and radiation dose among women treated for breast cancer. *J Natl Cancer Inst* 1994; **86**:983.

15. LeBeau MM, Albain KS, Larson RA, et al. Clinical and cytogenetic correlations in 63 patients with therapy-related myelodysplastic syndromes and acute nonlymphocytic leukemia; further evidence for characteristic abnormalities of chromosomes 5 and 7. *J Clin Oncol* 1986; **4**:325–32.

16. Rowley JD, Golomb HM, Vardiman JN. Nonrandom chromosome abnormalities in acute leukemia and dysmyelopoietic syndromes in patients with previously treated malignant disease. *Blood* 1981; **58**:759–63.

17. Detourmignies L, Castaigne S, Stoppa AM, et al. Therapy-related acute promyelocytic leukemia: a report on 16 cases. *J Clin Oncol* 1992; **10**:1430–6.

18. Pedersen-Bjergaard J, Sigsgaard TC, Nielsen D, et al. Acute monocytic or myelomonocytic leukemia with balanced chromosome translocation to band 11q23 after therapy with 4-epidoxorubicin and cisplatin or cyclophosphamide for breast cancer. *J Clin Oncol* 1992; **10**:1444–51.

19. Fisher B, Rockette H, Fisher ER, et al. Leukemia in breast cancer patients following adjuvant chemotherapy or postoperative radiation: The NSABP experience. *J Clin Oncol* 1985; **3**:1640–58.

20. Valagussa P, Moliterni A, Terenziani M, Zambetti M, Bonadonna G. Second malignancies following CMF-based adjuvant chemotherapy in resectable breast cancer. *Ann Oncol* 1994; **5**:803–8.

21. Curtis RE, Boice JD Jr, Stovall M, et al. Dose-dependent leukemia risk after drug and radiation treatment for breast cancer. *N Engl J Med* 1992; **326**:1745–51.

22. Cole MP, Jones CT, Todd ID. A new anti-oestrogenic agent in late breast cancer. An early clinical appraisal of ICI46474. *Br J Cancer* 1971; **25**:270–75.

23. Stewart HJ. The Scottish trial of adjuvant tamoxifen in node-negative breast cancer. Scottish Trials Breast Group. *Monogr Natl Cancer Inst* 1992; **11**:117–20.

24. Fisher B, Costantino J, Redmond C, et al. Endometrial cancer in Tamoxifen-treated breast cancer patients: findings from the National Surgical Adjuvant Breast and Bowel Project (NSABP) B-14. *J Natl Cancer Inst* 1994; **86**:527–37.

25. Rutqvist LE, Johansson H, Signomklao U, et al. Adjuvant tamoxifen therapy for early stage breast cancer and primary malignancies. *J Natl Cancer Inst* 1995; **87**:645–51.

26. Ribeiro G, Swindell R. The Christie Hospital adjuvant tamoxifen trial. *Monogr Natl Cancer Inst* 1992;**11**:121–5.

27. Miké V, Currie VE, Gee TS. Fatal neutropenia associated with long-term tamoxifen therapy (letter). *Lancet* 1994; **344**:541–2.

28. Kedar RP, Bourne TH, Powles TJ, et al. Effects of tamoxifen on uterus and ovaries of postmenopausal women in a randomised breast cancer prevention trial. *Lancet* 1994; **343**:1318–21.

29. Fornander T, Rutqvist L, Cedermark B, et al. Adjuvant tamoxifen in early breast cancer: occurrence of new primary cancers. *Lancet* 1989; **i**:117–20.

30. Andersson M, Storm HH, Mouridsen HT. Incidence of new primary cancers after adjuvant tamoxifen therapy and radiotherapy for early breast cancer. *J Natl Cancer Inst* 1991; **83**:1013–17.

31. Castiglione M, Gelber RD, Goldhirsch A. Adjuvant systemic therapy for breast cancer in the elderly. *J Clin Oncol* 1990; **8**:519–26.

32. Boccardo F, Rubagotti A, Amoroso D, et al. Chemotherapy versus tamoxifen versus chemotherapy plus tamoxifen in node-positive oestrogen-receptor positive breast cancer patients. An update at 7 years of the 1st GROCTA Trial. *Eur J Cancer* 1992; **28**:673–80.

33. DeMuylder X, Neven P, de Sommer M, et al.

Endometrial lesions in patients undergoing tamoxifen therapy. *Int J Gynaecol Obstet* 1991; **36:**127.

34. Mignotte H, Rodier JF, Lesur A, et al. Endometrial carcinoma associated with adjuvant tamoxifen therapy for breast cancer: a French multi-centre analysis of 89 cases. *The Breast* 1995; **4:**200–2.

35. van Leeuwen FE, Benraadt J, Coebergh JW, et al. Risk of endometrial cancer after tamoxifen treatment of breast cancer. *Lancet* 1994; **343:** 448–52.

36. Sasco AJ, Chaplain G, Saez S, et al. Case-control study of endometrial cancer following breast cancer effect of tamoxifen and radiotherapeutic castration [abstract]. *Epidemiology* 1996; **7:**9.

37. Ewertz M, Macado SG, Boice JD Jr, Jenson OM. Endometrial cancer following treatment for breast cancer: a case control study in Denmark. *Br J Cancer* 1984; **50:**687–92.

38. Hardell, L. Tamoxifen as risk factor for carcinoma of corpus uteri. *Lancet* 1988; **1:**563.

39. Hardell, L. Endometrial cancer and tamoxifen. *Lancet* 1994; **343:**978.

40. Magriples U, Naftolin F, Schwartz PE, et al. High-grade endometrial carcinoma in tamoxifen-treated breast cancer patients. *J Clin Oncol* 1993; **IIXX:**485–90.

41. Fornander T, Hellström AC, Moberger D. Descriptive clinicopathologic study of 17 patients with endometrial cancer during or after adjuvant tamoxifen in early breast cancer. *J Natl Cancer Inst* 1993; **85:**1850–5.

42. Lahti E, Blanco G, Kauppila A, et al. Endometrial changes in postmenopausal breast cancer patients receiving tamoxifen. *Obstet Gynecol* 1993; **81:**660–4.

43. Barakat RR. The effect of tamoxifen on the endometrium. *Oncology* 1995; **9:**129–34.

44. Cohen RJ, Wiernik PH, Walker MD. Acute non-lymphocytic leukemia associated with nitrosurea chemotherapy: Report of two cases. *Cancer Treat Rep* 1976; **60:**1257–66.

45. Billingham ME, Mason GW, Bristow MR, et al. Antracycline cardiomyopathy monitored by morphologic changes. *Cancer Treat* 1978; **62:**865–72.

14

Supportive care: chemotherapy-induced emesis and cancer pain

Makoto Ogawa, Yutaka Ariyoshi

CONTENTS • **Emetogenic potential** • **Antiemetic therapy** • **Cancer pain**

Various anticancer drugs, including alkylating agents, antimetabolites, anti-tumour antibiotics and plant alkaloids, are effective against breast cancer, but these agents have no ability to cure breast cancer on their own.

Thus, various combination regimens have been used to enhance anti-tumour activity; response rates exceeding 50% can be obtained using these combinations.

Chemotherapy has been commonly employed in two treatment strategies: one is adjuvant chemotherapy which has aimed at prolongation of relapse-free survival and length of overall survival after curative surgery; the other is chemotherapy for advanced disease in order to prolong survival duration.

As most anticancer drugs induce various grades of chemotherapy-induced emesis, it is extremely important to control this emesis because it is the most distressing toxicity for patients.

This chapter describes the emetogenic potential of single agent and combination regimens, and the treatment of chemotherapy-induced emesis.

EMETOGENIC POTENTIAL

The emetogenic potential of monotherapy with various anticancer drugs commonly employed in chemotherapy for breast cancer is given in Table 14.1.

Cisplatin, one of the most potent drugs[1,2] to induce emesis, has rarely been used in first-line chemotherapy for breast cancer. Among the drugs employed in first-line chemotherapy, anthracyclines[2,3] and cyclophosphamide can induce emesis of moderate grade in about 60–90%, including 10–20% above grade 3 in severity.

Table 14.1 Emetogenic potential of monotherapy

Moderate (≥3)	Mild (1–2)	Modest (<1)
Doxorubicin	5-Fluorouracil	Vincristine
Epirubicin	Methotrexate	Vinblastine
Cyclophos-phamide	Mitomycin C	Vindesine
	Mitozantrone	Vinorelbine
	Paclitaxel	
	Docetaxel	

5-Fluorouracil, methotrexate, mitomycin C, mitozantrone[4] and taxanes[5,6] induce emesis of WHO grade 1–2 in 30–40%, but emesis above grade 3 is rare. Vinca alkaloids[2,7] induce modest emesis (<1).

The use of single-agent chemotherapy against breast cancer is rare; therefore, the emesis that occurs in combination regimens is summarized in Table 14.2.

Original CMF[8–10,13] (oral cyclophosphamide, intravenous methotrexate and 5-fluorouracil) induced emesis in 57–92%, but incidence of severe emesis above WHO grade 3 was relatively low.

Intravenous CMF,[10] which has been commonly employed in the adjuvant setting, induced emesis in almost 100%, and about one-third of patients experienced severe emesis above grade 3. CMFP,[9,13] which is the original CMF plus oral prednisone, induced emesis in 35–77%, but severe emesis was relatively rare. CMFVP[11] (in which V is vincristine) induced a similar incidence and severity of emesis to the original CMF.

CAF[10–12] (cyclophosphamide, doxorubicin [Adriamycin], 5-fluorouracil) showed higher incidence of emesis than CMFP or CMFVP, and AC[13] (doxorubicin [Adriamycin], cyclophosphamide) showed a similar tendency to CAF. Overall, doxorubicin-containing regimens induced more profound emesis compared with CMF-type regimens.

Chemotherapy-induced emesis occurs via stimulation of both the emetic centre located in

Table 14.2 Emesis with combination regimens

Regimen	No. of patients	Emesis (%)			Reference
		Mild	Severe	Total	
CMF(p.o.)	62	65	3	68	Engelsman et al[9]
R CMF(p.o.)	116	63	28	92	
R CMF(i.v.)	122	60	36	96	Cummings et al[10]
R CMFP(p.o.)	76	30	7	37	
R CAF	79	38	17	56	Smalley et al[11]
R CMFVP	130	33	8	42	
R CAF	135	41	14	55	Hortobagyi et al[12]
R High-dose CAF	32	59	22	88	
R CAF	27	59	19	85	Tormey et al[13]
CMF p.o.	79	48	9	57	
R CMFP p.o.	86	30	5	35	Buser et al[14]
AC	166	58	15	73	

p.o., per oral. C, cyclophosphamide; M, intravenous methotrexate; F, 5-fluorouracil; P, prednisone; V, vincristine; A, doxorubicin (Adriamycin).

the dorsolateral reticular formation of the medulla, through the chemoreceptor trigger zone, and the emetic centre located in the stomach.

Chemotherapy-induced emesis[1] is divided into three types: the first and most common type is acute emesis which starts within 24 hours of the administration of chemotherapy. In most patients emesis starts within several hours but subsides within 24 hours with appropriate antiemetic therapy. The second type is classified as delayed emesis, which occurs more than 24 hours after initiation of chemotherapy, lasting 5–7 days in some patients. The mechanism for inducing this type of emesis is unknown, but female sex, cisplatin doses exceeding $100\,mg/m^2$ and poor initial control of acute emesis are risk factors that induce delayed emesis. The third type is classified as anticipatory emesis which begins before chemotherapy and this type usually occurs when emesis was poorly controlled after previ-

ous cycles of chemotherapy. Anticipatory emesis occurs in almost 25% of patients receiving several cycles of chemotherapy.

ANTIEMETIC THERAPY

Antiemetics used for chemotherapy-induced emesis are summarized in Table 14.3.

The management of emesis induced by chemotherapy demands appropriate use of various classes of antiemetic drugs. A main principle in the use of antiemetic therapy is the prophylactic application of antiemetic drugs by a convenient route of administration, although antiemetic drugs are also used to control emesis that has already developed.

Before the wide use of cisplatin, which is the most emetogenic drug, antiemetic therapy used a single dopamine inhibitor such as metoclopramide, or combined use of metoclopramide and diazepam.

Table 14.3 Antiemetics used for chemotherapy-induced emesis

Classification	Drug	Mechanism of action	Type of emesis controlled
Dopamine inhibitors	Prochlorperazine Chlorpromazine Haloperidol Metoclopramide	Act on chemotrigger zone	All types of emesis
Benzodiazepines	Diazepam Lorazepam	Act centrally by depressing the central cortex or emetic centre	Anticipatory emesis
Corticosteroids	Dexamethasone	Unknown	Effective in combination with other antiemetic drugs
Cannabinoids	Dronabinol	Unknown	
Serotonin antagonists	Granisetron Ondansetron Tropisetron	Bind to type 3 serotonin receptor (5-hydroxtryptamine or 5-HT$_3$)	Most effective for acute emesis

During the 1980s, however, research into new antiemetic drugs with more potential to control emesis was carried out and the serotonin (5-HT) antagonists were developed. In general, serotonin antagonists are the most effective drugs for controlling chemotherapy-induced emesis.

Oral ondansetron[14] at a dose of 8 mg three times a day for 15 days was administered for emesis induced by oral CMF, and complete control was noted in 74% for days 1–7 and in 60% for days 1–5, respectively, whereas using placebo complete control was 50% for days 1–7 and 35% for days 1–15 respectively (which is statistically significant). Major adverse events were headaches in 19% and constipation in 12%.

Another report[15] compared the efficacy of three serotonin antagonists given by intravenous administration to patients who received non-platinum combination regimens. Of 166 patients, 107 were patients with breast cancer who were treated with CMF, FAC or FEC (5-fluorouracil, epirubicin, cyclophosphamide). Overall, ondansetron, tropisetron and granisetron obtained complete and partial control of emesis in 85–94% of patients, and headaches were the only adverse event.

Thus, the use of intravenous serotonin antagonists for moderate and severe emesis is very effective. However, if the serotonin antagonists are not effective enough, the use of an intravenous serotonin antagonist in association with corticosteroids and other antiemetic adjuvants, such as lorazepam, is more effective than an intravenous serotonin antagonist alone.

For moderate and modest emesis oral serotonin antagonists are usually effective and sufficient; in addition, treatment with lorazepam, metoclopramide or prochlorperazine is a very good choice for mild and modest emesis and these drugs are probably less expensive than the serotonin antagonists.

Anticipatory emesis, which relates to previously poor control of emesis, occurs in about 25% of patients receiving several cycles of chemotherapy. Although the prevalence of this symptom may be reduced by the prophylactic administration of benzodiazepines, or a combination of benzodiazepines and oral serotonin antagonists, it is crucial to provide the best antiemetic control from the first cycle of chemotherapy to prevent anticipatory emesis.

CANCER PAIN

Cancer pain is one of the most common and unpleasant symptoms for patients with cancer. When cancer pain is intolerable, it is said that suicide[16] can enter a patient's mind. Thus, the control of cancer pain is the most important medical treatment for patients. All physicians who manage cancer pain should understand that pain associated with cancer includes both physiological and psychological profiles. Thus, careful assessment of pain should be carried out before the management is decided on, with the goal being to provide patients total relief and to improve their quality of life. To achieve this goal physicians should be concerned about the control of pain and should do their best to establish trust with their patients.

Incidence

The overall incidence of pain in various malignancies is in about 50% of patients at all stages of disease;[17] also about a quarter of patients at late phases of their illness have pain that requires the use of opioids. If this type of pain is not relieved sufficiently, daily activities, as well as the quality of life, are affected. In fact, several reports[16–19] suggested that adequate pain control was not given to a number of cancer patients in non-hospice setting as a result of the lack of knowledge of the physician about pain management.

Table 14.4 indicates the incidence of cancer pain according to tumour types when in an advanced stage.[17] Malignancies for which prevalence exceeds 70% include bone tumours, pancreatic cancer, gastric cancer, cervical cancer, lung cancer, breast cancer and prostate cancer. In haemopoietic malignancies the prevalence of pain is relatively low.

Table 14.4 Prevalence of cancer pain

Tumour type (advanced stage)	Prevalence (%)*
Bone tumour	75–80 (70–85)
Pancreatic cancer	79 (72–100)
Stomach cancer	75 (67–77)
Uterine/cervical cancer	75 (40–100)
Lung cancer	72 (58–85)
Breast cancer	72 (56–94)
Prostate cancer	70 (55–80)
Colon cancer	69 (47–95)
Lymphoma	58 (20–69)
Leukaemia	52 (5–58)
All	
All stage	50 (11–75)
Advanced stage	71 (52–96)

*The range is given in parentheses. Modified from Bonica.[17]

Aetiology

Tumour involvement is a major cause of cancer pain and this can include metastasis to the bones, invasion to neural structures, obstruction of a hollow viscus, mucous membrane ulceration, etc.

Cancer pain resulting from tumour metastasis to the bone is experienced most frequently. Pathological fractures with intolerable pain occur with a high incidence. According to the analysis of the relationship between primary lesions and bone metastasis,[20] in 1967 cases with various cancers, bone metastases were seen in 32.4% for prostate cancer, 21.9% for breast cancer, 16.4% for renal cancer, 11.7% for thyroid cancer, 10.9% for lung cancer and 11.2% for testicular tumours, respectively. The role of bone metastasis in melanoma, head and neck cancer, bladder cancer and rectal cancer ranged from 5% to 7%, and that in uterine cervical cancer, ovarian cancer and gastric cancer was less than 3% in incidence. More recent studies have shown that 30–40% of patients with metastatic breast cancer have bone involvement as their first metastasis. In addition, postmortem studies have revealed that, in patients with metastatic breast cancer, the incidence of bone metastases increases to 70–85%. For the actual sites of bone metastasis, these were 68.8% in vertebra, 40% in the pelvis and sacral bone, 25.2% in the femur, 25.1% in the ribs and 13.9% in the skull, respectively. Cancer pain[16] associated with direct tumour involvement is summarized in Table 14.5.

Cancer-induced syndromes, such as paraneoplastic syndromes, debility, postherpetic neuralgia, etc., may also produce pain, but the incidence[21] is likely to be 10% or less.

Table 14.5 Pain syndromes associated with direct tumour involvement

Tumour infiltration of bone
Metastases to the cranial vault
Metastases to the base of the skull:
    Jugular foramen syndrome
    Clivus metastases
    Sphenoid sinus metastases
Vertebral body syndromes:
    Fracture of the odontoid
    C7–T1 metastases
    Sacral syndromes
Tumour infiltration of viscera
Infiltration of pleura
Small and large bowel obstruction
Infiltration of pelvis and bladder wall
Tumour infiltration of nerve
Peripheral nerve:
    Peripheral neuropathy
    Intercostal neuropathy
Plexus:
    Brachial plexopathy
    Lumbosacral plexopathy
    Coeliac plexopathy
Root:
    Radiculopathy
    Leptomeningeal metastases
Spinal cord:
    Epidural spinal cord compression
    Intramedullary metastases

Venipuncture, bone marrow aspiration, biopsy and lumbar puncture are frequently employed diagnostic procedures which are accompanied by pain. Surgery is associated with postoperative pain. Chronic pain syndromes are often seen after radical neck resection, mastectomy or amputation of extremities, and are difficult to control. Pain after breast cancer surgery[22] is observed in around 5% of operated cases. Chemotherapy can produce postchemotherapy pain syndromes, such as peripheral neuropathy induced by plant alkaloids, mucositis-induced oral pain from fluoropyrimidine or methotrexate, various cytokine-induced headaches, abdominal pain caused by fluoropyrimidines, or vinca alkaloid-induced ileus. Mucositis, local skin reactions, enteritis and proctitis accompanied by radiotherapy also predispose to painful symptoms. Postradiation pain syndromes resulting from radiation fibrosis of the brachial plexus are also a form of cancer pain.

Assessment of cancer pain

The first step for the optimal management of cancer pain is the precise assessment of the pain of which the patient is complaining. Pain assessment[23] includes a detailed history of pain, oncological history, medical history, personal and social history, physical examination, review of medical information or laboratory data, differential diagnosis or therapy, and reassessment. Careful attention should be paid to each to avoid misjudgement.

The approach to the detailed history of pain is an initial evaluation of the pain. After receiving information about the location and number of sites of pain, its type and intensity must be analysed by the physician.

Pain usually consists of three types:[16] somatic, visceral and neuropathic. Metastatic bone pain, postsurgical pain and musculoskeletal pain are somatic. Visceral pain derives from infiltration, compression or extension of the viscera into the thorax or abdomen. Pain resulting from peritonitis carcinomatosa or pancreatic cancer is of the visceral type. In this case the patient sometimes cannot give an accurate location for the pain; the pain is also often accompanied by autonomic dysfunction, such as nausea and vomiting. Neuropathic pain occurs in cases of injury to the peripheral or central nervous system resulting from infiltration or compression of the tumour.

Metastatic- or treatment-induced neuropathies cause pain. These three types of pain sometimes occur in the same patient, and they respond differently to different therapeutic management.

On the whole cancer pain is somatic or visceral. The measurement of the intensity of that pain is also important, but it is very difficult to analyse because pain is a very subjective feeling and depends on the individual patient. According to the report by Tearnan et al,[24] 129 different words were used to describe pain by patients with cancer. Adequate assessment of the intensity of pain is, however, essential for optimal pain control, and to measure this intensity objectively, a validated method should be used. Several assessment instruments have already been established: the McGill Pain Questionnaire,[25] the Memorial Pain Assessment Card[26] and the Wisconsin Brief Pain Questionnaire.[27] These methods can be used by clinicians in the practice setting.

Management of cancer pain

Management of cancer pain can be conducted using two main strategies: one is antineoplastic therapy and the other direct analgesic therapy. The former can provide analgesia if it reduces tumour burden which affects the neural, visceral or skeletal tissues; the latter includes pharmacological management by analgesic medication, regional analgesia or neuroablative procedures.

Antineoplastic therapy
Irradiation to the origin of the pain resulting from cancer involvement is the treatment of choice for most patients with localized pain. According to the report by the Radiation

Therapy Oncology Group (RTOG),[27] 90% of patients with pain caused by solitary or multiple bone metastases experienced some relief of pain through irradiation and 54% eventually achieved complete pain relief. In addition, patients with pain caused by prostate or breast cancer showed complete relief more frequently, compared with those with lung or other primaries. Complete or minimum pain relief occurred in 96% of patients within 2 weeks of the initiation of treatment. This suggests that irradiation is a useful treatment modality for bone pain in breast and other cancers.

Patients with advanced disease who have been exposed to various anticancer drugs in previous treatment sessions might be refractory to chemotherapy, although it could still be the choice in the control of cancer pain if patients had sufficient organ function and relatively good performance status. It should be remembered that breast cancer is sensitive to chemotherapy. When patients are anthracycline naive but refractory to CMF-type regimens, combination regimens containing doxorubicin or epirubicin are worth while trying. If CAF-type regimens are not effective, paclitaxel (Taxol) could be an alternative drug. Paclitaxel[29] is a new drug that is very active against breast cancer; it also overcomes pleiotrophic drug resistance clinically.

Hormonal therapy is also effective for cancer pain caused by breast cancer: the administration of medroxyprogesterone acetate[30,31] was reported to lessen cancer pain in 75–95% of patients.

Pharmacological management
The most common management of cancer pain is pharmacological. In almost 85% of patients[32,33] with cancer, pain can be partially or completely relieved with oral analgesic drugs, including non-opioids, opioids and adjuvant analgesics, such as corticoids, antidepressants or anticonvulsants. The World Health Organization's three-step analgesic ladder[34] portrays the progression in the doses and types of analgesic drugs that are used for optimal management of cancer pain. This is a non-invasive approach, and is also the most recommended

strategy for controlling cancer pain. Until it becomes evident that this approach is not effective, intravenous or subcutaneous administration of these drugs, or alternative modalities such as regional analgesia or neuroablative procedures, should not be chosen.

According to the WHO ladder, aspirin, paracetamol or non-steroidal anti-inflammatory agents (NSAIDs) are the initial analgesic step; these drugs are best for mild-to-moderate pain. If pain relief is obtained, drug administration should continue. If pain persists after reassessment, weak opioids are used for moderate pain, such as codeine, in the second step.

For severe pain not relieved by the above-mentioned drugs, strong opioids should be considered for moderate-to-severe pain, with or without non-opioids and/or adjuvant analgesics. If patients need a strong opioid as the initial therapy as a result of severe cancer pain, it can be given initially for rapid pain relief.

Opioids are the major class of analgesics used for cancer pain that is unmanageable. They produce their analgesic activity via binding to specific receptors. These opioid analgesics include the full agonists (morphine, hydromorphone, codeine, oxycodone, hydrocodone, methadone, levorphanol and fentanyl), partial agonists (buprenorphine etc.), or mixed agonist–antagonist (pentazocine or butorphanol tartrate). Among them morphine is the most commonly used opioid for moderate-to-severe pain because of its availability in a wide range of dosages, various administrative routes, its well-known pharmacology and its cost-effectiveness.

The oral route is the preferred route of administration for morphine. Oral morphine is available in immediate and controlled-release forms (MS Contin, Oramorph). In controlled-release tablets the drug is immediately released on crushing. Such short-acting preparations provide great flexibility for pain control.

Almost 85% of patients[32] with moderate or severe pain can achieve pain control with oral morphine, and adequate prescription of morphine is essential for cancer pain control.

Morphine is classified as a full agonist with no ceiling effect. This drug is best administered on an 'around the clock' schedule for pain control. In addition, oral morphine should be used on a regular schedule rather than only 'as needed'. The dose given should be adjusted for each patient, to find out the best daily dosing requirement for complete pain relief. If the side effects are acceptable, the optimal daily dose for pain relief can reach several hundred milligrams in total.

The addition of adequate adjuvant medication can provide excellent palliation for most patients with cancer pain. These include corticosteroids, anticonvulsants, antidepressants, neuroleptic agents or muscle relaxants. As adjuvant drugs to opioids they enhance their analgesic efficacy and treat concurrent symptoms that exacerbate pain.

Side effects of morphine include constipation, nausea, confusion, sedation and respiratory depression. If constipation or nausea occurs, laxatives or antiemetics should be tried without cessation of morphine. If side effects do not allow the optimal utilization of morphine, changing to a different opioid is quite often successful. Each approximate equianalgesic dose of several oral opioids is: 30 mg every 3–4 hours (for morphine); 90–120 mg every 12 hours (for controlled-release morphine – MS Contin); 7.5 mg every 3–4 hours (for hydromorphone); 4 mg every 6–8 hours (for levorphanol); 20 mg every 6–8 hours (for methadone); 60 mg every 3–4 hours (for codeine); or 10 mg every 3–4 hours (for oxycodone). Transdermal fentanyl is an alternative option.

When there is a need to increase dose requirements to maintain pain relief, this is called 'tolerance'. This term is occasionally confused with psychological dependence. Both are expected with long-term use for pain relief. The confusion sometimes leads to ineffective treatment, so clinicians need to be able to differentiate tolerance from psychological dependence. The addition of adequate adjuvant medication can provide excellent palliation for most patients with cancer pain.

REFERENCES

1. Mitchell EP, Gastrointestinal toxicity of chemotherapeutic agents. *Semin Oncol* 1992; **19**:566–79.
2. Ghaddar H, Fraschini G. Antiemetic therapy. In: *Medical Oncology. A Comprehensive Review* (Pazdur R, ed.). Huntington: PRR, 1993:475–84.
3. Taguchi T, Ogawa M, Izuo M, Terasawa T, Yoshida M, Nakajima M. A prospective randomized trial comparing epirubicin and doxorubicin in advanced or recurrent breast cancer. *Jpn J Cancer Chemother* 1986; **13**:3498–507.
4. Shenkenberg TD, Von Hoff DD. Mitoxantrone: A new anticancer drug with significant clinical activity. *Ann Intern Med* 1986; **105**:67–81.
5. Cortes JE, Pazdur R. Docetaxel. *J Clin Oncol* 1995; **13**:2643–55.
6. Holmes FA, Walters RS, Theriault RL, et al. Phase II trial of taxol, an active drug in the treatment of metastatic breast cancer. *J Natl Cancer Inst* 1991; **83**:1797–805.
7. Weber BL, Vogel C, Jones S, et al. Intravenous vinorelbine as first-line and second-line therapy in advanced breast cancer. *J Clin Oncol* 1995; **13**:2722–30.
8. Nomura Y, Tominaga T, Adachi I, Koyama H, Fukami A. Clinical evaluation of cyclophosphamide, methotrexate and 5-fluorouracil (CMF) on advanced and recurrent breast cancer. *Jpn J Cancer Chemother* 1994; **21**:1949–56.
9. Engelsman E, Klijn JCM, Rubens RD, et al. 'Classical' CMF versus a 3-weekly intravenous schedule in postmenopausal patients with advanced breast cancer. An EORTC Breast Cancer Co-operative Group Phase III Trial (10808). *Eur J Cancer* 1991; **27**:966–70.
10. Cummings FJ, Gelman R, Horton J. Comparison of CAF versus CMFP in metastatic breast cancer: Analysis of prognostic factors. *J Clin Oncol* 1985; **3**:932–40.
11. Smalley RV, Lefante J, Bartolucci A, Carpenter J, Vogel C, Krauss S. A comparison of cyclophosphamide, Adriamycin and 5-fluorouracil (CAF) and cyclophosphamide, methotrexate. 5-fluorouracil, vincristine, and prednisone (CMFVP) in patients with advanced breast cancer. *Breast Cancer Res Treat* 1983; **3**:209–20.
12. Hortobagyi GN, Bodey GP, Buzdar AU, et al. Evaluation of high-dose versus standard FAC chemotherapy for advanced breast cancer in protected environment units: A prospective randomized study. *J Clin Oncol* 1987; **5**:354–64.

13. Tormey DC, Gelman R, Band PR, et al. Comparison of induction chemotherapies for metastatic breast cancer. *Cancer* 1982; **50**:1235–44.

14. Buser KS, Joss RA, Piquet D, et al. Oral ondansetron in the prophylaxis of nausea and vomiting induced by cyclophosphamide, methotrexate and 5-fluorouracil (CMF) in women with breast cancer. Results of a prospective, randomized, double-blind, placebo-controlled study. *Ann Oncol* 1993; **4**:475–9.

15. Jantunen IT, Muhonen TT, Kataja VV, Flander MK, Teerenhovi L. 5-HT$_3$ receptor antagonists in the prophylaxis of acute vomiting induced by moderately emetogenic chemotherapy – A randomized study. *Eur J Cancer* 1993; **29A**:1669–72.

16. Foley KM. Supportive care and the quality of life of the cancer patient. In: *Cancer Principles & Practice of Oncology*, 4th edn (DeVita Jr VT, Hellman S, Rosenberg SA, eds). Philadelphia: JB Lippincott Co., 1993:2417–48.

17. Bonica JJ. Treatment of cancer pain: Current status and future needs. In: *Advances in Pain Research and Therapy* (Field HL, Dubner R, Cervero F, eds). Vol. 9. *Proceedings of the Fourth World Congress on Pain*. New York: Raven Press, 1985:589–616.

18. Levin D, Cleeland CS, Dar R. Public attitudes toward cancer pain. *Cancer* 1982; **56**:2337–9.

19. Cleeland CS, Cleeland LM, Dar R, Rinehardt LC. Factors influencing physician management of cancer pain. *Cancer* 1986; **58**:796–800.

20. Clain A. Secondary malignant disease of bone. *Br J Cancer* 1965; **19**:15–25.

21. Grossman SA, Sheidler VR. Pain. In: *Clinical Oncology* (Abeloff MD, Armitage JO, Lichter AS, Niederhuber JE, eds). New York: Churchill Livingstone, 1995:357–71.

22. Vecht CJ. Arm pain in the patient with breast cancer. *J Pain Sympt Manag* 1990; **5**:109–19.

23. Grossman SA. Cancer pain assessment: a continual challenge. *Support Care Cancer* 1994; **2**:105–10.

24. Tearnan J, Blake II, Cleeland CS. Unaided use of pain descriptors by patients with cancer pain. *J Pain Sympt Manag* 1990; **5**:228–32.

25. Graham C, Bond SS, Gertrovitch MM, Cook MR. Use of the McGill Questionnaire in the management of cancer pain – replicability and consistency. *Pain* 1980; **8**:377–84.

26. Fishman B, Pasternak S, Wallerstein SL, et al. The Memorial Pain Assessment Card: A valid instrument for the assessment of cancer pain. *Cancer* 1986; **60**:1151–7.

27. Baut RL, Cleeland CS, Flanery RC. The development of the Wisconsin Brief Pain Questionnaire to assess pain in cancer and other disease. *Pain* 1983; **17**:197–210.

28. Tong D, Gillick L, Hendrickson, FR. The palliation of symptomatic osseous metastases. Final Results of the study by the Radiation Therapy Oncology Group. *Cancer* 1982; **50**:893–9.

29. Slichenmyer WJ, Von Hoff DD. Taxol: a new and effective anti-cancer drug. *Anti-Cancer Drug* 1991; **2**:519–30.

30. Cavalli F, Goldhirsch A, Jungi F, Martz G, Mermillod B, Alberto P, for the Swiss Group for Clinical Cancer Research. Randomized trial of low-versus high-dose medroxyprogesterone acetate in the induction treatment of postmenopausal patients with advanced breast cancer. *J Clin Oncol* 1984; **2**:414–19.

31. Pannuti F, Martoni A, Lenza GR, Piana E, Nanni P. A possible new approach to the treatment of metastatic breast cancer: Massive doses of medroxyprogesterone acetate. *Cancer Treat Rep* 1978; **62**:499–504.

32. Cleeland CS. The impact of pain in patients with cancer. *Cancer* 1984; **54**:2635–41.

33. Foley KM. The treatment of cancer pain. *N Engl J Med* 1985; **313**:84–5.

34. World Health Organization. *Cancer Pain Relief.* Geneva: WHO, 1986.

15

Two decades of psychosocial research: an overview for the practitioner

Barbara F Rabinowitz

CONTENTS • The dynamics • The interventions

Over the greater part of the twentieth century, more of the research conducted on behalf of the women (now more than 180 000 each year) who develop breast cancer is in the arena of the physiological rather than the psychological. In the past two decades there has been increasing research emphasis as well as clinical reports aimed at expanding our understanding of the social, psychological and sexual impact of breast cancer diagnosis and treatments, as well as interventions that could help to mitigate those effects.

THE DYNAMICS

Emotional issues

Every woman who receives a diagnosis of breast cancer is at some risk for emotional complications.[1-3] Renneker and Cutler were among the earliest to focus attention on the psychological adjustment to breast cancer and encouraged physicians to be sensitive to the emotional adjustment to the diagnosis and to the loss of the breast.[4] This early clinical focus gave way to later research on these topics.[5-11] Research by Taylor et al found a variety of illness and treatment-based psychological problems in the breast cancer population that they studied.[12]

After effects of depression, anxiety and hostility have been described in the clinically based literature.[13-17] There has also been decreased self-esteem[10,15,18,19] and a decreased sense of personal control.[6,15,20] Mood disturbances and more generalized disturbances in quality of life have been found associated with specific physical effects of breast cancer or its treatments such as lymphedema[21] and pain.[22] Researchers have found depression, hostility, hopelessness, denial and alienation in women with breast cancer.[7,23,24] As anticipated, increased mood disturbances have been found among mastectomy patients compared with benign breast biopsy controls.[25-27] Statistically more psychological distress was found for women with mastectomy compared with other groups (healthy, those undergoing cholecystectomy or benign biopsy).[28] Both breast cancer patients and their spouses were found to have poorer psychosocial adjustment than that found in a non-cancer population.[29] Studying women with mastectomy and those with lumpectomy, Fallowfield found both groups to experience 'psychiatric morbidity'.[11] In addition, women may have to cope with a sense of illness and/or treatment-related fatigue, making it difficult to concentrate.[30] It is clear that a great many adjustments have to be faced by those having a diagnosis of breast cancer.[31]

Impact on emotional status is apparently not equally experienced by all. Payne and Massie[32] report a likelihood that 10–25% of all women with breast cancer develop a level of depression that will require treatment. In Royak-Shaler's review, women undergoing surgery for breast cancer were found to show depression twice that of a cancer-free population,[17] whereas others have reported that emotional reactions for women with breast cancer are less like robust psychopathology and more like a strong adjustment reaction.[33] For some as yet not clearly defined subset of women, there does appear to be a spontaneous decrease in preliminarily experienced anxiety and depression.[34]

Researchers have broadened their scope from reaction to the diagnosis and surgery to include investigation of the impact of chemotherapy.[35] Frequently, women receiving chemotherapy report an increase in depression and anxiety.[36] Budin found that those women receiving chemotherapy had significantly more adjustment difficulties and reported more symptom distress.[37] In spite of advances brought forward to control some side effects of chemotherapy, women continue to report a strong negative emotional reaction to hair loss, weight gain, skin changes and other physiological chemotherapy-induced effects.[38] Although some women relate that they are able to continue to feel fairly stable emotionally through this experience, many others report a sense that their lives revolve around chemotherapy treatments and the resultant after effects.

Depression and anxiety are not infrequently found in women receiving radiotherapy.[39] Women often report feeling demoralized as a reaction to the profound fatigue that is a normal effect of radiotherapy. Although skin changes in the radiotherapy target area are generally well controlled, some women find it difficult to manage the thickening and varying degrees of skin discoloration. In circumstances in which tattoos are employed as the marker for the treatment area, many report a period of emotional turmoil at having been 'branded'.

There was early anticipation that patients who underwent breast-conservation therapy (BCT) would experience less negative emotional impact than women receiving modified radical mastectomy (MRM). One research group did report that women who had a lumpectomy were found to be significantly less anxious, less sad, to have less sexual difficulty and to feel more in control of their lives, compared with women who had an MRM.[40] Others, both clinically and empirically, have found no difference between the groups on measures of anxiety, depression and other quality of life indicators.[11,34,41,42] There are reports of some psychological sequelae for both groups.[43–45]

Fear of recurrence is frequently cited by women as a constant companion, especially around the time of annual examinations. Some have described this fear of recurrence as their major concern.[46] It had been hypothesized that women who received MRM would experience less fear than women who underwent BCT, but a recent study did not find this to be the case.[47] Women report with great frequency that all illnesses or minor physical discomforts are first and foremost feared as a sign that their disease has returned. Although there may be some diminution of this focus as years go by, this anxiety-tainted awareness is most often reported as lifelong.

Although there has been great variety to the research regarding emotional sequelae of breast cancer and its treatments, it is important to acknowledge that most studies have been conducted with white women.[48] Little empirically derived information has been presented regarding these issues for women in other ethnic groups. Care should be taken not to presume that findings for one ethnic group are equally applicable to others. In response to this underrepresentation, the National Cancer Institute and other funders of cancer research have added requirements that minority groups be well represented in current and future studies.

Psychosexual issues

Later researchers have added sexual issues to their investigations of the impact of breast cancer.[43,49,50] Understanding of sexual difficulties for the cancer survivor is frequently complicated, because sexual problems are often multiply determined.[51] The cancer, the emotional reactions to the diagnosis and the treatment effects can often interact in a way that decreases sexual feelings.[52] The physical effects of chemotherapy, as well as depression and anxiety, may all impact on the ability of a woman to feel sexually attractive and to relate sexually to her partner.[53] Although underacknowledged by health care providers, recent research has shown that some of the most persistent problems faced by women with breast cancer are those related to sexuality.[43,50] Women often report decreased personal sense of attractiveness, belief that they are no longer attractive to their partner, lessened sexual desire, decrease in frequency of intercourse, and increased difficulty with arousal, lubrication and orgasm. In addition to frank sexual dysfunction, women also note difficulty in talking with their partners about their feelings, their fears and the future. This is unfortunate in the face of the potentially salutary impact of open communication. One recent study reported improved sexual function for those who could share intimate and even frightening feelings.[54]

Some earlier studies showed less negative sexual consequences for BCT patients compared with those with MRM. However, more recent studies have found both groups experiencing similar difficulties.[11,33,55] It has been postulated that the variable of choice has resulted in the more recently reported levelling out of impact on sexuality between the two groups.[56] Schover et al's study of women with BCT compared with women with MRM and immediate reconstruction found equal distribution of sexual problems.[57] As anticipated, research continues to report that women with BCT maintain greater satisfaction with body image.[3,47,58]

There is some evidence of physiological genesis for decreased sexual desire and loss of capacity for orgasm resulting from chemotherapeutically induced diminished ovarian function which causes decreased androgen levels.[59] Women frequently report a significant negative effect of chemotherapy on sexuality.[55,57]

Although women on hormonal treatment with tamoxifen are not reported to experience the problems with lubrication reported by women receiving chemotherapy, which results from the apparent estrogenic effect of tamoxifen, they frequently report that irregular menses, vaginal discharges and vaginal soreness dramatically impact on their sexual function.[60] Sexual problems may not surface immediately and may take 6–24 months to become apparent.[52] Therefore, it should not be expected that sexual difficulties have been avoided if they are not reported in the early stages of recovery.

Longer-term survivor issues

There is variability in longer-term emotional impact for women with breast cancer. One study of quality of life for long-term cancer survivors found generally good psychological status.[61] There were, however, variations in subsets in that study, with some women experiencing ongoing emotional difficulties. Additional studies have found that the emotional impact of cancer does linger for the long-term survivors.[62,63] Polinsky reported that most women in his study noted ongoing physical effects, anxiety, fear, anger and a variety of sexual difficulties.[62] However, women often stop discussing their long-lasting psychological sequelae, fearing that others have tired of hearing of their fears and sadness. When invited to address this, women will often report loneliness and a sense of disconnection from friends and family because they harbor these emotions in secret.

Both chemotherapy and radiotherapy patients were found to have unremitting problems with continuing negative impact on quality of life 2–10 years after treatment.[64] Greater difficulties with stamina were reported by survivors of radiotherapy whereas chemotherapy patients described lingering smell aversions as troublesome. Both groups reported ongoing depression and anxiety. This and other clinical reports are contrary to the frequent expectation that these patients are most often free of ongoing emotional difficulties once treatment is completed.

For some of these longer-term survivors, their fear of recurrence then becomes a reality that they must face. Increased depression with recurrence is frequent.[49,65] Women often report guilt and remorse regarding past treatment decisions, chasms in communication with friends and family regarding the recurrence, additional physical changes and increased emotional distress.[49] Although there is little research to date on psychological sequelae for bone marrow transplant (BMT) survivors, one study of BMT survivors, 6–18 years after treatment for a variety of cancer diagnoses, found that survivors, having transcended the early difficult times, reported the quality of their lives to be the same or better than before BMT.[66] However, that was not true for everyone in the study, with a small group found to be living lives of emotional anguish which included, isolation, unemployment and disability.

Family impact of breast cancer

In addition to the emotional impact on the women with the breast cancer diagnoses, it has become clear that family members are affected emotionally and require support.[9,29,67–70] Partners report the stress of living with uncertainty, the emotional impact of increased home-based roles, decreases in communication, loneliness, confusion about what to tell the children, and guilt about feelings of concern that they have for themselves.[71] Northouse et al. found husbands of women with recurrence to report psychosocial role problems similar to the women with breast cancer, with husbands' role difficulties focused mainly on social/leisure activities and sexuality.[69] A review article regarding the impact of breast cancer on spouses and children clearly makes the point that family members experience emotional distress which includes anxiety, depression and mood swings.[72] Unfortunately, these realities get in the way of the ability of family members to support the woman with breast cancer.

Very little of the available research has been conducted with a focus on single women. One preliminary study found that these women experience more emotional difficulty than their married counterparts and found significant emotional impact on their offspring.[73] Women in the study reported feelings of isolation, more pressure related to their illness and higher levels of depression. Decreased feelings of self-worth and lessened sense of social acceptance were found in their children. Another study of unmarried women reported relatively low levels of psychosocial adjustment problems in the late postoperative recovery phase.[37] Clearly more research is needed on this topic.

In addition to the emerging body of research on quality of life, there is a growing literature based on the impact of psychological status and psychosocial intervention on survival. Social support was found to be a 'significant and independent predictor' of survival in one study.[74] Studying patients with cancer at three different sites, Ell and colleagues found 'emotional support from primary network members to be protective with respect to survival ... at all stages for women with breast cancer'.[75] In a widely reported study, Spiegel et al found significant added survival for women with breast cancer who had received the program-based psychosocial intervention.[76] A review of other studies did not find significance for impact of psychosocial intervention on survival.[77] In their review, Cella and Holland relate that methodological problems continue in research regarding the impact of psychological state on survival.[78] Many have noted the need for further study in this arena.[79–82] Science will have to await future research to break through continuing controversy regarding the impact of psychological status on survival.[83]

THE INTERVENTIONS

Social and professional support

Early and ongoing research has found 'support' to be an important ingredient for healthy living and for recovery from disease.[24,84–89] Support may consist of 'verbal and/or non verbal information or advise, tangible aid, or action that is offered by social intimates or inferred by their presence that has beneficial emotional and behavioral effects on the recipient'.[90] Professional support is defined similarly but is offered by the healthcare provider rather than by social intimate. Patients frequently discuss the importance of support in their recovery process.

There have been a great variety of instruments designed for use in the study of support.[91] In spite of the lack of consistency in instruments employed, there is, nevertheless, a large enough body of literature to offer validity to the impact of this variable on psychosocial recovery for women with breast cancer.

Studying a variety of healthy populations, support was found related to depression,[92,93] anxiety,[94] psychological maladjustment[95,96] and general mental health status.[97] Researchers have found social support to impact significantly on recovery from alcoholism,[98] adaptation to multiple sclerosis,[99] hope and self-esteem for spinal cord-injured patients,[100] adaptation to ostomies[101] and level of functioning for chronic obstructive pulmonary disease patients.[102] Investigating impact of support for cancer patients, Peck and Boland found information/communication support to be important to the overall psychological well-being of radiotherapy patients.[103] Support from the family was found to correlate with less fear and pain for cancer patients.[104] Advanced cancer patients, in one study who underwent group counseling, showed a significant improvement in self-concept.[105] In yet another study, those patients who were found to be interested in receiving more information from their medical team were significantly more hopeful.[106] In a study of women with gynecological cancer, social support was found to have a salutary impact on adjustment.[107]

Some preliminary research has shown an association between social support and survival for women with breast cancer.[24,108] Although there are those who are convinced that there is a strong correlation, others remain unconvinced and there are strong supporters for both sides of the issue.[79,80,83] Although acknowledging progress in psychoneuroimmunology, caution has been forwarded that oversimplification into 'suggestions that cancer can be cured by having the right attitude' should be resisted.[109]

There is strong evidence that support can positively impact on the quality of life. Among the earliest studies, a descriptive retrospective study of 12 mastectomy patients suggested that the extent of emotional problems experienced by the breast cancer patients depended in part on support from friends and family.[110] Mastectomy patients who had received counseling and information from an interdisciplinary team showed increased perceptions of self-efficacy compared with the non-counseled controls.[28] In an outcome study for a support group for metastatic breast cancer patients, the treatment group was found to be less phobic than the control group, to have fewer maladaptive coping mechanisms and to have significantly lower mood disturbance scores.[111] In a number of studies, breast cancer patients who noted their emotional recovery as very good related that they perceived significantly more understanding and emotional support from family and health professionals than those women who did not report good emotional recovery.[6,112,113]

Satisfaction with surgery was found to be enhanced in women who received preoperative information,[114] whereas patients in another study who felt that they received inadequate support related problems in adjustment.[115] Bloom predicted that support would improve the ability of breast cancer patients to adjust and found that to be so.[85] Those patients receiving nurses' counseling showed greater social recovery and better adaptation to their mastectomy.[26] Fewer difficulties with psychosocial adjustment were found for breast cancer patients and their spouses who reported higher levels of support.[29] Perceived or expected social support surfaced as the variable predictor for level of social functioning of post-mastectomy women.[116] One recent study has shown that support has a salutary impact on healthier behaviors.[89] Higher levels of support have been found to be positively associated with lessened anxiety and depression,[117] increased self-esteem and emotional balance.[118] Hoskins reported that emotional adjustment of women with breast cancer could be predicted, in part, based on marital support and support from other adults.[119]

In this still evolving arena of social research, it is important to note that sample size was often small, with populations not consistently well matched for age, social condition and ethnicity. Measures of social support varied as did definition of emotional/psychosocial/psychological/quality of life recovery, although each was usually well defined within the body of each study. Statements about any attempt to control for confounding variables or regarding whether studies were prospective or randomized were often lacking in the earlier research. There does, nevertheless, appear to be worthy clinical and empirical evidence of an interaction between support and psychological recovery for the breast cancer patient.

Importance of physician/patient relationship

The relationship of the physician with the patient is of great importance.[120–122] Trust and confidence in the relationship have been postulated as impacting on women's ability to manage the emotional reaction to the cancer diagnosis.[120] Investigations of the needs of women with breast cancer found that women desired health professionals who showed interest, respect and understanding, and who were committed to 'caring, not only curing'.[113,123] Women report monitoring the quality of the relationship that they have with their physician; they are very sensitive to any nuances, because they feel that their lives are in their doctors' hands.[124] This wish for a quality relationship is not always fulfilled. Eighty-four percent of breast cancer survivors in one study reported difficulties understanding their physicians, expressing themselves to their physicians and asking them questions.[125] In addition, findings from this study suggest that patients' perceptions about communication with their healthcare team had an impact on psychological adjustment. Effort directed to effective communication can help patients to grasp information relayed by the physician, increase patient satisfaction, decrease patient anxiety, foster better compliance with treatment regimens and contribute to improved quality of life for patients.[126] Professional support in one study was found to be positively correlated with how women felt in general and with how they felt about themselves.[127] Although most studies regarding physician/patient relationship have been conducted related to initial diagnosis, both clinical reports and one recent study have noted decreased feelings of comfort with and acceptance by their physicians and nurses after recurrence.[49] It seems clear that patients continue to need the support of healthcare professionals at the time of recurrence as much as they did earlier.

Sense of caring and adequate information are two types of support often cited as vital in the psychosocial recovery of breast cancer patients.[49,122,124,128] Timing of information provision is an important variable because women generally want to know of potential difficulties before they occur.[121] Most patients in one recent study wanted detailed information about the cancer and the treatment plan.[129] Women have reported that, although the diagnosis leaves them feeling out of control, information often helps them regain some sense of that control.[124] Women can experience some emotional relief from the physical symptoms (weight gain, hair loss, pain), changes in intimate and sexual relationships, and in relationships with friends, family and co-workers, as well as changes in how women feel about themselves (self-esteem, self-worth) from a physician who can help to normalize common effects.[62] Spouses also have a need to receive information directly from the physician and may themselves adjust better to their partner's experience when they receive it.[69]

Assessment and referral represent important interventions for physicians regarding patients' psychosocial status. Although it is expected that patients will experience a great range of emotions, it is essential that physicians monitor and evaluate patients for appropriate intervention.[32,124] There are recognized indicators of women who are at greater than average psychological risk. Schover et al recommend psychological screening as a routine for women who report a troubled marital relationship, who feel unattractive and dissatisfied with their sexual relationship, who are less educated or who have undergone chemotherapy.[57] Chemotherapy stands out as a greater risk for sexual difficulty than type of surgery. Others have recommended previous psychiatric problems or poor social support as additional indicants of risk for psychological distress and inquiry should be made about both.[121,130,131] In addition, inquiry should be made regarding number of stressful events within the 5 years previous to the diagnosis, because women with higher numbers of such events are also at greater psychoemotional risk.[132] Although it is not always easy for the physician to differentiate between grief reactions engendered by normal illness and depression, it is essential to refer for evaluation if there is concern.[3,32] Delay is to be avoided and early intervention should be recommended when risks are noted.[41] Bloch and Kissane encourage physicians to include psychosocial care as an 'integral part of good clinical management'.[133]

Assessment and referral activities should include the family[67,72,124] because family members are often experiencing their own emotional reaction and needs for psychosocial support.[70] Medical centers and hospitals often offer support groups for children of cancer patients, for spouses and family members, and for couples. Referral is a meaningful intervention which will often be taken most seriously when provided by a physician; it will often contribute to improved quality of life for the patient and the family.

Intimacy and sexuality appear to be the most neglected of post-diagnosis topics between physicians and patients.[59] What women might expect in this arena should be included in physician/patient pre-treatment discussions. Avoidance of the topic has been postulated as one of the greatest obstacles to sexual rehabilitation for cancer patients.[52] The following have been given as reasons for the avoidance: lack of time, feelings of inadequate background, discomfort caused by the sensitive nature of the topic and insecurity about what actions to recommend. Most of these barriers can be

overcome. Expectations of the amount of time that could be needed are often exaggerated. Recommending books in which the topic is addressed (Table 15.1) presents sexuality in a way that informs the woman that these are issues that may surface, that others have reported and successfully dealt with these issues, and that their physician would be available for more information. It is important that physicians inquire about any sexual difficulties, because patients will most often not introduce the topic. To facilitate this inquiry physicians can be aided by a brief evaluation instrument that is available[52] or questions included in Table 15.2. A listing of professionals who have been trained to work with issues of intimacy and sexuality can be obtained and will help to facilitate appropriate referral (Table 15.3 provides examples of American organizations).

Advocacy is a frequently under-represented physician support activity. Ganz defines physician advocacy as being a 'helper, counselor, or supporter who defends the best interest of the patient'.[122] Physicians could advocate for their patients with other members of the multidisciplinary team, insurers and others with whom patients are in contact during their treatment. Communication with employers on behalf of patients may be a most beneficial form of advocacy through information dissemination, and may help women maintain employment.[121]

Encouraging women to become involved in advocacy organizations, such as the National Breast Cancer Coalition and National Coalition for Cancer Survivorship in the USA, can often help women feel empowered and that they can make a difference – perhaps for themselves, and certainly for others. Encouraging women to reach out to other women who may have previously experienced similar symptoms may be helpful (e.g. Reach to Recovery is an American organization that can be contacted through the American Cancer Society). Likewise, fostering involvement of patients in support groups is important.[62,134] Although such groups provide women with the opportunity to receive meaningful support, not all women wish to take part in group programs.[109] Nevertheless, in the face of the oft-reported social isolation of breast

Table 15.1

Kahane DH, *No Less A Woman: Femininity, Sexuality, and Breast Cancer*. Hunter House, California, 1995

Kaye R, *Spinning Straw Into Gold: Your Emotional Recovery from Breast Cancer*. Simon & Schuster, New York, 1991

Dackman, L, *Upfront: Sex and The Postmastectomy Woman*. Viking Penguin, New York, 1990

Murcia A, Stewart B, *Man to Man: When the Woman You Love Has Breast Cancer*. St Martin's Press, New York, 1990

LaTour K, *The Breast Cancer Companion: From Diagnosis Through Treatment to Recovery: Everything You Need to Know For Every Step Along the Way*. William Morrow & Co., New York, 1993

When The Woman You Love Has Breast Cancer. Y-Me, Chicago, 1995
For Single Women With Breast Cancer. Y-Me, Chicago, 1995

Table 15.2

- Very often women feel some change in their intimate relationship after the breast cancer diagnosis. How has this been for you?
- People frequently feel some change sexually during this time. What have you noticed?
- Speaking to a counselor for a few sessions is often helpful because of the impact of this cancer diagnosis and the treatment on sexuality. Would you like a list of local counselors?

Table 15.3

American Association of Sex Educators, Counselors and Therapists (AASECT), PO Box 238, Mount Vernon, IA 52314-0238
American Association of Marriage and Family Therapists, 1133, 15th Street, North West, Suite 300, Washington, DC 20005

cancer patients,[124,135] encouraging women to attend a few sessions to evaluate the potential benefit for themselves is advice well given.

Physician researchers can make an important contribution by advocating for the inclusion of quality of life measures in all cancer research. The US Food and Drug Administration noted the importance of psychosocial sequelae in its 1985 declaration that quality of life is a 'cancer endpoint' equal in importance to survival.[136] Quality of life measures have even more recently been included in phase II trials.[137–139] Fallowfield calls for monitoring of quality of life as a mandatory part of all clinical trial follow-up;[140] however, up to 1995 only 15% of active trials in one national cooperative group included a quality of life component.[136]

Although some women move through the breast cancer diagnosis and treatment with little apparent emotional impact, more frequently there are at least transitional, and sometimes lifelong, emotional sequelae. Modern medicine is moving quickly to recognize the need for psychosocial support for patients and for 'an integrated approach to caring for the whole person at all stages of illness.'[141]

REFERENCES

1. Miller P. Mastectomy: a review of psychosocial research. *Health Soc Work* 1981; **6**:60–6.
2. Weinstock J. Breast cancer: psychosocial consequences for the patient. *Semin Oncol Nurs* 1991; **17**:207–15.
3. Andersen BL, Doyle-Mirzadeh S. Breast disorders and breast cancer. In: *Psychological Aspects of Women's Health Care: The Interface Between Psychology, Obstetrics and Gynecology* (Stewart DE, Stotland NL, eds). American Psychiatric Press, Inc., Washington D.C. 1993:425–46.
4. Renneker R, Cutler M. Psychological problems of adjustment to cancer of the breast. *JAMA* 1952; **148**:833–8.
5. Worden W, Weisman A. The fallacy in post-mastectomy depression. *Am J Med Sci* 1977; **273**:169–75.
6. Jamison KR, Wellisch DK, Pasnau RO. Psychosocial aspects of mastectomy: the woman's perspective. *Am J Psychiatry* 1978; **135**:432–6.
7. Greer S, Morris T, Pettingale KW. Psychological response to breast cancer: effect on outcome. *Lancet* 1979; **ii**:785–7.
8. Gerard D. Sexual functioning after mastectomy: life vs. lab. *J Sex Marital Ther* 1982; **8**:305–15.
9. Wood J, Tombrink J. Impact of cancer on sexuality and self image: a group program for patients and partners. *Soc Work Health Care* 1983; **8**:45–54.
10. Bloom J, Cook M, Fotopoulis S, et al. Psychological response to mastectomy. *Cancer* 1987; **59**:189–96.
11. Fallowfield LJ. Psychosocial adjustment after treatment for early breast cancer. *Oncology* 1990; **4**:89–97.
12. Taylor SE, Lichtman RR, Wood JV, et al. Illness-related and treatment-related factors in psychological adjustment to breast cancer. *Cancer* 1985; **55**:2506–13.
13. Lewis FM, Bloom JR. Psychosocial adjustment to breast cancer: a review of selected literature. *Int J Psychiatry Med* 1978; **9**:1–17.
14. Holland JC, Mastrovito R. Psychologic adaptation to breast cancer. *Cancer* 1980; **15**:1045–52.
15. Silberfarb PM. Psychiatric problems in breast cancer. *Cancer* 1984; **53**:820–4.
16. Wellisch DK. Implementation of psychosocial services in managing emotional stress. *Cancer* 1984; **53**:828–32.
17. Royak-Schaler R. Psychological processes in breast cancer: a review of selected research. *J Psychosoc Oncol* 1991; **9**:71–89.
18. Polivy J. Psychological effects of mastectomy on a woman's feminine self-concept. *J Nerv Mental Dis* 1977; **164**:77–87.
19. Small EC. Psychosocial issues in breast disease. *Clin Obstet Gynecol* 1982; **25**:447–54.
20. Schain W. Psychological impact of the diagnosis of breast cancer on the patient. In: *Breast Cancer* (Vaeth JM, ed.). Basel: Karger, 1976:68–89.
21. Woods M, Tobin M, Mortimer P. The psychosocial morbidity of breast cancer patients with lymphoedema. *Cancer Nursing* 1995; **18**:467–71.
22. Miaskowski C, Dibble S. The problem of pain in outpatients with breast cancer. *Oncol Nurs Forum* 1995; **22**:791–7.
23. Derogatis LR, Abeloff MD, Melisaratos N. Psychological coping mechanisms and survival time in metastatic cancer. *JAMA* 1979; **242**:1504–8.
24. Funch DP, Marshall J. The role of stress, social support and age in survival from breast cancer. *J Psychosom Res* 1983; **27**(1):77–83.

25. Morris T, Greer HS, White P. Psychosocial and social adjustment to mastectomy: a two year follow-up study. *Cancer* 1977; **40**:2381–7.

26. Maguire P, Brooke M, Tait A, et al. The effect of counseling on physical disability and social recovery after mastectomy. *Clin Oncol* 1983; **9**:319–24.

27. Gottschalk LA, Hoigaard-Martin J. The emotional impact of mastectomy. *Psychiatry Res* 1986; **17**:153–67.

28. Bloom J, Ross R, Burnell G. Effects of social support on patient adjustment after breast surgery. *Patient Counsel Health Educ* 1978; **1**:50–9.

29. Northouse L. Social support in patients' and husbands' adjustment to breast cancer. *Nurs Res* 1988; **37**:91–5.

30. Cimprich B. Attentional fatigue following breast cancer surgery. *Res Nurs Health* 1992; **15**:199–207.

31. Loveys B, Klaich K. Breast cancer: demands of illness. *Oncol Nurs Forum* 1991; **18**:75–80.

32. Payne DK, Massie MJ. Monitor patient's emotional adaptation to breast cancer. *Oncology News Int* 1995; **4**:32.

33. Wolberg WH, Romsaas EP, Tanner MA, et al. Psychosexual adaptation to breast cancer surgery. *Cancer* 1989; **63**:1645–55.

34. Goldberg JA, Scott RN, Davidson PM, et al. Psychological morbidity in the first year after breast surgery. *Eur J Surg Oncol* 1992; **18**:327–31.

35. Jacobsen PB, Bovbjerg DH, Schwartz MD, et al. Conditioned emotional distress in women receiving chemotherapy for breast cancer. *J Consult Clin Psychol* 1995; **63**:108–14.

36. Baider L, Amikam JC, Kaplan De-Nour A. Time-limited thematic group with post-mastectomy patients. *J Psychosom Res* 1984; **28**:323–30.

37. Budin W. The relations among primary treatment alternatives, symptom distress, perceived social support, and psychosocial adjustment to breast cancer in unmarried women. Unpublished Doctoral Dissertation, New York University, 1996.

38. Freedman TG. Social and cultural dimensions of hair loss in women treated for breast cancer. *Cancer Nurs* 1994; **17**:334–41.

39. Evans RL, Connis RT. Comparison of brief group therapies for depressed cancer patients receiving radiation treatment. *Public Health Rep* 1995; **10**:306–11.

40. Kemeny M, Wellisch D, Schain W. Psychosocial outcome in a randomized surgical trial for treatment of primary breast cancer. *Cancer* 1988; **62**:1231–7.

41. Ganz PA, Hirji K, Sim MS, et al. Predicting psychosocial risk in patients with breast cancer. *Med Care* 1993; **31**:419–31.

42. Levy SM, Herberman, RB, Lee JK, et al. Breast conservation versus mastectomy: distress sequelae as a function of choice. *J Clin Oncol* 1989; **7**:367–75.

43. Ganz P, Schag AC, Lee J, et al. Breast conservation versus mastectomy: is there a difference in psychological adjustment or quality of life in the year after surgery? *Cancer* 1992; **69**:1729–38.

44. Pozo C, Carver C, Noriega V, et al. Effects of mastectomy versus lumpectomy on emotional adjustment to breast cancer: a prospective study of the first year postsurgery. *J Clin Oncol* 1992; **10**:1292–8.

45. Omne-Ponten M, Holmberg L, Burns T, et al. Determinants of the psychosocial outcome after operation for breast cancer: results of a prospective comparative interview study following mastectomy and breast conservation. *Eur J Cancer* 1992; **28A**:1062–7.

46. Fredette SL. Breast cancer survivors: concerns and coping. *Cancer Nurs* 1995; **18**:35–46.

47. Lasry JCM, Margolese RG. Fear of recurrence, breast-conserving surgery, and the trade-off hypothesis. *Cancer* 1992; **69**:2111–5.

48. Powell DR. Social and psychological aspects of breast cancer in African–American women. *Ann NY Acad Sci* 1994; **736**:131–9.

49. Mahon SM, Casperson DS. Psychosocial concerns associated with recurrent cancer. *Cancer Pract* 1995; **3**:372–80.

50. Schag CAC, Gans PA, Polinsky ML, et al. Characteristics of women at risk for psychosocial distress in the year after breast cancer. *J Clin Oncol* 1993; **11**:783–93.

51. Welch-McCaffrey D, Hoffman B, Leigh SA, et al. Surviving adult cancers. Part 2: psychosocial implications. *Ann Intern Med* 1989; **111**:517–24.

52. Auchincloss SS. Sexual dysfunction in cancer patients: brief clinical evaluation and treatment guidelines. *Proceedings of the Workshop How Psychosexual Reproductive Issues Affect Patients' Cancer?* American Cancer Society Atlanta, GA, 1987:122–8.

53. Maldonado R. Mastectomy and sexual identity: the reconstruction of self-image. *Trends Health Care Law Ethics* 1995; **10**:45–52.

54. Ghizzani A, Pirtoli L, Bellezza A, et al. The evaluation of some factors influencing the sexual

life of women affected by breast cancer. *J Sex Marital Ther* 1995; **21:**57–63.

55. Wilmoth CM, Townsend J. A comparison of the effects of lumpectomy versus mastectomy on sexual behaviors. *Cancer Pract* 1995; **3:**279–85.

56. Lopchinsky RA, Engel D, Hrycyszhyn H. Effect of choice on the psychologic impact of mastecomy. *Breast Dis* 1992; **5:**259–66.

57. Shover LR, Yetman RJ, Tuason LJ, et al. Partial mastectomy and breast reconstruction. A comparison of their effects on psychosocial adjustment, body image, and sexuality. *Cancer* 1995; **75:**54–64.

58. Mock V. Body image in women treated for breast cancer. *Nurs Res* 1993; **42:**153–7.

59. Kaplan HS. A neglected issue: the sexual side effects of current treatments for breast cancer. *J Sex Marital Ther* 1992; **18:**3–19.

60. Kaplan HS, Owett T. The female androgen deficiency syndrome. *J Sex Marital Ther* 1993; **19:**3–24.

61. Kurtz ME, Wyatt G, Kurtz JC. Psychological and sexual well-being, philosophical/spiritual views, and health habits of long-term cancer survivors. *Health Care Women Int* 1995; **16:**253–62.

62. Polinsky ML. Functional status of long-term breast cancer survivors: demonstrating chronicity. *Health Soc Work* 1994; **19:**165–73.

63. Ferrell BR, Hassay-Dow K, Leigh S, et al. Quality of life in long-term cancer survivors. *Oncol Nurs Forum* 1995; **22:**915–22.

64. Berglund G, Bolund C, Fornander R, Rutqvist LE, Sjoden PO. Late effects of adjuvant chemotherapy and postoperative radiotherapy on quality of life among breast cancer patients. *Eur J Cancer* 1991; **27:**1075–81.

65. Jenkins PL, May VE, Hughes LE. Psychological morbidity associated with local recurrence of breast cancer. *Int J Psychiatry* 1991; **21:**149–55.

66. Haberman M, Bush N, Young K, et al. Quality of life of adult long-term survivors of bone marrow transplantation: a qualitative analysis of narrative data. *Oncol Nurs Forum* 1993; **20:**1545–53.

67. Lewis FM. Strengthening family supports. Cancer and the family. *Cancer* 1990; **65:**752–9.

68. Adler D. Breast cancer in the family: critical issues in adaptation. *Innovations in Breast Cancer Care* 1996; **1:**70–4.

69. Northouse L, Dorris G, Charron-Moore C. Factors affecting couples' adjustment to recurrent breast cancer. *Soc Sci Med* 1995; **41:**69–76.

70. Lewis FM. Balancing our lives: a study of the married couple's experience with breast cancer recurrence. *Oncol Nurs Forum* 1995; **22:**943–53.

71. Vess JD, Moreland JR, Schwebel AI, et al. Psychosocial needs of cancer patients: learning from patients and their spouses. *J Psychosoc Oncol* 1988; **6:**31–51.

72. Northouse LL. The impact of cancer in women on the family. *Cancer Pract* 1995; **3:**134–42.

73. Lewis FM, Zahlis EH, Shands ME, et al. The functioning of single women with breast cancer and their school-aged children. *Cancer Pract* 1996; **4:**15–24.

74. Waxler-Morrison N, Hislop G, Mears B, et al. Effects of social relationships on survival for women with breast cancer: a prospective study. *Soc Sci Med* 1991; **33:**177–83.

75. Ell K, Nishimoto R, Mediansky L, et al. Social relations, social support and survival among patients with cancer. *J Psychosom Res* 1992; **36:**531–41.

76. Spiegel D, Bloom J, Kraemer H, Gottheil E. Effect of psychosocial treatment on survival of patients with metastatic breast cancer. *Lancet* 1989; **ii:**888–91.

77. Gellert G, Maxwell R, Siegel B. Survival of breast cancer patients receiving adjunctive psychosocial support therapy: a ten year follow-up study. *J Clin Oncol* 1993; **11:**66–9.

78. Cella D, Holland J. Methodological considerations in studying the stress-illness connection in women with breast cancer. In *Stress and Breast Cancer* (Cooper CL, ed.). Chichester: John Wiley & Sons, 1988:197–214.

79. LeShan L. A new question in studying psychosocial interventions and cancer. *Advances* 1991; **7:**69–71.

80. Greenwood B. Cancer, conventional medical treatment, and psychosocial effects on healing processes. *Advances* 1992; **8:**2–3.

81. Fox B. LeShan's hypothesis is provocative, but is it plausible? *Advances* 1992; **8:**82–4.

82. Achterberg-Lawlis J. Human research and studying psychosocial interventions for cancer. *Advances* 1992; **8:**2–4.

83. Dreher H. Mind–body research and its detractors. *Advances* 1993; **9:**59–62.

84. House J, Robbins C, Metzner H. The association of social relationships and activities with mortality: prospective evidence from the Tecumseh Community health study. *Am J Epidemiol* 1982; **116:**123–40.

85. Bloom JR. Social support, accommodation to

stress and adjustment to breast cancer. *Soc Sci Med* 1982; **16**:1329–38.

86. Blazer DG. Social support and mortality in an elderly community population. *Am J Epidemiol* 1982; **115**:684–94.

87. Funch DP, Mettlin C. The role of support in relation to recovery from breast surgery. *Soc Sci Med* 1982; **16**:91–8.

88. Nelles W, Blanchard C, McCaffrey R, et al. Social supports and breast cancer: a review. *J Psychosoc Oncol* 1991; **9**:21–34.

89. Franks P, Campbell T, Shields C. Social relationships and health: the relative roles of family functioning and social support. *Soc Sci Med* 1992; **34**:779–88.

90. Gottlieb B. Social networks and social support in community mental health. In: *Social Networks and Social Support*. (Gottlieb B, ed.). Beverly Hills: Sage Publications, 1981:11–42

91. Cohen S, Syme SL. Issues in the study and application of social support. In: *Social Support and Health*. New York: Academic Press, 1985 3–22.

92. Cohen S, Sherrod D, Clark M. Social skills and the stress-protective role of social support. *J Personal Soc Psychol* 1986; **50**:963–73.

93. Lin N, Dean A, Ensel W. Social support scales; a methodological note. *Schizophr Bull* 1981; **7**:73–89.

94. Abbey A, Abramis D, Caplan R. Effects of different sources of social support and social conflict on emotional well-being. *Basic Appl Soc Psychol* 1985; **6**:111–29.

95. Holahan C, Moos R. Social support and psychological distress: a longitudinal analysis. *J Abnormal Psychol* 1981; **90**:365–70.

96. Ross CE, Mirowsky J. Explaining the social patterns of depression: control and problem solving or support and talking. *J Health Soc Behav* 1989; **30**:206–19.

97. Kessler R, McLeod J. Social support and mental health in community samples. In: *Social Support and Health*. New York: Academic Press, 1985 219–40.

98. Booth BM, Russell DW, Soucek S, et al. Social support and outcome of alcoholism treatment: an exploratory analysis. *Am J Drug Alcohol Abuse* 1992; **18**:87–101.

99. Wineman N. Adaptation to multiple sclerosis: the role of social support, functional disability, and perceived uncertainty. *Nurs Res* 1990; **39**:294–9.

100. Piazza D, Holcombe J, Foote A, et al. Hope, social support and self esteem of patients with spinal cord injuries. *J Neurosci Nurs* 1991; **23**:224–30.

101. Rheaume A, Gooding B. Social support, coping strategies, and long term adaptation to ostomy among self-help group members. *J Enterostomal Ther* 1991; **18**:11–15.

102. Lee RN, Graydon JE, Ross E. Effects of psychological well-being, physical status, and social support on oxygen-dependent COPD patients' level of functioning. *Res Nurs Health* 1991; **14**:323–8.

103. Peck A, Boland J. Emotional reactions to radiation treatment. *Cancer* 1977; **40**:180–4.

104. Weidman-Gibbs H, Achterberg-Lawlis J. Spiritual values and death anxiety: implications for counseling with terminal cancer patients. *J Counsel Psychol* 1978; **25**:563–9.

105. Ferlic M, Goldman A, Kennedy BJ. Group counseling in adult patients with advanced cancer. *Cancer* 1979; **43**:760–6.

106. Cassileth BR, Zupkis RV, Sutton-Smith K, et al. Information and participation preferences among cancer patients. *Ann Intern Med* 1980; **92**:832–6.

107. Mishel M, Braden C. Uncertainty: a mediator between support and adjustment. *West J Nurs Res* 1987; **9**:43–57.

108. Morgenstern H, Gellert GA, Walter SD, et al. The impact of a psychological support program on survival with breast cancer: the importance of selection bias in program evaluation. *J Chron Dis* 1984; **37**:273–82.

109. Williams TR, O'Sullivan M, Snodgrass SE, Love N. Psychosocial issues in breast cancer. Helping patients get the support they need. *Postgrad Med* 1995; **98**:97–9, 103–4, 107–8.

110. Ervin Q. Psychologic adjustment to mastectomy. *Med Aspects Human Sex* 1973; **7**:42–61.

111. Bloom J, Spiegel D. The relationship of two dimensions of social support to the psychological well-being and social functioning of women with advanced breast cancer. *Soc Sci Med* 1984; **19**:831–7.

112. Pistrang N, Barker C. The partner relationship in psychological response to breast cancer. *Soc Sci Med* 1995; **40**:789–97.

113. Palsson MBE, Norberg A. Breast cancer patients' experiences of nursing care with the focus on emotional support: the implementation of a nursing intervention. *J Adv Nurs* 1995; **21**:277–85.

114. Dunkel-Schetter C, Wortman C. The interper-

sonal dynamics of cancer: problems in social relationships and their impact on the patient. In: *Interpersonal Issues in Health Care.* (Friedman S, DiMatteo MR, eds.). New York: Academic Press, 1982 69–100.

115. Peters-Golden H. Breast cancer: varied perceptions of social support in the illness experience. *Soc Sci Med* 1982; **16**:483–91.

116. Penman D, Bloom J, Fotopoulis S, et al. *The Impact of Mastectomy on Self-Concept and Social Function: A Combined Cross-Sectional and Longitudinal Study with Comparison Groups. Women's Health,* 1987 **3/4**:101–30.

117. Neuling SJ, Winefield HR. Social support and recovery after surgery for breast cancer: frequency and correlates of supportive behaviors by family, friends, and surgeon. *Soc Sci Med* 1988; **27**:385–92.

118. Dunkel-Schetter C. Social support and coping with cancer. Unpublished Doctoral Dissertation, Northwestern University, 1981.

119. Hoskins CN. Patterns of adjustment among women with breast cancer and their partners. *Psychol Rep* 1995; **77**:1017–8.

120. Barber HR. Psychosocial aspects of chemotherapy. *Loss Grief Care* 1987; **1**:11–18.

121. Bloom JR. Softening the psychological sequelae of mastectomy. *Primary Care Cancer* 1989; 13–16.

122. Ganz PA. Advocating for the woman with breast cancer. *CA Cancer J Clin* 1995; **45**:114–26.

123. Roberts CS, Cox CE, Reintgen DS, et al. Influence of physician communication on newly diagnosed breast patients' psychologic adjustment and decision-making. *Cancer* 1994; **74**:336–41.

124. Spiegel D. Facilitating emotional coping during treatment. *Cancer* 1990; **66**:1422–6.

125. Lerman C, Daly M, Walsh WP, et al. Communication between patients with breast cancer and health care providers. *Cancer* 1993; **72**:2612–20.

126. Siminoff LA. Improving communication with cancer patients. *Oncology(Huntingt)* 1992; **6**:83–7.

127. Rabinowitz B. Measurement of the effect of social/informal and professional/formal support with women receiving treatment for breast cancer. Unpublished Doctoral Dissertation, Rutgers, The State University, 1993.

128. Ganz P. Patient education as a moderator of psychological distress. *J Psychosoc Oncol* 1988; **6**:181–99.

129. Hack TF, Degner LF. Relationship between preferences for decisional control and illness information among women with breast cancer: a quantitative and qualitative analysis. *Soc Sci Med* 1994; **39**:279–89.

130. Glanz K, Lerman C. Psychosocial impact of breast cancer: A critical review. *Ann Behav Med* 1992; **14**:204–12.

131. Rowland JH, Holland JC, Ghaglassian T, Kinne D. Psychological response to breast reconstruction. Expectations for and impact on postmastectomy functioning. *Psychosomatics* 1993; **34**:241–50.

132. Maunsell E, Brisson J, Deschenes L. Psychological distress after initial treatment of breast cancer. Assessment of potential risk factors. *Cancer* 1992; **70**:120–5.

133. Bloch S, Kissane DW. Psychosocial care and breast cancer. *Lancet* 1995; **346**:1114–5.

134. Spiegel D. Commentary. How do you feel about cancer now? – survival and psychosocial support. *Public Health Rep* 1995; **110**:298–300.

135. Muzzin LJ, Anderson NJ, Figueredo AT, Gudelis SO. The experience of cancer. *Soc Sci Med* 1994; **38**:1201–8.

136. Cella D, Bonomi A. Measuring quality of life. In: *Cancer Management: A Multidisciplinary Approach*, vol. 39 (Pazdur R, Boia LR, Hoskins WJ, Wagman LD, eds). 1996:773–87.

137. Seidman AD, Portenoy R, Yao TJ, et al. Quality of life in phase II trials: a study of methodology and predictive value in patients with advanced breast cancer treated with paclitaxel plus granulocyte colony-stimulating factor. *J Natl Cancer Inst* 1995; **87**:1316–22.

138. Dieras V, Marty M, Tubiana N, et al. Phase II randomized study of paclitaxel versus mitomycin in advanced breast cancer. *Semin Oncol* 1995; **22**:33–9.

139. Seidman AD, Hudis CA, Norton L. Memorial Sloan–Kettering Cancer Center experience with paclitaxel in the treatment of breast cancer: from advanced disease to adjuvant therapy. *Semin Oncol* 1995; **22**:3–8.

140. Fallowfield L. Assessment of quality of life in breast cancer. *Acta Oncol* 1995; **34**:689–94.

141. Ashby MA, Kissane DW, Beadle, Rodger A. Psychosocial support, treatment of metastatic disease and palliative care. *Med J Aust* 1996; **164**:43–9.

16

New chemotherapy drugs

Luca Gianni, Giuseppe Capri

CONTENTS • **Tubulin-active drugs** • **Antimetabolites** • **Anthracyclines** • **Conclusions**

For almost three decades after the classic CMF regimen (cyclophosphamide, methotrexate and fluorouracil), the most substantive advance in new chemotherapy drugs for breast cancer treatment was the introduction of doxorubicin and epirubicin.[1] The design of adequate multi-disciplinary strategies, including recent approaches with high-dose and high-density chemotherapy, has allowed full exploitation of the therapeutic potential of that limited set of drugs.

Drug development has been very productive in the last few years, and new cytotoxic agents that may significantly improve current treatment options in women with breast cancer are actively being investigated. Interestingly, a number of the new cytotoxic agents under investigation in breast cancer patients have mechanisms of action that differ from those of the ingredients of CMF or AC (doxorubicin [Adriamycin] and cyclophosphamide), expanding the diversity of intracellular targets and the chance of more substantial therapeutic effects (Fig. 16.1). Available results justify the continuous

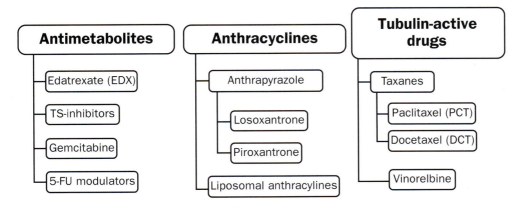

Figure 16.1 Flow chart of the new anticancer drugs for breast cancer.

effort devoted to their development, and their implementation in current treatment strategies for women with breast cancer is a welcome and exciting challenge.[2]

TUBULIN-ACTIVE DRUGS

The taxanes, paclitaxel and docetaxel, and the semisynthetic vinca alkaloid, vinorelbine, disrupt the tubulin microtubule cellular system via different mechanisms, and are the most promising new cytotoxic drugs in breast cancer (Figure 16.1).

Paclitaxel

Preclinical and clinical pharmacology
Paclitaxel is the prototype compound of a new class of antineoplastic drugs which target microtubules. It specifically binds to the β-subunit of tubulin,[3] enhances the polymerization of tubulin monomers and stabilizes tubulin polymers, increasing the fraction of cells in the G_2 or M phase of the cell cycle.[4,5] Phase specificity is consistent with the observation that paclitaxel is more cytotoxic and more potent on long than on short exposure in leukaemia cell lines,[5] and in MCF-7 breast cancer cells.[6] It also indicates a theoretical advantage for using long duration of infusions in humans. However, cell-cycle block is observed in sensitive as well as in resistant cell lines,[5,7] and microtubule bundle and aster formation induced by paclitaxel occurs in human tumour cells regardless of sensitivity to the drug.[7] Induction of apoptosis, a mechanism that has been shown for paclitaxel,[8,9] may give an alternative explanation to cytotoxicity in susceptible cells.

Preclinical pharmacology of paclitaxel clearly demonstrated its involvement in pleiotropic drug resistance.[10,11] Based on this mechanism, clinical cross-resistance should be expected between paclitaxel and other drugs affecting multidrug resistance, most notably the anthracyclines.[12] Also, in this case, preclinical studies indicated that long rather than short duration of exposure was an effective way to overcome

cross-resistance in breast cancer and lymphoma cells.[13] In addition to this common mechanism, resistance to paclitaxel may also arise from specific mutations of tubulin that prevent microtubule stabilization.[14,15] The clinical relevance of this mechanism has yet to be ascertained.

The combination of paclitaxel with other drugs is associated in vitro with cytotoxic synergism or antagonism which depends on the sequence of administration of the taxane and the combined drug. This effect was initially demonstrated for the combination of paclitaxel and cisplatin,[16] and has a precise clinical counterpart in that tolerability of the combination is better when cisplatin is given before paclitaxel than the other way around.[16] Sequence dependency now appears to be a feature that is also common to the use of paclitaxel by infusion over at least 24 hours in combination with anthracyclines, cyclophosphamide and antimetabolites. In all these cases, with the notable exception of the combination with cyclophosphamide, the sequence effect is associated with pharmacokinetic interference.

A clinical observation that has not, as yet, received a mechanistic explanation is that patients with breast cancer over-expressing the human epidermal growth factor receptor 2 (HER2) are more sensitive to treatment with paclitaxel than patients with HER2-negative tumours.[17] Over-expression of HER2 is a feature common to about one-third of patients with breast cancer, and is associated with a poor prognosis.[18] Collateral sensitivity to paclitaxel is a welcome feature in the perspective of exploiting synergism between the taxane and new biological therapy targeted at the HER2, such as the recombinant human monoclonal antibody that targets the protein product of the *HER*2 gene, i.e. p185[HER2].[19]

The clinical pharmacology of paclitaxel has been the subject of extensive investigation aimed at the characterization of its disposition as well as at the definition of pharmacokinetic/ pharmacodynamic relationships. Paclitaxel follows non-linear pharmacokinetics,[20–22] and plasma concentrations can be fitted to a three-compartment model in which non-linearity results from saturable distribution, saturable metabolism and saturable elimination.[22] The non-linear disposition is more pronounced with short infusions. As paclitaxel can safely be administered by a variety of schedules, the effects of non-linearity may have clinical relevance. For any given schedule, dose adjustments may result in plasma concentrations and exposure to the drug that are not proportional to the dose modification. Lack of proportionality entails the risk of excessive toxicity with dose increments, and of unpredictable decrease of anti-tumour activity with dose reductions.[22] As a result of non-linearity, short infusions of paclitaxel are associated with a larger area under the time × concentration curve (area under the curve, AUC) than observed after administration of an identical dose over 24 hours or longer. However, the haematological toxicity of short infusions is lower.[23] This apparent inconsistency results from the fact that a haematological toxicity is linked to the time that paclitaxel spends above a given threshold concentration in plasma.[20,22] The time spent above the threshold concentration for neutropenia with the 3-hour infusion is shorter than with the 24-hour infusion of paclitaxel, thus explaining the lower bone marrow toxicity observed when the drug is infused over 3 hours.[20,22] Duration of exposure above a threshold concentration is possibly relevant to other pharmacological effects of paclitaxel, such as those at different targets of anti-tumour response, so that anti-tumour activity of different infusion schedules of paclitaxel may be different for different tumour types.[22]

Finally, the predominant hepatic elimination of paclitaxel involves the problem of dose adjustments in patients with liver alterations. Reports indicate that plasma disposition of paclitaxel is indeed affected by concomitant liver alterations.[24,25] However, a definite set of guidelines for dose modification in the presence of altered liver function tests has not yet been defined and validated.

Another relevant feature of paclitaxel pharmacology is related to its clinical formulation in Cremophor EL (CEL) (polyoxyl 20 castor oil). The vehicle of paclitaxel plays a major role in triggering hypersensitivity reactions, which sig-

nificantly slowed the pace of the drug in early clinical development.[26] At concentrations that can be reached with a 3-hour infusion of paclitaxel, CEL is a revertant of multidrug resistance.[27] In mice, non-linearity of paclitaxel pharmacokinetics is caused by CEL,[28] and Cremophor also causes the persistence of high plasma concentrations of anthracyclines in mice and humans.[29] This effect may explain why the toxicity of the combination is worse when paclitaxel (for 24 hours) is given before doxorubicin than when in the opposite sequence.[30] The clinical implications of the biological and pharmacokinetic effects of CEL are potentially not minor. Although they are still unclear, it is important to realize that administration of paclitaxel involves the concomitant infusion of another active compound. This is also relevant to the ongoing search and development of analogues of the taxane with better water solubility and no need for formulation in CEL; they may be better tolerated, but they may also lose some of the clinical advantages observed with paclitaxel.

Clinical results

Major hypersensitivity reactions during the early clinical development of paclitaxel prompted the concomitant routine use of prophylactic medication with antihistamines and glucocorticoids, and of infusions over 24 hours.[31] After premedication alone was proved effective and sufficient to prevent serious hypersensitivity reactions,[23] paclitaxel was tested using various schedules. The choice between paclitaxel infusions over 1, 3, 24, 96 and 120 hours every 3 weeks[32–35] is now largely based on the potentially different therapeutic merits of each schedule. As already discussed, efficacy should be better with longer infusion, as supported by the phase specificity of the drug. However, for the time being, an 'optimal' therapeutic schedule of paclitaxel has not been defined, and is possibly different in different tumour types.[36]

The toxicity of paclitaxel has been thoroughly investigated and described[4] (Table 16.1). With premedication, serious hypersensitivity reactions may occur in about 1–2% of patients, and are no longer viewed as a limiting factor for the use of the drug.[23,31] Of note, infusions of paclitaxel over 72, 96 or 120 hours do not require premedication at all.[26,35,37] Neutropenia, peripheral neuropathy and stomatitis, which are the more common clinical side effects of the taxane, are also schedule dependent. Severe neutropenia is typically brief, rarely associated with thrombocytopenia, and less frequent with 3-hour than with 24-hour infusions,[23] although it limits the dose of paclitaxel to 120–140 mg/m² with infusions of 72–120 hours[26,35,37] compared with the maximum tolerated dose of 250 mg/m² defined for the 3- and 24-hour infusion.[38,39] A reversible, dose-dependent and cumulative peripheral neuropathy[4,40] is also schedule dependent and more severe with the 3-hour than the 24-hour infusion schedule.[38] The latter feature has been attributed to the larger AUC achieved with the shorter infusion schedule.[38]

Two neurological signs associated with short infusion of paclitaxel deserve special mention. The drug administration is often associated with pruritus, which often has a palmar and plantar distribution and may be very disturb-ing. In addition, scotomata and loss of visual acuity have been reported.[39,41] The reversibility of these neuro-optic manifestations is still uncertain and should be carefully investigated in view of the planned and ongoing use of the drug in adjuvant and neoadjuvant trials in breast cancer. Original reports of paclitaxel-induced cardiac toxicity[4,42] have more recently found a distinct ultrastructural counterpart,[43] but initial concerns are now discounted as a result of the non-malignant and asymptomatic nature of the cardiac effects of single-agent paclitaxel. Nausea and vomiting are not frequent and rarely require the use of antiemetics, probably because of the glucocorticoids used for premedication. Finally, a reversible paclitaxel-induced total body alopecia is common to all schedules.

Paclitaxel is one of the most active anti-tumour agents currently available to women with breast cancer, and responses have been reported in all disease sites.[4] Table 16.2 shows that response rates for paclitaxel ranged from about 60% to about 20%.[25,33,34,44–59] The large variability may depend in part on the different

---

Table 16.1 Main toxicities of paclitaxel

- Hypersensitivity reactions (type I) (1–2.3% severe with premedication):
  Probably caused by Cremophor EL; premedication with H_1 or H_2-receptor blockers and steroids required with short–intermediate duration of infusion (1–24 hours), but not with long infusion (≥72 hours)

- Neutropenia (40–70% at <500 ANC/µl):
  Dose limiting; short lived; reversible
  Schedule dependent (more pronounced with infusion ≥24 hours)

- Peripheral neuropathy (20–40% at grade II or III):
  Reversible, dose dependent and *cumulative*
  Schedule dependent (more pronounced with 3- than with 24-hour infusion)

- Stomatitis/mucositis (0–10% at grade II or III):

ANC, absolute neutrophil count.

doses and schedules used in different trials. However, differences in host tolerability, tumour characteristics and number of sessions and type of prior chemotherapy also have a major impact on the probability of response. The anti-tumour efficacy of the drug is lower in more heavily pre-treated patients, indicating some degree of cross-resistance with conventional chemotherapy (Table 16.2). In view of the widespread use of doxorubicin and epirubicin for all stages of breast cancer, it is important to note that paclitaxel still induced major objective responses in 20–40% of women who failed prior treatment with anthracyclines.[34,46,47,51–53,60] As mentioned above, preclinical pharmacology indicated that long rather than short infusions should be used in anthracycline-resistant patients. However, lack of complete clinical cross-resistance between anthracyclines and paclitaxel was observed with 3-, 24- and 96-hour infusions of the taxane.[34,39,45] Interestingly, the responses observed with the 96-hour infusion were independent of the expression of the multidrug resistance phenotype,[34] suggesting

Table 16.2 Efficacy of paclitaxel given by different doses and infusion durations in women with different prior number and type of treatment for metastatic breast cancer

Reference	n	Prior therapy for stage IV	Dose (mg/m2)	Infusion (h)	G-CSF	OR (%)	CR (%)	OR in anthracycline resistant (%)
Reichman[44]	26	No	250	24	Yes	62	12	
Seidman[45]	25	1	250	24	Yes	44	0	
Holmes[46]	25	1	250	24	No	56	12	33
Seidman[45]	51	≥2	200	24	Yes	28	0	
Abrams[47]	172	≥2	135–175	24	No	23	2	24
Davidson[48]	26	No	225	3	No	54	0	
Seidman[49]	25	No	250	3	No	32	4	
Bishop[50]	50	No	200	3	No	31	0	
Bonneterre[51]	101	No	225	3	No	44	6	44
Gianni[52]	50	1	175–225	3	No	38	14	37
Nabholtz[53]	236	1	135	3	No	22	2	13
Nabholtz[53]	235	1	175	3	No	29	5	26
Geyer[54]	74	1	210	3	No	18	3	
Riccio[55]	28	1	140–200	3	No	36	4	
Seidman[49]	24	≥2	175	3	No	21	0	
Vermorken[25]	33	≥2	250–300	3	Yes	6	0	
Greco[33]	17	≥2	135	1	No	35	0	
Wilson[34]	33	≥2	140	96	No	48	0	50
Seidman[56]	26	1	120–140	96	No	27	0	27

n, number; G-CSF, granulocyte colony-stimulating factor; OR, overall response; CR, complete response; anthracycline resistance as indicated in the original reference.

that clinical resistance to anthracyclines and subsequent response to paclitaxel are not necessarily influenced by this mechanism.

A clear definition of the best infusion duration in women with breast cancer should also take into account that paclitaxel over 96 hours has shown activity in patients resistant to the taxane given by either the 3-hour or the 24-hour schedule,[61,62] even though another study did not support the finding.[63] An ongoing study comparing 3- versus 96-hour infusion at similarly tolerable doses will provide an answer about the role of exposure duration on anti-tumour efficacy in breast cancer patients.[64] Finally, paclitaxel can be administered at high intensity on days 1 and 8 every 3 weeks at a maximum dose of $350 \, \text{mg/m}^2$ cycle with high response rate (64%), but increased severity of neurotoxicity (L Gianni, unpublished results). In a second and still ongoing study, paclitaxel is being administered twice weekly.[65] In summary, paclitaxel used as a single agent in metastatic breast cancer is active at all doses and all schedules. The probability of response is lower in pre-treated patients, but efficacy is maintained in women with anthracycline-resistant tumours. A number of randomized trials are now ongoing to define the dose–response relationship of paclitaxel in breast cancer, to assess its optimal dose and schedule, and to compare its activity and safety profile with other anticancer agents (for a review see the literature[66]). At the present time, until these aspects can be clarified, there is no clear indication that paclitaxel should be used at doses higher than $175 \, \text{mg/m}^2$ every 3 weeks. In addition, the short infusion over 3 or even 1 hour can be conveniently given as an outpatient procedure and is safe, and there is no solid criticism to challenge its widespread use.

The very good anti-tumour response in metastatic breast cancer has justified the conduct of a growing number of studies of paclitaxel combined with several other anticancer agents.[67–89] Tables 16.3 and 16.4 summarize the most relevant of these studies. As mentioned above, the use of paclitaxel in combination is complicated by the need to ascertain the effect of sequence of administration on tolerability.

The combination of paclitaxel and doxorubicin has been the focus of several pilot studies aimed at exploiting the high therapeutic potential of the two drugs[46,67–78,90–92] (Table 16.3). In four reported studies, the trial design was different with regard to the duration of paclitaxel and doxorubicin infusion. The study conducted at the National Cancer Institute (NCI) used a simultaneous 72-hour infusion of the two drugs and did not address the question of the effect of sequence on the tolerability of the combination. Neutropenia, typhlitis and thrombocytopenia were the dose-limiting toxicities.[67] At the MD Anderson Cancer Center, paclitaxel was used by 24-hour and doxorubicin by 48-hour infusion. In this study, the sequence of paclitaxel followed by doxorubicin was significantly more toxic than the opposite sequence.[90,93] The more toxic sequence was also associated with significantly higher doxorubicin and doxorubicinol concentrations than the opposite sequence,[30] thus establishing a pharmacokinetic rationale for the observed difference of tolerability.

The Eastern Cooperative Oncology Group (ECOG) study also used a 24-hour infusion of paclitaxel whereas doxorubicin was given by intravenous bolus.[69] Also, in this case, the sequence of paclitaxel followed by doxorubicin was more toxic than the opposite sequence. To define a combination regimen that could be used as an outpatient procedure, the National Cancer Institute of Milan designed a study in which doxorubicin was given by bolus 15 minutes before the start or after the end of paclitaxel given over 3 hours.[70,91] The order of drug administration was found to have no effect on the tolerability of the combination. The latter study showed a very high level of anti-tumour activity (94% major response; 41% complete response), as well as a high incidence of cardiac toxicity (20%). These results may be caused by therapeutic and toxic synergism between paclitaxel and doxorubicin. Indeed, a pharmacokinetic interference between doxorubicin and paclitaxel leads to increased plasma concentrations of the anthracycline.[30,94] As mentioned above, this effect can be caused by Cremophor EL.[29] The exposure of tumour and myocardial

Table 16.3 Efficacy of paclitaxel/anthracycline combinations in women previously untreated for metastatic breast cancer

Reference	n	Anthracycline treatment		Paclitaxel treatment				OR (%)	CR (%)
		Dose (mg/m²)	Infusion (h)	Dose (mg/m²)	Infusion (h)	G-CSF	Sequence effect		
Fisherman[67]	39	60	72	180	72	Yes	NA	72	8
Buzdar[68]	31	48–60	48	125–150	24	Yes	Yes	64	6
Sledge[69]	12	75	Bolus	200	24	Yes	NA	58	25
Sledge[69]	12	50–60	Bolus	150–175	24	Yes	Yes	42	17
Gianni[70]	32	60	Bolus	125–200	3	No	No	94	41
Dombernowsky[71]	29	50–60	0.50	155–200	3	No	NA	83	24
Frassinetti[72]	25	50	Bolus	130–250	3	No	NA	79	32
Schwartsmann[73]	25	60	Bolus	250	3	Yes	NA	80	28
Cazap[74]	27	60	Bolus	200	3	No	NA	48	4
Catimel[75]	25	Epi 50–60	Bolus	110–250	3	No	NA	44	
Conte[76]	18	Epi 90	Bolus	135–225	3	No	NA	83	17
Luck[77]	41	Epi 60	1	175–225	3	No	NA	68	17
Di Costanzo[78]	23	MTZ 10–14	Bolus	175	3	No	NA	65	17

G-CSF, granulocyte colony-stimulating factor; OR, overall response; CR, complete response; Epi, epirubicin; MTZ, mitozantrone; NA, not assessed.

Table 16.4 Efficacy of paclitaxel in combination with anticancer drugs other than anthracyclines in women with metastatic breast cancer

| Author | n | Prior therapy for stage IV | Combined drug | Paclitaxel treatment | | | | |
				Dose (mg/m²)	Infusion (h)	OR (%)	CR (%)	G-CSF
Wasserheit (as cited in Tolcher[79])	41	No	CDDP	200	24	49	12	Yes
Browne (as cited in Tolcher[79])	15	No	CDDP	135	24	53	13	No
Gelmon[80]	27	No	CDDP	90	3	85	11	No
Sparano[81]	14	No	CDDP	90	3	21		No
McCaskill-Stevens[82]	25	No	CDDP	90	3	60	12	No
Tolcher[83]	42	2	CTX	160	72	55	2	Yes
Kennedy[84]	34	1	CTX	135–200	24	29	6	Yes
Murad[85]	22	≥2	IFX	175	3	50	9	No
Klaassen[86]	35	1–2	5FU, LV	135–175	3	19	8	No
Paul[87]	34	33%	5FU, LV	175	3	62	9	No
Nicholson[88]	34	33%	5FU, LV	175	3	62	9	No
Hainsworth[89]	45	36%	5FU, LV, MTZ	135	1	51	4	No

CDDP, cisplatin; CTX, cyclophosphamide; 5FU, 5-fluorouracil; LV, folinic acid (leucovorin); MTZ, mitozantrone; see Table 16.3 for other abbreviations; IFX, ifosfamide.

cells to higher anthracycline concentrations than would be expected in the absence of paclitaxel could explain, in simple quantitative terms, the anti-tumour activity and the incidence of cardiac toxicity of that trial.[70] As the efficacy of paclitaxel and doxorubicin given as a 72-hour infusion was of the order of 70% and no cardiac toxicity was reported in patients with previously untreated metastatic breast cancer,[67] the results of the Milan study may be the consequence of the schedule of infusion of doxorubicin and paclitaxel rather than of their combination and their doses. The very good response rate and high incidence of cardiac effects of the combination designed by the Milan group were confirmed by another study that used similar doses and schedules of doxorubicin and paclitaxel.[71] The two studies cannot address the question of whether the high response rate may also significantly increase the time to treatment failure and overall survival of patients with metastatic breast cancer. These data will be made available by ongoing multicentre trials of the combination now being performed by the Southwest Oncology Group (SWOG) and ECOG in the USA. In the latter trial, dexroxazone was to be added to decrease the incidence of cardiac events. In an attempt to optimize the combination according to in vitro observations, doxorubicin and paclitaxel were administered in sequence with an interval of 16 hours with high anti-tumour activity and no clinical cardiac toxicity.[72] Other studies have adopted epirubicin to decrease the incidence of cardiac events, and preliminary results confirm the general impression that the combination of paclitaxel and anthracyclines is very active (Table 16.3).

Other combinations of paclitaxel are at a more preliminary stage[78–89] (Table 16.4), with the exception of those trials addressing the feasibility and efficacy of the use of paclitaxel and cisplatin.[79–82] A study in which the two drugs were administered twice weekly showed good anti-tumour activity (85%) in patients who had all received prior anthracyclines.[80] The reported efficacy has prompted other investigators to design similar combinations that would offer significant palliation for women who already failed prior therapy with anthracyclines. These second-generation studies (Table 16.4) gave generally poorer results in terms of anti-tumour efficacy, and consistently reported a high incidence of neurological toxicity, with asthenia and fatigue often being limiting.[79] The possibility that the anti-tumour activity observed with two-weekly cisplatin and paclitaxel resulted from the frequent administration of the taxane rather than from the synergistic effects of the combined use of cisplatin is now being tested.[65]

The anti-tumour activity of paclitaxel, its novel mechanism of action and its good tolerability have justified its incorporation into adjuvant or neoadjuvant regimens. The Cancer and Leukemia Group B (CALGB) has randomized patients to receive paclitaxel single agent (175 mg/m^2) for four cycles or no treatment after an initial randomization to three different doses of doxorubicin and cyclophosphamide. At Memorial Sloan Kettering Cancer Center, based on the feasibility and encouraging preliminary results of the rapid sequential administration of doxorubicin and high-dose cyclophosphamide in patients with resectable stage II/III breast cancer and four or more involved axillary lymph nodes,[95] paclitaxel (250 mg/m^2 over 24 hours of infusion) was incorporated for three cycles after doxorubicin and before or concomitant with high-dose cyclophosphamide in regimens for women with breast cancer of similar risk category.[96] Finally,

the very promising results reported with use of the combination of paclitaxel over 3 hours of infusion and bolus doxorubicin[70] has motivated an ongoing trial in which patients with primary breast cancer of diameter larger than 2 cm are randomized to receive adjuvant doxorubicin for four cycles followed by CMF, or adjuvant doxorubicin plus paclitaxel followed by CMF, or to the same paclitaxel-containing regimen administered as primary chemotherapy.[2]

The many studies now ongoing and soon to be designed will provide important answers about the optimal use of paclitaxel as a single agent and in combination, and about its actual merits in the treatment of women with different stages of breast cancer.

Docetaxel

Preclinical and clinical pharmacology

Docetaxel is a semisynthetic analogue of paclitaxel with a higher affinity for microtubules, higher intracellular accumulation and higher anti-tumour potency.[97–99] Docetaxel and paclitaxel have the same mechanism of action, and have similar in vitro cytotoxicity. However, preclinical studies showed that cross-resistance between the analogue and paclitaxel is not complete.[97,100] As reviewed by Arbuck and Blaylock,[101] docetaxel is a phase-specific drug that blocks cells in the M phase of the cell cycle. This would suggest that it should be used by schedules that allow for prolonged exposure, as also indicated by experiments with tumour cells in vitro.[102] However, the tolerability in mice was schedule independent.[103] An important difference of the pharmacology of docetaxel in respect of paclitaxel is that the analogue follows linear pharmacokinetics in mice. As non-linearity of paclitaxel pharmacokinetics in mice has been attributed to Cremophor,[28] this important difference between the two analogues could be the result of their different formulation. In humans, docetaxel disposition can be described by a three-compartment model that is independent of dose and schedule of administration.[104] The large population analysis of this report has shown that docetaxel clearance is significantly related to age, body surface area, plasma protein levels and liver enzymes.[104] In addition, the study indicated that the risk of grade IV neutropenia is strongly related to a slow clearance of docetaxel.[104] This very important pharmacological study could be used for individualizing the dose of docetaxel, and has already been used to justify dose reductions in the presence of altered liver function.

Clinical studies

Phase I trials of docetaxel tested a more limited set of schedules than in the case of paclitaxel, and found that neutropenia, mucositis and skin reactions were the dose-limiting toxicities.[105–110] Table 16.5 is a compilation of the toxicity profiles of docetaxel from the studies available in the literature. The maximum tolerated dose was defined in a range of 80–115 mg/m², confirming in humans that tolerability of the new taxane was schedule independent, as reported in mice.[103]

Docetaxel is formulated in polysorbate 80 instead of Cremophor. The different vehicle of the clinical formulation led to the expectation that premedication would not be required, as it is for paclitaxel because of the Cremophor vehicle. However, acute hypersensitivity reactions were noted in about 30% of patients during phase I and phase II trials, even though the occurrence of serious reactions was lower (about 2%) than that reported with paclitaxel. The observation raises the possibility that acute reactions with administration of paclitaxel and docetaxel are actually the result of the taxane structure itself, even though a causative role for polysorbate 80 cannot be ruled out in the case of docetaxel. The reactions have also justified the use of routine premedication with antihistamine and glucocorticoids,[111,112] or with glucocorticoids alone.[113]

The most frequent dose-limiting toxicity of docetaxel was neutropenia, which was of grade IV severity in about 70–80% of patients, and led

---

Table 16.5 Main toxicities of docetaxel

- Hypersensitivity reactions (type I) (2% severe without premedication):
  Premedication with steroids and/or H_1- and H_2-receptor blockers required

- Neutropenia (70–80% at <500 ANC/µl):
  Dose limiting; short lived; reversible

- Peripheral neuropathy (6–10% at grade II or III):
  Reversible, generally milder than with paclitaxel

- Stomatitis (10–20% at grade II or III)

- Skin and nail toxicity (10–12% at grade III)

- Fluid retention (capillary leak syndrome?):
  Cumulative, dose dependent, limiting normal life
  50% risk after median 400 mg/m² without premedication, 800 mg/m² with premedication
  Slowly reversible, responsive to diuretics

ANC, absolute neutrophil count.

to frequent episodes of febrile neutropenia and infection. Other toxicities caused by docetaxel were peripheral neuropathy, similar to that caused by paclitaxel but less frequent and less severe, stomatitis and total body alopecia. Two other toxicities are unique to docetaxel and unusual. The taxane causes a syndrome of fluid retention which was noted in the phase I trials; it is common in about 50% of patients, as noted from the collected phase II experience in breast cancer patients.[111–115] This syndrome is characterized by oedema (localized, pulmonary, peripheral or generalized) which can be associated with weight gain and pleural effusions in about 20% of patients. Its appearance is related to the cumulative administered dose of docetaxel. Fluid retention is observed in 50% of patients after a total dose of docetaxel 400 mg/m². However, the use of dexamethasone 8 mg orally or equivalent doses of other glucocorticoids for eight administrations, starting one day before and ending 2 days after docetaxel, delays the onset of the syndrome so

that the risk of fluid retention is about 50% after 800 mg/m² of the drug.[113] Fluid retention is not life threatening, but has an impact on the quality of life of patients by limiting their ability to cope with daily chores, and causes treatment discontinuation in as many as 20% of cases. For this reason, the toxicity may represent a problem for the prolonged use of docetaxel, as it may be sought in responding patients with metastatic breast cancer. Finally, a skin and nail toxicity characterized by generalized erythroderma, erythrodisestesia and onycholysis (of grade II and III severity) is also unique to the analogue in as many as 10% of patients.[116]

The development of docetaxel in breast cancer is at an earlier stage than that of paclitaxel. The drug has been used at 100 mg/m² over one hour of infusion every 3 weeks, and showed very good anti-tumour activity. Table 16.6 summarizes the results of several trials.[112,113,115–120] It is especially attractive that docetaxel has a high efficacy not only in previously untreated patients, but also in women who already failed

Table 16.6 Efficacy of single-agent docetaxel in women with metastatic breast cancer

Reference	n	Prior therapy for stage IV	Prior anthracycline (n)	Docetaxel dose (mg/m²)	OR (%)	CR (%)	OR in anthracycline resistant (%)
Ravdin[113]	35	Yes	35	100	57	9	54
Valero[115]	34	Yes	34	100	53		53
Trudeau[112]	32	No		100	63	9	
Trudeau[112]	15	No		75	40	6	
Chevallier[114]	31	No	10	100	68	16	
ten Bokkel[116]	32	Yes	22	100	53	6	
Dieras[117]	34	No		75	50	15	
Trandafir[118]	224	Yes	224	70–100	19		28
Valero[119]	26	Yes	26	100	11	4	
Fumoleau[120]	37	No	21	100	68	5	

n, number; OR, overall response; CR, complete response.

one or more lines of chemotherapy (Table 16.6). In addition, the response rate and the quality of response were similar for all sites of metastatic dissemination, including liver and lung metastases. Of note, all trials consistently indicated that clinical resistance to anthracyclines, often defined as progression while receiving treatment,[115] did not appear to influence the probability of response (Table 16.6). In a small trial, Valero et al[119] also reported three major responses (one complete) in 26 patients who already failed prior anthracycline as well as paclitaxel treatment.[119] Although this observation can indicate the lack of complete cross-resistance between the two taxanes, it should also be noted that paclitaxel is recommended at doses that are far from the maximum tolerated dose (MTD), whereas docetaxel is mostly used at a near-MTD dose. Response to docetaxel in patients progressing after paclitaxel can therefore be the result of a dose–response effect for taxanes rather than of lack of cross-resistance between the two drugs.

The same consideration should also be kept in mind when evaluating the reported overall anti-tumour activity of docetaxel in breast cancer, which is remarkable and apparently superior to that of paclitaxel. At the recommended dose (100 mg/m² by infusion over 1 hour every 3 weeks), docetaxel causes bone marrow toxicity so frequent and severe as to make the design of combination regimens difficult. In two trials, toxicity concerns justified protocol amendments to deliver a dose of docetaxel of 75 mg/m².[111,112] Results were still very good (Table 16.6). However, a larger experience of the actual dose–response relationship in breast cancer patients would be appropriate in order to define the optimal therapeutic potential of this analogue.

Based on their activity as single agents, combination regimens of docetaxel with doxorubicin,[121] epirubicin and cyclophosphamide,[122] and vinorelbine[123] are now in progress. Initial results indicate the need for a substantial decrease in the dose of docetaxel when used together with doxorubicin.[121] The concern about the incidence of severe toxicities has not been cleared up based on available preliminary

results (88% of grade IV neutropenia and 15% of patients with febrile neutropenia require hospitalization).

Vinorelbine

Preclinical and clinical pharmacology

Vinorelbine is a semisynthetic vinca alkaloid which is also the first analogue of its family to bear a chemical substitution on the catharanthine ring, rather than on the vindoline portion of the molecule.[124] The reaction of vinorelbine with tubulin is similar to that of other vinca alkaloids, and causes microtubule depolymerization while blocking their formation.[125] In this respect, the action of vinorelbine and the other vinca alkaloids is opposite to that of the taxanes. A detailed investigation of the interaction with microtubules showed that, among all vinca alkaloids, vinorelbine had the weakest affinity for axonal microtubules, while maintaining a very strong affinity for spindle tubulin.[126] This led to the expectation that the new alkaloid had a higher therapeutic index and was less neurotoxic. Similar to other vincas, vinorelbine is also involved in glycoprotein P-related multidrug resistance.[127] In vitro, resistance may also arise from alterations in α- and β-tubulin proteins causing decreased drug binding or resistance to microtubule disassembly.[128]

The plasma disposition of vinorelbine has been thoroughly investigated in a series of studies conducted with newer analytical techniques which no longer depend on measurements of total blood or plasma radioactivity after injection of the radiolabelled drug.[129–132] The metabolism of vinorelbine is predominantly hepatic; the drug disappears from plasma with a triphasic decay, has a high total body clearance that approaches hepatic blood flow, and a terminal half-life of about 20–30 hours.[129–132] Vinorelbine is very lipophilic and absorbed by the oral route, but the formulation of powder-filled capsules, which were of clinically proven utility, was abandoned because of excessive risk to workers during the manufacturing process.[129] A recent characterization of the absorption of vinorelbine as a liquid-filled, soft gelatin capsule indicated that oral administration is associated with a large first-pass effect, average absorption of about 27% and moderate intraindividual variability.[129] The renewed availability of an oral formulation widens the clinical applicability of this anti-cancer agent.

In a series of phase I studies the recommended dose of vinorelbine has been defined at 30 mg/m[2] per week by slow intravenous administration. Other schedules, such as prolonged intravenous infusion, have also been tested.[133,134] The recommended oral dose with the new formulation is 100 mg/m[2] per week.[129] Table 16.7 has been compiled from the literature giving the main toxicities of the new vinca analogue. The drug is a mild vesicant, and local phlebitis or pain at the infusion site can occur in about 20–30% of patients.[135] Common to all schedules, the dose-limiting toxicity of vinorelbine is haematological. Myelosuppression is usually not cumulative and is mainly characterized by neutropenia.[136] This effect often limits the possibility of maintaining the planned weekly interval between administrations, and recent reports suggest the more feasible regimen of vinorelbine on days 1 and 8 of a 3-week cycle.[136] The other common toxicity of vinorelbine is neurological, characterized by paraesthesias and hyperaesthesias.[135] As predicted by the lower affinity for axonal microtubules, vinorelbine is less neurotoxic than other vinca compounds, with severe symptoms occurring in only about 2% of patients after protracted therapy. Constipation is common, but paralytic ileus is a rare occurrence. Stomatitis, nausea and vomiting, and constipation are the most common gastrointestinal side effects, and are usually more pronounced with the oral formulation.[129] An uncommon toxicity is pain of unspecified aetiology, and chest pain that can be associated with electrocardiographic changes consistent with ischaemia.[135] Importantly, the drug causes alopecia in only about 12% of patients.

Clinical studies

The clinical results of vinorelbine are impressive and suggest that this agent is the most important vinca alkaloid developed for several solid tumours, including breast cancer. Such favourable impression comes from the combination of its anti-tumour efficacy, manageable toxicity, low neurotoxic potential and feasibility for oral administration. Efficacy in breast cancer has been extensively investigated, and it is consistently in the range of 30–40% (Table 16.8).[134,136–150] Although efficacy is higher in patients treated with vinorelbine as first-line chemotherapy for stage IV disease (Table 16.8), significant anti-tumour activity has also been reported in women who had received and failed prior chemotherapy for metastastatic disease.[136,137,141] An important clue to the latter investigations, which showed an overall response rate of about 25–30%, is the demonstration that vinorelbine was not cross-resistant with CMF, and was also active in women who had prior exposure to anthracyclines or even clear-cut resistance to doxorubicin.[136,151] In addition, a recent trial showed that patients who failed treatment with paclitaxel were still responsive to vinorelbine and vice versa.[136] As

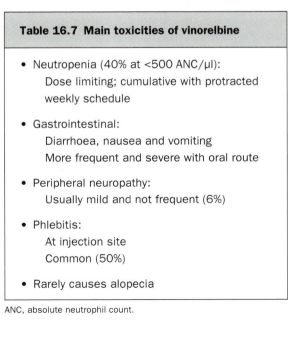

Table 16.7 Main toxicities of vinorelbine

- Neutropenia (40% at <500 ANC/µl):
  Dose limiting; cumulative with protracted weekly schedule

- Gastrointestinal:
  Diarrhoea, nausea and vomiting
  More frequent and severe with oral route

- Peripheral neuropathy:
  Usually mild and not frequent (6%)

- Phlebitis:
  At injection site
  Common (50%)

- Rarely causes alopecia

ANC, absolute neutrophil count.

vinorelbine is a phase-specific drug, an important attempt at increasing therapeutic efficacy is that of using prolonged infusion schedules. The results of a phase I/II trial indicated good activity (36%) in previously treated breast cancer patients, although the increased therapeutic index of this modality of administration was not conclusively shown in the report.[134]

A selected series of the most active combinations incorporating vinorelbine for breast cancer patients is shown in Table 16.9.[152–161] Efficacy of about 70% was commonly observed when the combinations were used as first treatment for stage IV disease. Of note, combinations with doxorubicin also produced very good overall and complete response rate in patients who failed prior adjuvant therapy containing anthracyclines.[158,160] In spite of the large body of evidence in favour of vinorelbine use in breast cancer, there is still no information on its use as adjuvant or neoadjuvant chemotherapy in earlier stages of the disease, a direction that was indicated recently and would indeed appear justified.[162]

ANTIMETABOLITES

Antimetabolites comprise chemotherapeutic agents that are traditionally employed in treatment of breast cancer, such as the antifolate methotrexate and the pyrimidine analogue 5-fluorouracil (5FU). Extensive research has identified several new analogues of these agents. In breast cancer, the new antifolate edatrexate and the deoxycytidine analogue gemcitabine are the ones with more promising preliminary results. New selective thymidylate

---

Table 16.8 Efficacy of vinorelbine by different schedules in women with stage IV breast cancer with different prior therapy

Reference	n	Prior therapy (n)			Dose (mg/m²)	Schedule	OR (%)	CR (%)
		Stage IV	Adjuvant	Anthracyclines				
Weber[137]	60	No	46	No	30	Weekly	35	15
Weber[137]	47	46	NA	NA	30	Weekly	32	6
Romero[138]	44	No	22	19	30	Weekly	41	7
Garcia-Conde[139]	50	No	33	27	30	Weekly	50	2
Fumoleau[140]	145	No	62	42	30	Weekly	41	7
Gasparini[141]	67	50	NA	30	20–25	Weekly	36	4
Vogel[142]	39	No	NA	20	30	Weekly	32	
Ranuzzi[143]	34	No	NA	24	25	Weekly	47	9
Degardin[144]	100	100	NA	100	30	Weekly	16	1
Toussaint[134]	30	30	NA	27	5.5–10	96 h	32	
Toussaint[134]	34	No	34	Yes	5.5–10	96 h	40	
Winer[145]	52	No	NA	NA	50–80	Oral	29	6
Spicer[146]	96	96		Yes	80–100	Oral	11	

n, number; OR, overall response; CR, complete response; NA, not assessed.

Table 16.9 Efficacy of vinorelbine in different combinations for metastatic breast cancer

Reference	n	Stage IV	Adjuvant	Anthracyclines	VNB dose (mg/m²)	Combined drug/dose (mg/m²)	Schedule	OR (%)	CR (%)
				Prior therapy					
Spielmann[160]	89	No	27	20	25	DOX/50	Days 1, 8	74	21
Hochster[152]	50	No	20	No	25	DOX/50	Days 1, 8	54	12
Ferrero[153]	37	No	14	12	25	MTZ/12	Days 1, 8	51	13
Kayitalire[154]	25	Yes	Yes	25	25	MTZ/10–12	Days 1, 8	36	
Scheithauer[155]	34	34		14	30	MTC/15	Days 1, 21	35	6
Dieras[156]	67	No	40	34	30	5FU/750 × 5	Days 1, 5	67	16
Norris[157]	267	Yes	Yes	No	25	DOX/50	Days 1, 8	35	
Costa[158]	22	No			25	DOX/25 days 1, 8	Days 1, 8	82	14
Leone[159]	43	No			35	IFO/2000 × 3	Days 1, 15	58	14

OR, overall response; CR, complete response; VNB, vinorelbine; DOX, doxorubicin; MTZ, mitozantrone; MTC, mitomycin C; 5FU, 5-fluorouracil; IFO, ifosfamide.

synthase inhibitors are still at a very early phase of development in breast cancer. The new possibility of modulating 5FU disposition and absorption with co-administration of ethinyluracil can open unsuspected new applications of this old drug in all sensitive tumours, including breast cancer.

Edatrexate

Edatrexate is an analogue that has the same mechanism of action as methotrexate.[163] It enters cells via the reduced folate carrier and is subsequently polyglutamated and retained intracellularly. Uptake and retention of edatrexate are superior to those of methotrexate in tumour cell lines, but not in normal tissues,[164] providing a rationale for an improved therapeutic index. The pharmacokinetic and toxicology profile of edatrexate in animals is similar to those of methotrexate.[165] However, important preclinical differences were reported. Even though the superiority of high-dose methotrexate over conventional doses has often been disputed, the use of edatrexate with folinic acid rescue proved to be far better than the same schedule of methotrexate against several metastatic solid tumours.[166] Another important feature emerging from preclinical evaluations is that edatrexate has synergistic cytotoxicity in combination with vinca alkaloids,[167] cisplatin[168] and paclitaxel.[169]

Phase I trials have defined a recommended dose of 80 mg/m^2 weekly or 100 mg/m^2 weekly for 3 weeks followed by a 2-week rest period.[170,171] The toxicity of edatrexate in humans is similar to that of methotrexate, with the relevant difference that the dose-limiting toxicity is stomatitis or generalized mucositis, which can be lethal in its more severe form associated with diarrhoea.

Three studies involving 101 patients reported significant anti-tumour efficacy of edatrexate in women with breast cancer (20–40%).[172–174] These studies confirmed the good bone marrow tolerability of edatrexate, but also showed that it is difficult to maintain the planned dose intensity of the weekly schedule, mainly because of mucositis. Combination regimens were planned, based on the reported results. In one combination study, edatrexate was administered before paclitaxel and has shown very promising activity mostly in pre-treated patients.[169] Given the better therapeutic index that emerged from preclinical studies and the good activity reported in the as yet limited experience in women with breast cancer, it is not unreasonable to consider the introduction of edatrexate in place of methotrexate in new as well as in established regimens, even though the superiority of the analogue should be assessed in a direct randomized comparison.

Gemcitabine

This is a fluorine-substituted analogue of deoxycytidine which has a very manageable toxicity profile.[175] Like cytarabine (cytosine arabinoside or Ara-C), it is activated by deoxycytidine kinase, for which it has a greater affinity than cytarabine.[176] Its lesser susceptibility to deamination and greater membrane permeability determine the prolonged maintenance of high intracellular levels.[177] Its mechanism of action involves the interference at different levels of the physiological cellular machinery,[178] which results in apoptosis in susceptible cells.[179,180] Once incorporated into DNA, it interferes with chain elongation. Furthermore, the triphosphate form also inhibits DNA polymerases, whereas the diphosphate is an inhibitor of ribonucleotide reductase.[175] This effect causes a reduction of the intracellular pools of the natural competing substrate deoxycytidine triphosphate.[181]

Gemcitabine was found to be active against a wide range of tumour cell lines.[182] Relevant to clinical application is the potent radiosensitizing effect observed in HT-29 cells.[183] Gemcitabine pharmacokinetics have been explored in several species including humans. A very important aspect of its disposition is that the drug is not protein bound, rapidly distributes into all body spaces and is largely excreted into the urine (about 80%) within 24 hours of administration.

Two important aspects of the early clinical evaluation of gemcitabine deserve attention, and have been reviewed concisely elsewhere.[184] Most phase II studies identified the recommended dose at 800 mg/m^2 in a 30-minute infusion weekly for 3 of every 4 weeks. However, less heavily pre-treated patients can tolerate much larger doses, and gemcitabine 1200 mg/m^2 is now recommended in previously untreated patients. The other important aspect was the observation that gemcitabine is cleared from the plasma 40% faster in men than in women.[185] This will require a reassessment of the toxicity data from initial studies which did not consider sex as a variable in their evaluation. Although the schedule indicated above is commonly used in most clinical investigations, the finding that formation of the active metabolite is saturable is renewing interest in schedules of prolonged infusion.[186]

The dose-limiting toxicity of gemcitabine is neutropenia.[184] Other toxicities are fatigue, 'flu-like symptoms and elevation of liver transaminases. Overall, the toxicity profile is that of a drug that can be combined easily into polychemotherapy regimens.

The above discussion about preclinical and clinical pharmacology is directly relevant to the two studies performed in breast cancer patients.[187,188] In the first, gemcitabine was used in pre-treated patients at relatively low doses (800 mg/m^2), even though the sex of the patients would discount the possibility of under-treatment. In this trial, in which only half the patients had already received chemotherapy for metastatic breast cancer, the response rate was 25%.[187] In another study of previously untreated patients gemcitabine at 1200 mg/m^2 induced a 46% response rate in women who had at most received prior adjuvant chemotherapy.[188] These studies support the validity of further exploitation of the use of gemcitabine in breast cancer, in view of the manageability of administration, the possible synergism with other drugs of proven efficacy, such as paclitaxel, and the attractive feature of exploiting another mechanism of tumour cytotoxicity which could result in modulation of the effects of other antimetabolites.

Ethinyluracil

5-Fluorouracil is a standard component of many chemotherapy regimens for breast cancer. Modulation of 5FU activity is actively pursued by concomitant use of folinic acid for full inhibition of thymidylate synthase. Another approach that may be as effective is that of protracted infusion of 5FU over several weeks to exploit the phase and cycle specificity of the drug. This approach can actually salvage patients who failed prior rapid administration regimens containing 5FU.[189] Another way of modulating 5FU is that of inhibiting dehydropyrimidine dehydrogenase (DPD), the rate-limiting enzyme responsible for drug catabolism and for about 80% of its total body clearance.[190,191] Ethinyluracil is such an inhibitor and has just completed phase I and pharmacological evaluation.[192–194] At doses that are completely non-toxic, it fully inhibits the catabolism of 5FU. Inhibition of catabolism not only decreases interpatient variability, it also significantly decreases, by a factor of 10–20, the total body clearance of 5FU, so the terminal half-life of the drug is about 5 hours in the presence of the inhibitor compared with about 10 minutes in its absence. The dose of 5FU must therefore be decreased accordingly. In addition to this dramatic pharmacokinetic effect, inhibition of catabolism may be an effective means of overcoming 5FU resistance. Indeed, responses were observed during phase I trials in patients who had failed prior 5FU therapy.[194] In addition, the drug availability after oral administration becomes complete in the presence of ethinyluracil. At an oral dose of 5FU 1.3 mg/m^2 for 28 days, in combination with ethinyluracil 10 mg twice a day, plasma concentrations of the antimetabolite are similar to those measured after continuous intravenous infusion of 5FU at 300 mg/m^2 per day. The use of the DPD inhibitor thus provides an alternative way of administering chronic fluorouracil reliably. The ease of such an approach would finally make it possible to explore fully the theoretical advantage of continuous 5FU therapy in women with breast cancer, and studies in this direction are ongoing.

ANTHRACYCLINES

The pivotal role of doxorubicin and epirubicin in the treatment of breast cancer, as well as in several other solid tumours and haematological malignancies, has justified extensive research for new analogues capable of inducing a similarly high response in the absence of the limiting cardiac toxicity of the classic anthracyclines. In spite of years of research and the testing of hundreds of compounds in preclinical studies and many in clinical evaluations, new and better anthracyclines are still missing. Of note in the case of breast cancer is the development of the anthrapyrazole losoxantrone which could have a better therapeutic index than the classic anthracyclines. In addition, doxorubicin formulated in liposomes may allow for a better exploitation of its substantial efficacy, as recently reviewed by Smith and Henderson.[195]

Losoxantrone

Losoxantrone is an anthrapyrazole with high efficacy in breast cancer patients. Anthrapyrazoles are a series of new agents synthesized in the attempt to overcome the cardiotoxic effects of classic anthracyclines resulting from their free radical-generating properties. This goal was achieved by modification of the structure of the chromophore, so that formation of semiquinone radicals is significantly reduced with respect to doxorubicin.[196] Three different anthrapyrazoles were selected for clinical development: teloxantrone, piroxantrone and losoxantrone. The first two showed modest anti-tumour effects while displaying a pattern of toxicity that discouraged their further evaluation. Of note, piroxantrone was cardiotoxic, and devoid of significant anti-tumour efficacy when tested in some patients with breast cancer.[196] Losoxantrone has been more extensively studied because of its favourable toxicity profile and the good activity reported in three phase II studies in breast cancer.[197,198] This anthrapyrazole causes dose-limiting neutropenia in 50–70% of patients, with a 4% incidence of febrile neutropenia at the maximum tolerated

dose of 55 mg/m². Alopecia and nausea appeared to be of a lesser degree than with comparable doses of doxorubicin. In women with metastatic disease and little or no prior exposure to chemotherapy, the response rate varied from 43% to 63%, whereas in women previously treated for metastatic breast cancer the reported efficacy was 35%.[197,198] According to the reported investigations, the cardiotoxic potential of losoxantrone is lower than that of the classic anthracyclines.[196] In summary, losoxantrone appears to be a very active new drug with potential use in breast cancer patients. Efficacy is similar to that of doxorubicin. The full pattern of toxicity and cardiotoxic potential requires extensive evaluation, even though so far the development of this new and potentially important anthracycline analogue has not been as expeditious as the preliminary data would have justified. It is especially interesting that losoxantrone is now being tested in combination with paclitaxel to assess whether similarly good therapeutic results could be achieved without causing the increased cardiac toxicity described for the combination of the taxane with doxorubicin.[199]

CONCLUSIONS

Pharmacological research in the past 5–10 years has provided an unprecedented wealth of new drugs for breast cancer patients. This comes at a time when the field of breast cancer treatment is rapidly evolving. New multidisciplinary approaches using high-dose, high-density or high-intensity chemotherapy for high-risk patients are becoming commonly accepted, if not as yet standard, treatment. Novel classes of 'biological' therapy such as monoclonal antibodies, tumour vaccines and gene therapy modalities are now moving into the early phase of clinical evaluation. New tumour tissue rather than tumour cell targets, such as neovascularization, have been identified and stimulated intensive preclinical research which is now providing clinicians with new classes of drugs. These different research leads will be competing for the human and economic resources of the clinical research community. The wide and somewhat sudden availability of new chemotherapy drugs calls, now more than ever before, for the definition of a precise strategy for their clinical development.

The classic approach to the development of new cytotoxic drugs in any neoplastic disease calls for definition of the toxicity profile, assessment of the optimal schedule of administration, evaluation of efficacy as single agents in patients pre-treated with chemotherapy and, in specific cases such as breast cancer, evaluation of efficacy after failure of the most active available conventional drug(s). This initial approach is followed by comparative studies to define the therapeutic advantage of the new drug over established treatments for the investigated disease. Finally, a similar approach of non-comparative and comparative studies is requested for potentially useful combinations of the new drugs that are needed before such combinations are adopted in those early stages of disease in which a maximum therapeutic advantage could be exploited. The full application of such a strategy for all new compounds is clearly very difficult, if not impossible, in any single neoplastic disease. This difficulty calls for the definition of alternative ways of investigating newly available drugs. Definition of such an alternative strategy is beyond the scope of a single chapter. However, some specific goals in the development of the new chemotherapy drugs described above can be of use.

The clinical results of paclitaxel and docetaxel clearly indicate that these taxanes represent a major addition to the treatment options for breast cancer. The incorporation of these drugs in combination regimens for breast cancer is an obvious goal for exploiting their full activity in the initial therapy of metastatic breast cancer, as well as in programmes of adjuvant or neoadjuvant chemotherapy. While this type of investigation is in progress, it is clear that the comparative role of the two drugs requires definite clarification. Comparison of results from phase II studies is always biased. In the case of the two taxanes, the bias is not only the result of the difficulty of comparing selection criteria, host tolerability and disease

extent, but also of the fact that the drugs have some apparent intrinsic differences. The toxicity and anti-tumour activity of paclitaxel are dose and schedule dependent, and the optimal dose and schedules have not as yet been defined.[36] Schedule dependency was not shown for docetaxel. For this reason docetaxel was consistently used at full therapeutic doses in most trials. However, it should be noted that its anti-tumour activity was observed with administration of doses that are very close to the maximum tolerated one. The key point is a definite clarification of the respective role and therapeutic index of the two taxanes. Such clarification requires prospective evaluation in a randomized study, in which the two drugs are used at doses and schedules that cause comparable toxicity. Such a trial is now ongoing in the USA. Another important aspect for both taxanes is the definition of the durability of therapeutic results in women with metastatic breast cancer, for whom the major therapeutic objective is palliation, which may require chronic treatment. Available data from phase II trials do not allow for conclusions about this important aspect because the usually small size of the patient populations, the bias of their selection and the lack of homogeneity of subsequent therapies prevent a meaningful analysis of overall survival and, quite often, of disease-free survival itself. Finally, it appears that the high toxicity associated with the best combinations of paclitaxel (e.g. doxorubicin for cardio-toxicity) calls for their use as induction therapy for a limited number of cycles (four to six) before other types of chemotherapy or other means of treatment to avoid long-term effects, especially in women who will receive the treatment as adjuvant or neoadjuvant chemotherapy for operable breast cancer.

The data available for use of vinorelbine in breast cancer reflect a somewhat uncertain development design, so that promising results indeed reflect the ingenuity of individual investigators rather than fitting into a general plan of development. A novel regimen that is generating much interest incorporates vinorelbine and paclitaxel.[200] The appealing feature of such a combination is that of disposing of a total microtubule toxin. Although their sequential administration is antagonistic, concurrent administration of vinorelbine and paclitaxel achieves synergistic cytotoxicity against MCF-7 and MDA-MB-231 breast cancer cells in vitro. Experiments have confirmed the synergism in vivo while demonstrating the feasibility of the combination in mice bearing P388 murine leukaemia cells.[201] Attempts to combine the two drugs are still at a preliminary stage.

Given the traditional role of antimetabolites and anthracyclines in the treatment of breast cancer, special emphasis should be given to studies evaluating new analogues of these classes. The difficulty of assessing the role of new analogues is multiple as a result of the high probability that the analogues are forcibly tested on patients already treated with the prototype drug who could possibly be resistant. In this case, rapid evaluation of the analogue should be performed in previously untreated patients to be able to test the new drug alone or in combination against conventional treatment containing the prototype drug. In this respect, the approach for evaluating the feasibility and efficacy of losoxantrone in combination with paclitaxel appears to be well planned and possibly capable of overcoming the usual slow progress of evaluation. Similar approaches are being followed in the case of edatrexate.

Other and probably better responses will be found through the ingenuity of investigators who face the unprecedented and fascinating challenge of defining the therapeutic role of a number of new drugs and new classes of drugs which could significantly change and improve the current treatment options in women with breast cancer.

REFERENCES

1. Henderson IC. Chemotherapy for metastatic disease. In: *Breast Diseases*, 2nd edn. (Harris JR, Hellman S, Henderson IC, Kinne DW, eds). Philadelphia: JB Lippincott Co., 1991:604–65.
2. Bonadonna G. Current and future trends in the multidisciplinary approach for high-risk breast cancer. The experience of the Milan Cancer Institute. *Eur J Cancer* 1996; **32A**:209–14.
3. Rao S, Krauss NE, Heerding JM, et al. 3'-(p-Azidobezamido)taxol photolabels the N-terminal 31 amino acids of β-tubulin. *J Biol Chem* 1994; **269**:3132–4.
4. Rowinsky EK, Donehower RC. Drug therapy: paclitaxel (Taxol). *N Engl J Med* 1995; **332**:1004–14.
5. Rowinsky EK, Donehower RC, Jones RJ, et al. Microtubule changes and cytotoxicity in leukemic cell lines treated with taxol. *Cancer Res* 1988; **48**:4093–100.
6. Capri G, Tarenzi E, Fulfaro F, et al. The role of taxanes in the treatment of breast cancer. *Semin Oncol* 1995; **23**: (suppl 2):68–75.
7. Roberts JR, Allison DC, Dooley WC, et al. Effects of taxol on cell cycle traverse: Taxol induced polyploidization as a marker for drug resistance. *Cancer Res* 1990; **50**:710–16.
8. Bhalla K, Ibrado AM, Tourkina E, et al. Taxol induces internucleosomal DNA fragmentation associated with programmed cell death in human myeloid leukemia cells. *Leukemia* 1993; **7**:563–8.
9. Gangemi RMR, Tiso M, Marchetti C, et al. Taxol cytotoxicity on human leukemia cell lines is a function of their susceptibility to programmed cell death. *Cancer Chemother Pharmacol* 1995; **36**:385–92.
10. Podda S, Ward M, Himelstein A, et al. Transfer and expression of the human multiple drug resistance gene into live mice. *Proc Natl Acad Sci USA* 1992; **89**:9676–80.
11. Perez RP, Hamilton TC, Ozols RF, et al. Mechanisms and modulation of resistance to chemotherapy in ovarian cancer. *Cancer* 1993; **71**:1571–80.
12. Hahn SM, Liebmann JE, Cook J, et al. Taxol in combination with doxorubicin or etoposide. Possible antagonism in vitro. *Cancer* 1993; **72**:2705–11.
13. Zhan Z, Kang Y-K, Regis J, et al. Taxol resistance: in vitro and in vivo studies in breast cancer and lymphoma [abstract]. *Proc Annu Meet Am Assoc Cancer Res* 1993; **34**:215.
14. Schibler MJ, Cabral F. Taxol-dependent mutants of Chinese hamster ovary cells with alterations in α- and β-tubulin. *J Cell Biol* 1986; **102**:1522–31.
15. Cabral F, Abraham I, Gottesman MM. Isolation of a Taxol-resistant Chinese hamster ovary cell mutant that has an alteration in α-tubulin. *Proc Natl Acad Sci USA* 1981; **78**:4388–91.
16. Rowinsky EK, Gilbert MR, McGuire WP, et al.

Sequence of taxol and cisplatin: a Phase I and pharmacologic study. *J Clin Oncol* 1991; **9:** 1692–703.

17. Seidman AD, Baselga J, Yao T-Y, et al. HER2-/*neu* over-expression and clinical taxane sensitivity: a multivariate analysis in patients with metastatic breast cancer [abstract]. *Proc Annu Meet Am Soc Clin Oncol* 1996; **15:**104.

18. Seshadri R, Firgaira FA, Horsfall DJ, et al. Clinical significance of HER-2/neu oncogene amplification in primary breast cancer. The South Australian Breast Cancer Study Group. *J Clin Oncol* 1993; **11:**1936–42.

19. Baselga J, Tripathy D, Mendelsohn J, et al. Phase II study of weekly intravenous recombinant humanized Anti-p185[HER2] monoclonal antibody in patients with HER2/*neu*-overexpressing metastatic breast cancer. *J Clin Oncol* 1996; **14:**737–44.

20. Huizing MT, Keung AC, Rosing H, et al. Pharmacokinetics of paclitaxel and metabolites in a randomized comparative study in platinum-pretreated ovarian cancer patients. *J Clin Oncol* 1993; **11:**2127–35.

21. Sonnichsen DS, Hurwitz CA, Pratt CB, et al. Saturable pharmacokinetics and paclitaxel pharmacodynamics in children with solid tumors. *J Clin Oncol* 1994; **12:**532–8.

22. Gianni L, Kearns CM, Giani A, et al. Nonlinear pharmacokinetics and metabolism of paclitaxel and its pharmacokinetic/pharmacodynamic relationships in humans. *J Clin Oncol* 1995; **13:** 180–90.

23. Eisenhauer EA, ten Bokkel Huinink W, Swenerton KD, et al. European-Canadian randomized trial of taxol in relapsed ovarian cancer: high vs. low dose and long vs. short infusion. *J Clin Oncol* 1994; **12:**2654–66.

24. Egorin M, Venook A, Jahan T, et al. Plasma pharmacokinetics and biliary excretion of paclitaxel in patients with hepatic dysfunction [abstract]. *Ann Oncol* 1994; **5** (suppl 5):196.

25. Vermorken JB, ten Bokkel Huinink WW, Mandjes IA, et al. High-dose paclitaxel with granulocyte colony-stimulating factor in patients with advanced breast cancer refractory to anthracycline therapy: a European Cancer Center trial. *Semin Oncol* 1995; **22:**16–22.

26. Weiss RB, Donehower RC, Wiernik PH, et al. Hypersensitivity reactions from taxol. *J Clin Oncol* 1990; **8:**1263–8.

27. Chervinsky DS, Brecher ML, Hoelcle MJ. Cremophor-EL enhances taxol efficacy in a multi-drug resistant C1300 neuroblastoma cell line. *Anticancer Res* 1993; **13:**93–6.

28. Sparreboom A, van Tellingen O, Nooijen WJ, et al. Nonlinear pharmacokinetics of paclitaxel in mice results from the pharmaceutical vehicle Cremophor EL. *Cancer Res* 1996; **56:**2112–15.

29. Millward LK, Cosson EJ, Stokes KH, et al. Cremophor EL changes the pharmacokinetics of doxorubicin [abstract]. *Proc Annu Meet Am Assoc Cancer Res* 1995; **36:**373.

30. Holmes FA, Madden T, Newman RA, et al. Sequence-dependent alteration of doxorubicin pharmacokinetics by paclitaxel in a Phase I study of paclitaxel and doxorubicin in patients with metastatic breast cancer. *J Clin Oncol* 1996; **14:**2713–21.

31. Fisherman J, McCabe M, Hillig M, et al. Phase I of taxol and doxorubicin with G-CSF in previously untreated metastatic breast cancer [abstract]. *Proc Annu Meet Am Soc Clin Oncol* 1992; **11:**54.

32. Hainsworth JD, Greco FA. Paclitaxel administered by 1-hour infusion. Preliminary results of a phase I/II trial comparing two schedules. *Cancer* 1994; **74:**1377–82.

33. Greco FA, Hainsworth JD. One-hour paclitaxel infusion schedules: a phase I/II comparative trial. *Semin Oncol* 1995; **22:**118–23.

34. Wilson WH, Berg SL, Bryant G, et al. Paclitaxel in doxorubicin-refractory or mitoxantrone-refractory breast cancer: a Phase I/II trial of 96-hour infusion. *J Clin Oncol* 1994; **12:**1621–9.

35. Spriggs DR, Tondini C. Taxol administered as a 120 hour infusion. *Invest New Drugs* 1992; **10:** 275–8.

36. Gianni L. Theoretical and practical aspects of paclitaxel scheduling [Editorial]. *Ann Oncol* 1995; **6:**861–3.

37. Wilson WH, Berg S, Kang YK, et al. Phase I/II study of taxol 96-hour infusion in refractory lymphoma and breast cancer: pharmacodynamics and analysis of multi-drug resistance (mdr-1) [abstract]. *Proc Annu Meet Am Soc Clin Oncol* 1993; **12:**134.

38. Schiller JH, Storer B, Tutsch K, et al. Phase I trial of 3-hour infusion of paclitaxel with or without granulocyte colony-stimulating factor in patients with advanced cancer [see comments]. *J Clin Oncol* 1994; **12:**241–8.

39. Gianni L, Munzone E, Capri G, et al. Paclitaxel in metastatic breast cancer: A trial of two doses by 3-hour infusion in patients with disease recurrence after prior therapy with anthracyclines. *J Natl Cancer Inst* 1995; **87:**1169–75.

40. Rowinsky EK, McGuire WP, Guarnieri T, et al. Cardiac disturbances during the administration of taxol. *J Clin Oncol* 1991; **9**:1704–12.

41. Capri G, Munzone E, Tarenzi E, et al. Optic nerve disturbances: a new form of paclitaxel neurotoxicity. *J Natl Cancer Inst* 1994; **86:** 1099–101.

42. Rowinsky EK, Chaudhry V, Cornblath DR, et al. Neurotoxicity of taxol. *Monogr Natl Cancer Inst* 1993; **15**:107–15.

43. Shek TW, Luk IS, Ma L, et al. Paclitaxel-induced cardiotoxicity. An ultrastructural study. *Arch Pathol Lab Med* 1996; **120**:89–91.

44. Reichman BS, Seidman AD, Crown JP, et al. Paclitaxel and recombinant human granulocyte colony-stimulating factor as initial chemotherapy for metastatic breast cancer. *J Clin Oncol* 1993; **11**:1943–51.

45. Seidman AD, Reichman BS, Crown JPA, et al. Paclitaxel as second and subsequent therapy for metastatic breast cancer: activity independent of prior anthracycline response. *J Clin Oncol* 1995; **13**:1152–9.

46. Holmes FA, Walters RS, Theriault RL, et al. Phase II trial of taxol, an active drug in the treatment of metastatic breast cancer. *J Natl Cancer Inst* 1991; **83**:1797–805.

47. Abrams JS, Vena DA, Baltz J, et al. Paclitaxel activity in heavily pretreated breast cancer: a National Cancer Institute treatment referral center trial. *J Clin Oncol* 1995; **13**:2056–65.

48. Davidson NG. Single-agent paclitaxel at first relapse following adjuvant chemotherapy for breast cancer. *Semin Oncol* 1995; **22** (suppl 14):2–6.

49. Seidman AD, Tiersten A, Hudis C, et al. Phase II trial of paclitaxel by 3-hour infusion as initial and salvage chemotherapy for metastatic breast cancer. *J Clin Oncol* 1995; **13**:2575–81.

50. Bishop JF, Dewar J, Tattersall MH, et al. A randomized phase III study of taxol (paclitaxel) vs CMFP in untreated patients with metastatic breast cancer [abstract]. *Proc Annu Meet Am Soc Clin Oncol* 1996; **15**:110.

51. Bonneterre J, Tubiana-Hulin M, Chollet P, et al. Taxol 225 mg/mq by 3-hour infusion without G-CSF as a first line therapy in patients with metastatic breast cancer [abstract]. *Proc Annu Meet Am Soc Clin Oncol* 1996; **15**:128.

52. Gianni L, Munzone E, Capri G, et al. Paclitaxel in metastatic breast cancer: a trial of two doses by a 3-hour infusion in patients with disease recurrence after prior therapy with anthracyclines. *J Natl Cancer Inst* 1995; **87**:1169–75.

53. Nabholtz JM, Gelmon K, Spielmann M, et al. Multicenter, randomized comparative study of two doses of paclitaxel in patients with metastatic breast cancer. *J Clin Oncol* 1996; **14**:1858–67.

54. Geyer Jr CE, Green SJ, Moinpour C, et al. A phase II trial of paclitaxel in patients with metastatic refractory carcinoma of the breast: a southwest oncology group (SWOG) study [abstract]. *Proc Annu Meet Am Soc Clin Oncol* 1996; **15**:107.

55. Riccio L, Hudis C, Holmes FA, et al. Phase II study of semisynthetic paclitaxel in patients with metastatic breast cancer previously treated with one chemotherapy regimen [abstract]. *Proc Annu Meet Am Soc Clin Oncol* 1996; **15**:119–20.

56. Seidman AD, Hochhauser D, Gollub M, et al. Ninety-six-hour paclitaxel infusion after progression during short taxane exposure: a phase II pharmacokinetic and pharmacodynamic study in metastatic breast cancer. *J Clin Oncol* 1996; **14**:1877–84.

57. Gelmon K, Nabholtz JM, Bontenbal M, et al. Randomized trial of two doses of paclitaxel in metastatic breast cancer after failure of standard therapy [abstract]. *Ann Oncol* 1994; **5** (suppl 5):198.

58. Seidman AD, Barrett S, Hudis C, et al. Three hour taxol infusion as initial and salvage chemotherapy of metastatic breast cancer [abstract]. *Proc Annu Meet Am Soc Clin Oncol* 1994; **13**:65.

59. Abrams JS, Vena DA, Baltz J, et al. Paclitaxel (taxol) activity in heavily treated metastatic breast cancer [abstract]. *Ann Oncol* 1994; **5** (suppl 5):199.

60. Wilke H. Foreword. *Semin Oncol* 1996; **23** (suppl 3):1–2.

61. Seidman AD, Hochhauser D, Yao T-J, et al. 96 hour paclitaxel after prior short taxane infusion: Phase II pharmacokinetic and pharmacodynamic study in metastatic breast cancer [abstract]. *Proc Annu Meet Am Soc Clin Oncol* 1995; **14**:113.

62. Riseberg D, Cowan K, Tolcher A, et al. 96-hour paclitaxel without and with r-verapamil in patients with metastatic breast cancer previously treated with 3- or 24-hour paclitaxel [abstract]. *Proc Annu Meet Am Soc Clin Oncol* 1995; **14**:180.

63. Chang AY, Boros L, Garrow G, et al. Paclitaxel by 3-hour infusion followed by 96-hour infusion on failure in patients with refractory malignant disease. *Semin Oncol* 1995; **22**:124–7.

64. Holmes FA, Valero V, Walters R, et al. Phase III

trial of paclitaxel administered over 3- or 96-hr for metastatic breast cancer [abstract]. *Proc Annu Meet Am Soc Clin Oncol* 1996; **15**:106.

65. Gelmon KA. Biweekly paclitaxel in the treatment of patients with metastatic breast cancer. *Semin Oncol* 1995; **22**:117–22.

66. Seidman AD. The emerging role of paclitaxel in breast cancer therapy. *Clin Cancer Res* 1995; **1**: 247–56.

67. Fisherman JS, Cowan KH, Noone M, et al. Phase I/II study of 72-hour infusional paclitaxel and doxorubicin with granulocyte colony-stimulating factor in patients with metastatic breast cancer. *J Clin Oncol* 1996; **14**:774–82.

68. Buzdar AU, Holmes FA, Hortobagyi GN. Paclitaxel in the treatment of metastatic breast cancer: M.D. Anderson Cancer Center experience. *Semin Oncol* 1995; **22** (suppl 6):101–4.

69. Sledge GW Jr, Robert N, Sparano JA, et al. Eastern Cooperative Oncology Group studies of paclitaxel and doxorubicin in advanced breast cancer. *Semin Oncol* 1995; **22**:105–8.

70. Gianni L, Munzone E, Capri G, et al. Paclitaxel by 3-hour infusion in combination with bolus doxorubicin in women with untreated metastatic breast cancer: high antitumor efficacy and cardiac effects in a dose-finding and sequence-finding study. *J Clin Oncol* 1995; **13**:2688–99.

71. Dombernowsky P, Gehl J, Boesgaard M, et al. Paclitaxel and doxorubicin, a highly active combination in the treatment of metastatic breast cancer. *Semin Oncol* 1996; **23** (suppl 1):13–18.

72. Frassineti GL, Zoli W, Tienghi A, et al. Phase I/II study of sequential combination of paclitaxel and doxorubicin in the treatment of advanced breast cancer (ABC) [abstract]. *Proc Annu Meet Am Soc Clin Oncol* 1996; **15**:109.

73. Schwartsmann G, Menke CH, Caleffi M, et al. Phase II trial of taxol (T), doxorubicin (D) plus G-CSF in patients (pts) with metastatic breast cancer (MBC) [abstract]. *Proc Annu Meet Am Soc Clin Oncol* 1996; **15**:126.

74. Cazap E, Ventriglia M, Rubino G, et al. Taxol (T) plus doxorubicin (D) the treatment of metastatic breast cancer (MBC) in ambulatory patients (pts) [abstract]. *Proc Annu Meet Am Soc Clin Oncol* 1996; **15**:146.

75. Catimel G, Spielmann M, Dieras V, et al. Phase I study of paclitaxel and epirubicin in patients with metastatic breast cancer: a preliminary report on safety. *Semin Oncol* 1996; **23** (suppl 1):24–7.

76. Conte PF, Michelotti A, Baldini E, et al. Activity and safety of epirubicin plus paclitaxel in advanced breast cancer. *Semin Oncol* 1996; **23** (suppl 1):28–32.

77. Luck H-J, Thomssen C, duBois A, et al. Interim analysis of a phase II study of epirubicin and paclitaxel as first-line therapy in patients with metastatic breast cancer. *Semin Oncol* 1996; **23** (suppl 1):33–6.

78. Di Costanzo F, Sdrobolini A, Bilancia D, et al. Phase I-II trial of mitoxantrone (M) and taxol (T) in advanced breast cancer (ABC) [abstract]. *Proc Annu Meet Am Soc Clin Oncol* 1996; **15**:139.

79. Tolcher WA. Paclitaxel couplets with cyclophosphamide or cisplatin in metastatic breast cancer. *Semin Oncol* 1996; **23** (suppl 1): 37–43.

80. Gelmon KA, O'Reilly SE, Tolcher AW, et al. Phase I/II trial of biweekly paclitaxel and cisplatin in the treatment of metastatic breast cancer. *J Clin Oncol* 1996; **14**:1185–91.

81. Sparano JA, Neuberg D, Glick J, et al. A phase II trial of biweekly paclitaxel and cisplatin in patients with advanced breast carcinoma; an Eastern Cooperative Oncology Group (ECOG) trial [abstract]. *Proc Annu Meet Am Soc Clin Oncol* 1996; **15**:114.

82. McCaskill-Stevens W, Ansari R, Fisher W, et al. Phase II study of biweekly cisplatin and paclitaxel in the treatment of metastatic breast cancer [abstract]. *Proc Annu Meet Am Soc Clin Oncol* 1996; **15**:120.

83. Tolcher AW, Cowan KH, Noone MH, et al. Phase I study of paclitaxel in combination with cyclophosphamide and granulocyte colony-stimulating factor in metastatic breast cancer patients. *J Clin Oncol* 1996; **14**:95–102.

84. Kennedy MJ, Zahurak ML, Donehower RC, et al. Phase I and pharmacologic study of sequences of paclitaxel and cyclophosphamide supported by granulocyte colony-stimulating factor in women with previously untreated metastatic breast cancer. *J Clin Oncol* 1996; **14**:783–91.

85. Murad AM, Tinoco LA, Schwartsmann G. Phase II trial of the use of taxol and ifosfamide in heavily pre-treated patients with metastatic breast cancer [abstract]. *Proc Annu Meet Am Soc Clin Oncol* 1996; **15**:97.

86. Klaassen U, Harstrick A, Wilke H, et al. Preclinical and clinical study results of the combination of paclitaxel and 5-fluorouracil/folinic acid in the treatment of metastatic breast cancer. *Semin Oncol* 1996; **23** (suppl 1):44–7.

87. Paul MD, Garrett AM, Meshad M, et al. Paclitaxel and 5-fluorouracil in metastatic breast cancer: the US experience. *Semin Oncol* 1996; **23** (suppl 1):48–52.

88. Nicholson B, Paul D, Hande KR, et al. A phase II trial of paclitaxel, 5-fluorouracil leucovorin in metastatic breast cancer [abstract]. *Proc Annu Meet Am Soc Clin Oncol* 1996; **15**:102.

89. Hainsworth JD, Jones SE, Mennel RG, et al. Paclitaxel with mitoxantrone, fluorouracil and high-dose leucovorin in the treatment of metastatic breast cancer: a phase II trial. *J Clin Oncol* 1996; **14**:1611–16.

90. Holmes FA, Frye D, Valero V, et al. Phase I study of taxol and doxorubicin with G-CSF in patients without prior chemotherapy for metastatic breast cancer [abstract]. *Proc Annu Meet Am Soc Clin Oncol* 1992; **11**:66.

91. Gianni L, Straneo M, Capri G, et al. Optimal dose and sequence finding study of paclitaxel by 3 h infusion combined with bolus doxorubicin in untreated metastatic breast cancer patients [abstract]. *Proc Annu Meet Am Soc Clin Oncol* 1994; **13**:97.

92. Sledge GW. Defining the roles of paclitaxel and doxorubicin in the treatment of breast cancer [abstract]. *Proceedings of the 8th International Congress on Senology* 1994.

93. Holmes FA, Valero V, Walters RS, et al. The M.D. Anderson Cancer Center experience with taxol in metastatic breast cancer. *Monogr Natl Cancer Inst* 1993; **15**:161–9.

94. Berg SL, Cowan KH, Balis FM, et al. Pharmacokinetics of Taxol and Doxorubicin administered alone and in combination by continuous 72-hour infusion. *J Natl Cancer Inst* 1994; **86**:143–5.

95. Hudis C, Lebwohl D, Crown J, et al. Dose intensive sequential crossover adjuvant chemotherapy for women with high risk node positive primary breast cancer. In: *Adjuvant Therapy of Cancer* (Salmon S, ed.) 7th edn. Philadelphia: Lippincott, 1993:214–19.

96. Seidman AD, Hudis CA, Fennelly D, et al. Memorial Sloan-Kettering Cancer Center experience with paclitaxel in the treatment of breast cancer. *Semin Oncol* 1995; **22**:108–16.

97. Ringel I, Horwitz SB. Studies with RP 56976 (taxotere): a semisynthetic analogue of taxol. *J Natl Cancer Inst* 1991; **83**:288–91.

98. Gelmon K. The taxoids: paclitaxel and docetaxel. *Lancet* 1994; **344**:1267–72.

99. Lavelle F, Bissery MC, Combeau C, et al. Preclinical evaluation of docetaxel (Taxotere). *Semin Oncol* 1995; **22** (2, suppl 4):3–16.

100. Hanauske AR, Degen D, Hilsenbeck SG, et al. Effects of Taxotere and taxol on in vitro colony formation of freshly explanted human tumour cells. *Anticancer Drugs* 1992; **3**:121–4.

101. Arbuck SG, Blaylock BA. Dose and schedule issues. In: *Paclitaxel in Cancer Treatment* (McGuire WP, Rowinsky EK, eds). New York: Marcel Dekker, Inc., 1995:151–73.

102. Hill BT, Whelan RD, Shellard SA, et al. Differential cytotoxic effects of docetaxel in a range of mammalian tumor cell lines and certain drug resistant sublines in vitro. *Invest New Drugs* 1994; **12**:169–82.

103. Bissery M-C, Guenard D, Gueritte-Voegelein F, et al. Experimental antitumor activity of Taxotere (RP 56976, NSC 628503), a Taxol analogue. *Cancer Res* 1991; **51**:4845–52.

104. Bruno R, Sanderink GJ. Pharmacokinetics and metabolism of Taxotere (docetaxel). *Cancer Surv* 1993; **17**:305–13.

105. Tomiak E, Piccart MJ, Kerger J, et al. A phase I study of taxotere (RP 56976, NSC 628503) administered as a one hour intravenous infusion on a weekly basis [abstract]. *Eur J Cancer* 1991; suppl 2:1184.

106. Extra JM, Rousseau F, Bruno R, et al. Phase I and pharmacokinetic study of Taxotere (RP 56976; NSC 628503) given as a short intravenous infusion. *Cancer Res* 1993; **53**:1037–42.

107. Bissett D, Setanoians A, Cassidy J, et al. Phase I and pharmacokinetic study of taxotere (RP 56976) administered as a 24-hour infusion. *Cancer Res* 1993; **53**:523–7.

108. Pazdur R, Newman RA, Newman BM, et al. Phase I trial of Taxotere: five-day schedule. *J Natl Cancer Inst* 1992; **84**:1781–8.

109. Tomiak E, Piccart MJ, Kerger J, et al. Phase I study of docetaxel administered as a 1-hour intravenous infusion on a weekly basis. *J Clin Oncol* 1994; **12**:1458–67.

110. Burris H, Irvin R, Kuhn J, et al. Phase I clinical trial of taxotere administered as either a 2-hour or 6-hour intravenous infusion. *J Clin Oncol* 1993; **11**:950–8.

111. Hudis CA, Seidman AD, Crown JP, et al. Phase II and pharmacologic study of docetaxel as initial chemotherapy for metastatic breast cancer. *J Clin Oncol* 1996; **14**:58–65.

112. Trudeau ME, Eisenhauer EA, Higgins BP, et al. Docetaxel in patients with metastatic breast cancer: a Phase II study of the National Cancer

Institute of Canada-Clinical Trials Group. *J Clin Oncol* 1996; **14:**422–8.

113. Ravdin PM, Burris HA, Cook G, et al. Phase II trial of docetaxel in advanced anthracycline-resistant or anthracenedione-resistant breast cancer [see comments]. *J Clin Oncol* 1995; **13:**2879–85.

114. Chevallier B, Fumoleau P, Kerbrat P, et al. Docetaxel is a major cytotoxic drug for the treatment of advanced breast cancer: a phase II trial of the Clinical Screening Cooperative Group of the European Organization for Research and Treatment of Cancer. *J Clin Oncol* 1995; **13:**314–22.

115. Valero V, Holmes FA, Walters RS, et al. Phase II trial of docetaxel: a new, highly effective antineoplastic agent in the management of patients with anthracycline-resistant metastatic breast cancer [see comments]. *J Clin Oncol* 1995; **13:**2886–94.

116. ten Bokkel Huinink WW, Prove AM, Piccart M, et al. A phase II trial with docetaxel (Taxotere) in second line treatment with chemotherapy for advanced breast cancer. A study of the EORTC Early Clinical Trials Group. *Ann Oncol* 1994; **5:**527–32.

117. Dieras V, Fumoleau P, Chevallier B, et al. Second EORTC-clinical screening group (CSG) phase II trial of taxotere as first line chemotherapy in advanced breast cancer [abstract]. *Proc Annu Meet Am Soc Clin Oncol* 1994; **13:**78.

118. Trandafir L, Chahine A, Spielman M, et al. Efficacy of taxotere in advanced breast cancer patients not eligible for further anthracyclines [abstract]. *Proc Annu Meet Am Soc Clin Oncol* 1996; **15:**105.

119. Valero V, Burris III HA, Jones SE, et al. Multicenter pilot study of taxotere in taxol-resistant metastatic breast cancer [abstract]. *Proc Annu Meet Am Soc Clin Oncol* 1996; **15:**107.

120. Fumoleau P, Chevallier B, Kerbrat P, et al. A multicenter phase II study of the efficacy and safety of docetaxel as first-line treatment of advanced breast cancer: report of the Clinical Screening Group of the EORTC. *Ann Oncol* 1996; **7:**165–71.

121. Bourgeois H, Gruia G, Dieras V, et al. Docetaxel in combination with doxorubicin as 1st line CT of metastatic breast cancer a phase I dose finding study [abstract]. *Proc Annu Meet Am Soc Clin Oncol* 1996; **15:**148.

122. ten Bokkel Huinink W, Dubbelman R, Hiemstra A, et al. Phase I study of docetaxel alternating with epirubicin and cyclophosphamide in an escalated and accelerated schedule by the comcomitant use of lenograstim [abstract]. *Proc Annu Meet Am Soc Clin Oncol* 1996; **15:**141.

123. Fumoleau P, Delacroix V, Perrocheau G, et al. Docetaxel in combination with vinorelbine as 1st line CT in PTS with metastatic breast cancer: final results [abstract]. *Proc Annu Meet Am Soc Clin Oncol* 1996; **15:**142.

124. Mangeney P, Andriamialisoa RZ, Lallemand J-Y, et al. 5'-Nor-anhydrovinblastine, prototype of a new class of vinblastine derivatives. *Tetrahedron* 1979; **35:**2175–79.

125. Fellous A, Ohayon R, Vacassin T, et al. Biochemical effects of navelbine on tubulin and associated proteins. *Semin Oncol* 1989; **16** (2, suppl 4):9–14.

126. Binet S, Fellous A, Lataste H, et al. In situ analysis of the action of navelbine on various types of microtubules using immunofluorescence. *Semin Oncol* 1989; **16** (suppl 4):5–8.

127. Adams DJ, Knick VC. P-glycoprotein mediated drug resistance to 5'-nor-anhydrovinblastine (Navelbine®). *Invest New Drugs* 1995; **13:**13–21.

128. Cabral FR, Barlow SB. Mechanisms by which mammalian cells acquire resistance to drugs that affect microtubule assembly. *FASEB J* 1989; **3:**1593–601.

129. Rowinsky EK, Noe DA, Trump DL, et al. Pharmacokinetic, bioavailability, and feasibility study of oral vinorelbine in patients with solid tumors. *J Clin Oncol* 1994; **12:**1754–63.

130. Rahmani R, Bruno R, Iliadis A, et al. Clinical pharmacokinetics of the new antitumor drug navelbine (5'-noranhydrovinblastine). *Cancer Res* 1987; **47:**5796–9.

131. Marquet P, Lachatre G, Debord J, et al. Pharmacokinetics of vinorelbine in man. *J Clin Pharmacol* 1992; **32:**1096–8.

132. Krikorian A, Rahmani R, Bromet M, et al. Pharmacokinetics and metabolism of navelbine. *Semin Oncol* 1989; **16** (suppl 4):21–5.

133. Cvitkovic E, Izzo J. The current and future place of vinorelbine in cancer therapy. *Drugs* 1992; **44** (suppl 4):36–45.

134. Toussaint C, Izzo J, Spielmann M, et al. Phase I/II trial of continuous infusion vinorelbine for advanced breast cancer. *J Clin Oncol* 1994; **12:**2102–12.

135. Hohneker JA. A summary of vinorelbine (Navelbine) safety data from North American clinical trials. *Semin Oncol* 1994; **21:**42–7.

136. Terenziani M, Demicheli R, Brambilla C, et al. Vinorelbine: an active, non cross-resistant drug

in advanced breast cancer. Results of a Phase II study. *Breast Cancer Res Treat* 1997; in press.

137. Weber BL, Vogel C, Jones S, et al. Intravenous vinorelbine as first-line and second-line therapy in advanced breast cancer. *J Clin Oncol* 1995; **13**:2722–30.

138. Romero A, Rabinovich MG, Vallejo CT, et al. Vinorelbine as first-line chemotherapy for metastatic breast carcinoma. *J Clin Oncol* 1994; **12**:336–41.

139. Garcìa-Conde J, Lluch A, Martin M, et al. Phase II trial of weekly IV vinorelbine in first-line advanced breast cancer chemotherapy. *Ann Oncol* 1994; **5**:854–7.

140. Fumoleau P, Delgado FM, Delozier T, et al. Phase II trial of weekly intravenous vinorelbine in first-line advanced breast cancer chemotherapy. *J Clin Oncol* 1993; **11**:1245–52.

141. Gasparini G, Caffo O, Barni S, et al. Vinorelbine is an active antiproliferative agent in pretreated advanced breast cancer patients: a phase II study. *J Clin Oncol* 1994; **12**:2094–101.

142. Vogel C, O'Rourke M, Winer E, et al. A clinical trial of intravenous navelbine for first line treatment of women ≥60 years of age with advanced breast cancer [abstract]. *Proc Annu Meet Am Soc Clin Oncol* 1996; **15**:101.

143. Ranuzzi M, Nisticò C, Garufi C, et al. Vinorelbina in weekly schedule with G-CSF in patients with advanced breast cancer [abstract]. *Proc Annu Meet Am Soc Clin Oncol* 1996; **15**:125.

144. Degardin M, Bonneterre J, Hecquet B, et al. Vinorelbine (navelbine) as a salvage treatment for advanced breast cancer. *Ann Oncol* 1994; **5**:423–6.

145. Winer EP, Chu L, Spicer DV. Oral vinorelbine (navelbine) in the treatment of advanced breast cancer. *Semin Oncol* 1995; **22** (suppl 5):72–9.

146. Spicer D, McCaskill-Stevens W, Oken M, et al. Oral navelbina (NVB) in women with previously treated advanced breast cancer (ABC): a US multicenter phase II trial [abstract]. *Proc Annu Meet Am Soc Clin Oncol* 1994; **13**:76.

147. Fumoleau P, Delgado FM, Delozier T, et al. Phase II trial with navelbine (NVB) in advanced breast cancer: preliminary results [abstract]. *Proc Am Soc Clin Oncol* 1990; **9**:21.

148. Degardin M, Bonneterre J, Hecquet B, et al. Vinorelbine (navelbine) as a salvage treatment for advanced breast cancer. *Ann Oncol* 1994; **5**:423–6.

149. Fumoleau P, Delgado FM, Delozier T, et al.

Phase II trial of weekly intravenous vinorelbine in first-line advanced breast cancer chemotherapy. *J Clin Oncol* 1993; **11**:1245–52.

150. Fumoleau P, Delozier T, Extra JM, et al. Vinorelbine (Navelbine) in the treatment of breast cancer: the European experience. *Semin Oncol* 1995; **22** (suppl 5):22–9.

151. Jones S, Winer E, Vogel C, et al. A multicenter randomized trial of IV vinorelbine vs. IV alkeran in patients with anthracycline-refractory advanced breast cancer [abstract]. *Proc Annu Meet Am Soc Clin Oncol* 1994; **13**:103.

152. Hochster H, Vogel C, Blumenreich M, et al. A multicenter phase II study of navelbine (NVB) and doxorubicin (DOX) as first line chemotherapy of metastatic breast cancer [abstract]. *Proc Annu Meet Am Soc Clin Oncol* 1994; **13**:100.

153. Ferrero JM, Pivot X, Namer M, et al. Association mitoxantrone-vinorelbine en première ligne thérapeutique dans le cancer du sein métastatique. *Bull Cancer* 1995; **82**:202–7.

154. Kayitalire L, Spielmann M, Brain E, et al. Salvage chemotherapy (CT) with combination of mitoxantrone (MTZ) and vinorelbine (VRB) in resistant to anthracyclines advanced breast cancer (ABC) [abstract]. *Proc Annu Meet Am Soc Clin Oncol* 1993; **12**:90.

155. Scheithauer W, Kornek G, Haider K, et al. Effective second line chemotherapy of advanced breast cancer with navelbine and mitomycin C. *Breast Cancer Res Treat* 1993; **26**:49–53.

156. Dieras V, Pierga Y-Y, Extra JM, et al. Results of combination of navelbine (NVB) and fluorouracil (FU) in advanced breast cancer (ABC) with a group of sequential design (GSD) [abstract]. *Ann Oncol* 1992; **3** (suppl 5):178.

157. Norris B, Pritchard K, James K, et al. A phase III comparative study of vinorelbine combined with doxorubicin versus doxorubicin alone in metastatic/recurrent breast cancer: a National Cancer Institute of Canada (NCIC CTG) study [abstract]. *Proc Annu Meet Am Soc Clin Oncol* 1996; **15**:98.

158. Costa MA, Cabral-Filho S, Correa M, et al. Phase II study of sequential navelbine and doxorubicin for the treatment of metastatic breast cancer: preliminary results [abstract]. *Proc Annu Meet Am Soc Clin Oncol* 1996; **15**:100.

159. Leone B, Vallejo C, Romero A, et al. Ifosfamide and vinorelbine as first-line chemotherapy for metastatic breast cancer: final results [abstract]. *Proc Annu Meet Am Soc Clin Oncol* 1996; **15**:102.

160. Spielmann M, Dorval T, Turpin F, et al. Phase II trial of vinorelbine/doxorubicin as first-line therapy of advanced breast cancer. *J Clin Oncol* 1994; **12**:1764–70.

161. Hochster HS. Combined doxorubicin/vinorelbine (navelbine) therapy in the treatment of advanced breast cancer. *Semin Oncol* 1995; **22** (suppl 5):55–60.

162. Hortobagyi GN. Future directions for vinorelbine (navelbine). *Semin Oncol* 1995; **22** (suppl 5):80–7.

163. DeGraw JI, Brown VH, Tagawa H, et al. Synthesis and antitumour activity of 1-alkyl, 10-deaza-aminopterin: a convenient synthesis of 10-deaza-aminopterin. *J Med Chem* 1982; **25**: 1227–9.

164 Jolivet J, Jansen G, Peters GJ, et al. Leucovorin rescue of human cancer and bone marrow cells following edatrexate or methotrexate. *Biochem Pharmacol* 1994; **47**:659–67.

165. Grant SC, Kris MG, Young CW, et al. Edatrexate, an antifolate with antitumor activity: a review. *Cancer Invest* 1993; **11**:36–45.

166. Sirotnak FM, Otter GM, Schmid FA. Markedly improved efficacy of edatrexate compared to methotrexate in high dose regimen with leucovorin rescue against metastatic solid tumors. *Cancer Res* 1993; **53**:587–93.

167. Otter GM, Sirotnak FM. Effective combination therapy of metastatic murine solid tumors with edatrexate and the vinca alkaloids, vinblastine, navelbine and vindesine. *Cancer Chemother Pharmacol* 1994; **33**:286–90.

168. Perez EA, Hack FM, Webber LM, et al. Schedule-dependent synergism of edatrexate and cisplatin in combination in the A549 lung-cancer cell line as assessed by median-effect analysis. *Cancer Chemother Pharmacol* 1993; **33**: 245–50.

169. Fennelly D, Gilewski T, Hudis C, et al. Phase I trial of sequential edatrexate followed by paclitaxel: a design based on in vitro synergy in patients with advanced breast cancer [abstract]. *Proc Annu Meet Am Soc Clin Oncol* 1995; **14**:105.

170. Kris MG, Kinahan JJ, Gralla RJ, et al. Phase I trial and clinical pharmacological evaluation of 10-ethyl-10-deazaaminopterin in adult patients with advanced cancer. *Cancer Res* 1988; **48**:5573–9.

171. Tan C, Meyers P, Steinherz P, et al. Phase I clinical and pharmacologic study of 10-ethyl-10-deaza-aminopterin (10-edam) in children with advanced cancer [abstract]. *Proc Annu Meet Am Assoc Cancer Res* 1988; **29**:A914.

172. Schornagel J, van der Vegt S, Verweij J, et al. Phase II study of 10-ethyl-10-deazaaminopterin (10-EDAM) in chemotherapy naive patients with metastatic breast cancer [abstract]. *Ann Oncol* 1990; **1**:22.

173. Booser DJ, Dye CA, Clements SB, et al. Edatrexate (10-EDAM) for metastatic breast cancer: phase II study [abstract]. *Proc Annu Meet Am Soc Clin Oncol* 1994; **13**:109.

174. Vandenberg TA, Pritchard KI, Trudeau ME, et al. Phase II study of weekly edatrexate as first-line chemotherapy for metastatic breast cancer: a National Cancer Institute of Canada Clinical Trials Group Study. *J Clin Oncol* 1993; **11**: 1241–4.

175. Chabner BA. Cytidine analogues. In: *Cancer Chemotherapy and Biotherapy – Principles and Practice*, 2nd edn. (Chabner BA, Longo DL, eds). Philadelphia: Lippincott, 1995: 213–33.

176. Plunkett W, Huang P, Gandhi V. Preclinical characteristics of gemcitabine. *Anti-Cancer Drugs* 1995; **6**:7–13.

177. Heinemann V, Xu Y-Z, Chubbs S, et al. Cellular elimination of 2′,2′-difluorodeoxycitidine 5′-triphosphate: a mechanism of self potentiation. *Cancer Res* 1992; **52**:533–9.

178. Heinemann V, Schultz L, Issels RD, et al. Gemcitabine: a modulator of intracellular nucleotide and deoxynucleotide metabolism. *Semin Oncol* 1995; **22** (suppl 11):11–18.

179. Huang P, Plunkett W. Induction of apoptosis by gemcitabine. *Semin Oncol* 1995; **22** (suppl 11):19–25.

180. Huang P, Plunkett W. Fludarabine- and gemcitabine-induced apoptosis: incorporation of analogs into DNA is a critical event. *Cancer Chemother Pharmacol* 1995; **36**:181–8.

181. Plunkett W, Huang P, Xu Y-Z, et al. Gemcitabine: metabolism, mechanisms of action, and self-potentiation. *Semin Oncol* 1995; **22** (suppl 11):3–10.

182. Csoka K, Liliemark J, Larsson R, et al. Evaluation of the cytotoxic of gemcitabine in primary cultures of tumor cells from patients with hematologic or solid tumors. *Semin Oncol* 1995; **22** (suppl 11):47–53.

183. Shewach DS, Lawrence TS. Radiosensitization of human tumor cells by gemcitabine in vitro. *Semin Oncol* 1995; **22** (suppl 11):68–71.

184. Kaye SB. Gemcitabine: current status of Phase I and II trial [Editorial]. *J Clin Oncol* 1994; **12**: 1527–9.

185. Allerheiligen S, Johnston R, Hatcher C, et al. Gemcitabine pharmacokinetics are influenced by gender, body surface area, and duration of infusion [abstract]. *Proc Annu Meet Am Soc Clin Oncol* 1994; **13**:136.

186. Grunewald R, Abruzzese JL, Tarassoff P, et al. Saturation of 2',2' difluorodeoxycitidine 5'-triphosphate accumulation by mononuclear cells in a phase I trial of gemcitabine. *Cancer Chemother Pharmacol* 1991; **27**:258–63.

187. Carmichael J, Possinger K, Phillip P, et al. Advanced breast cancer: a phase II trial with gemcitabine. *J Clin Oncol* 1995; **13**:2731–6.

188. Blackstein M, Vogel CL, Ambinder R, et al. Phase II study of gemcitabine in patient with metastatic breast cancer [abstract]. *Proc Annu Meet Am Soc Clin Oncol* 1996; **15**:117.

189. Chang AYC, Most C, Pandya KJ. Continuous intravenous infusion of 5-fluorouracil in the treatment of refractory breast cancer. *Am J Clin Oncol* 1989; **12**:453–5.

190. Harris BE, Carpenter JT, Diasio RB. Severe 5-fluorouracil toxicity secondary to dihydropyrimidine dehydrogenase deficiency. A potentially more common pharmacogenetic syndrome. *Cancer* 1991; **68**:499–501.

191. Milano G, Etienne MC. Dihydropyrimidine dehydrogenase (DPD) and clinical pharmacology of 5-fluorouracil (review). *Anticancer Res* 1994; **14**:2295–7.

192. Adjei AA, Doucette M, Spector T, et al. 5-ethynyluracil (776C85), an inhibitor of dihydropyrimidine dehydrogenase, permits reliable oral dosing of 5-fluorouracil and prolongs its half-life [abstract]. *Proc Annu Meet Am Soc Clin Oncol* 1995; **14**:459.

193. Baker SD, Diaso R, Lucas VS, et al. Phase I and pharmacologic study of oral 5-fluorouracil on a chronic 28-day schedule in combination with the dehydropyrimidine dehydrogenase inactivator 776C85 [abstract]. *Proc Annu Meet Am Soc Clin Oncol* 1996; **15**:486.

194. Burris H, Schilsky R, Fields S, et al. Initial Phase I trial of the dihydropyrimidine dehydrogenase inactivator 5-ethynyluracil (776C85) plus 5-fluorouracil [abstract]. *Proc Annu Meet Am Soc Clin Oncol* 1995; **14**:171.

195. Smith G, Henderson G. New treatment for breast cancer. *Semin Oncol* 1996; **23**:506–28.

196. Gogas H, Mansi JL. The anthrapyrazoles. *Cancer Treat Rep* 1995; **21**:541–52.

197. Talbot DC, Smith IE, Mansi JL, et al. Anthrapyrazole CI 941: A highly active new drug agent in the treatment of advanced breast cancer. *J Clin Oncol* 1991; **9**:2141–7.

198. Calvert H, Smith I., Jones A, et al. Phase II study of losoxantrone in previously treated and untreated patients with advanced breast cancer (CA) [abstract]. *Proc Annu Meet Am Soc Clin Oncol* 1994; **13**:71.

199. Cobb P, Burris H, Peacock N, et al. Phase I trial of losoxantrone plus paclitaxel given every 21 days [abstract]. *Proc Annu Meet Am Soc Clin Oncol* 1995; **14**:476.

200. Chang AY, Garrow GC. Pilot study of vinorelbine (Navelbine) and paclitaxel (Taxol) in patients with refractory breast cancer and lung cancer. *Semin Oncol* 1995; **22**:66–70.

201. Knick VC, Eberwein DJ, Miller CG. Vinorelbine tartrate and paclitaxel combinations: enhanced activity against in vivo P388 murine leukemia cells. *J Natl Cancer Inst* 1995; **87**:1072–7.

17

New hormones

Manfred Kaufmann, Gunter von Minckwitz

CONTENTS • New anti-oestrogens • New aromatase inhibitors • Gonadotrophin-releasing hormone analogues • Antiprogestins • Conclusion and perspectives

As breast cancer is the most common malignant disease in women, the potential impact of endocrine treatment is tremendous. This therapeutic option is, to date, unique in comparison to other common malignancies. Endocrine therapy, as compared with chemotherapy, is active against tumour cells through distinct and highly selective mechanisms. This selectivity of action has a strong inverse correlation with unwanted side effects. The detection of oestrogen receptors and the working mechanism of different hormones, especially tamoxifen, therefore represent milestones in the treatment of breast cancer. Endocrine treatment was the first effective palliative treatment.[1] Endocrine adjuvant therapy has been shown to improve survival rates of primary breast cancer patients.[2]

Patients with metastatic disease, who have previously responded to endocrine treatment, have a high probability that their tumour will regress through a second or even third episode of different endocrine therapy; in this way the use of chemotherapy can be postponed. Hormone sequences for palliative treatment have been recommended according to the activity of the drugs and their side effects.[3] They have also been evaluated for the adjuvant setting. As a result of the large number of new

endocrine treatments being developed, these sequences will not be standardized in the near future.

Four groups of compounds can be defined in which there are new developments. The first are derivatives of tamoxifen, with different receptor binding activity and varying intranuclear responses; second are the highly selective inhibitors of aromatase, the key enzyme in oestrogen production in postmenopausal women; third are the recently introduced gonadotrophin-releasing hormone (GnRH) analogues and their recently synthesized antagonists; and fourth are the antiprogestins, the mechanism of action of which is based on a completely new mechanism.

NEW ANTI-OESTROGENS

Background and mechanism

There are two reasons for developing new compounds with anti-oestrogenic activity. First, resistance to tamoxifen, and therefore a progression of disease, appears in almost all patients with advanced breast cancer and about half of the patients being treated with tamoxifen in the adjuvant setting. Second, long-term use of tamoxifen may increase the risk for secondary primaries in the endometrium and perhaps other organs.[4]

For both these cases, the partial oestrogenic activity of the drug is thought to be, at least in part, responsible. Binding of tamoxifen to oestrogen receptors can be modified so that oestrogenic activity predominates over anti- oestrogenic activity, allowing oestrogen-dependent growth of tumour cells to occur. After drug withdrawal, tumour regression is sometimes observed. There can also be a varying effect of tamoxifen on other tissues, e.g. it acts on the endometrium more like oestrogen so that hyperplasias or endometrial cancer can develop. These substances, which have different effects on hormone-dependent organs, are called site-specific oestrogen receptor-modulating substances.[5]

Molecular studies have clarified two independent domains of transcriptional activation for the oestrogen receptor: one at the amino end (TAF1) and one at the carboxy end (TAF2). It is assumed that these two regions influence the assembly and efficient operation of the transcriptional complex. As receptor function is not the same in all cells, gene response to oestrogen is determined by both the differentiated nature of the cell and promoter context.[6] It is assumed that the relative strength of TAF1 and TAF2 could determine the partial agonist activity of anti-oestrogens. In cases where TAF2 is dominant, tamoxifen would be expected to act as an antagonist. The partial agonist activity observed in vivo would correspondingly depend on the activity of TAF1 (Figure 17.1).[7]

Compounds

Toremifene

This second-generation anti-oestrogen is a triphenylethylene derivative that is structurally very close to tamoxifen. It is absorbed from the gastrointestinal tract with a bioavailability of close to 100%. It is then metabolized in the liver and eliminated with the faeces after a half-life of 5–6 days.[8] The compound was registered in late 1996 and the recommended dose for treatment of postmenopausal metastatic breast cancer is 60 mg/day.

Toremifene shows a similar site-specific oestrogen receptor modulation to tamoxifen, regarding bone metabolism, serum lipid values but not the uterotropic effect.

Five phase III studies have been carried out which included 1869 patients. Different doses of toremifene have been compared with different doses of tamoxifen. An overview of the first three trials is given in Table 17.1.[9–11] One of these trials, the Nordic Study with 415 oestrogen receptor-positive or unknown patients, was double-blind and compared tamoxifen 40 mg/day with toremifene 60 mg/day. The results showed a slightly higher response rate and a significantly longer time to treatment failure for tamoxifen. When only oestrogen receptor-positive patients were analysed, the difference between the two treatments disappeared.[11] However, in a meta-analysis including 1420 patients, no difference was found in response rate, time to treatment failure and overall survival between tamoxifen and toremifene. Toremifene was generally well tolerated. Discontinuation of treatment was necessary in only 3% of patients. The toxicity profile was comparable to tamoxifen, including hot flushes, nausea and vertigo. A decrease in antithrombin III and prolactin plasma level and an increase in SHBG (sex hormone binding globulin) were generally found.[12] However, it is of interest, especially for use of anti-oestrogens as chemopreventive agents, that toremifene does not cause formation of DNA adducts because of the chlorine atom which stabilizes the electron structure of this molecule. In a 2-year carcinogenicity study, toremifene did not induce hepatocellular carcinomas.[13] On the other hand, it has shown effects in non-endocrine-dependent malignancy, which is suspected to be caused by an induction of apoptosis and manipulation of oncogene expression. This has been demonstrated on a mouse uterine sarcoma model and in a preliminary study on advanced renal carcinoma. In this study, using a dose of 300 mg/day objective remissions accounted for 16% and stable disease for 28%.[14]

Due to its non-carcinogeneity, toremifene represents an interesting drug for chemopreventive trials.

(a) Former design of steroid function

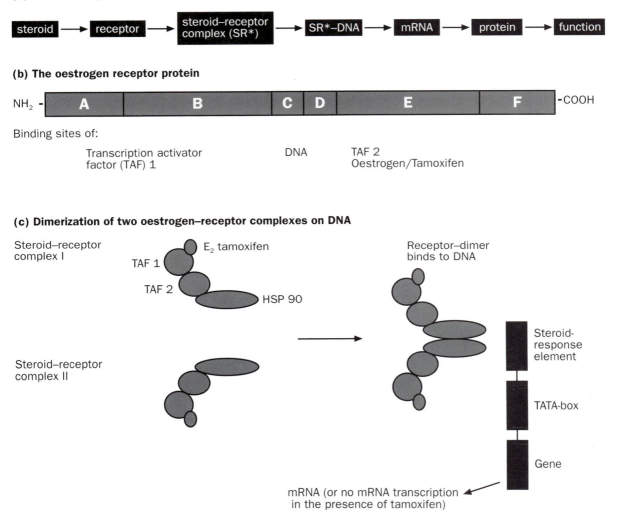

(b) The oestrogen receptor protein

Binding sites of:

Transcription activator   DNA   TAF 2
factor (TAF) 1   Oestrogen/Tamoxifen

(c) Dimerization of two oestrogen–receptor complexes on DNA

Figure 17.1 Change of the hypothesis of oestrogen receptor function.

Raloxifene

Raloxifene hydrochloride (LY 139481-HCl), a non-steroidal anti-oestrogen derived from benzothiophene, has been developed primarily for prevention and treatment of osteoporosis. Raloxifene hydrochloride undergoes first-pass hepatic metabolism with the principal circulating form being the glucuronide. It is almost completely eliminated in the faeces.[15] In comparison with tamoxifen, it shows a greater affinity for the oestrogen receptor, and has a different oestrogenic/anti-oestrogenic profile. In an ovariectomized rat model it has more extensive effects on hypolipidaemia and against bone resorption.[16] It elicits an extremely high degree of anti-oestrogenicity on the uterus, even in the presence of low-dose oestrogen.[17]

Raloxifene has been investigated for the

Table 17.1 Phase III clinical trials on toremifene in comparison to tamoxifen in metastatic breast cancer[9-11]

Trial	Response rates (%)			Time to treatment failure (months)	Median duration of survival (months)
	CR	RR	PR		
Erbamont I Trial					
(n = 648 patients)					
Tamoxifen 20 mg	5		19	5.8	31.1
Toremifene 60 mg	6		18	5.5	37.5
Toremifene 200 mg	5		19	5.5	29.6
Russian Baltic Trial					
(n = 463 patients)					
Tamoxifene 40 mg	2		19	5.0	23.4
Toremifene 60 mg	4.5		16	4.9	25.4
Toremifene 240 mg	4.5		24	6.1	23.8
Nordic Trial					
(n = 415 patients)					
Tamoxifen 40 mg		37.3		10.2	38.7
Toremifene 60 mg		31.3		7.3*	33.0

CR, complete response; PR, partial response; RR, response rate = CR + PR; *$p < 0.05$.

treatment of osteoporosis in two major trials. In a double-blind, placebo-controlled trial, a total of 251 patients were treated with raloxifene 200 mg/day, raloxifene 600 mg/day or Premarin (conjugated oestrogens) 0.625 mg/day. No difference was shown in the three treatment groups, compared with the placebo group, when markers of bone metabolism and low-density lipoprotein cholesterol (LDL-C) were assessed. Uterine biopsies revealed a significant suppression by raloxifene of oestrogenic effects on the endometrium compared with the oestradiol arm (Table 17.2). Raloxifene was safe and well tolerated, with no detectable or significant clinical or laboratory abnormalities.[18]

In animal experiments, raloxifene was shown to inhibit the growth of dimethylbenzanthracene (DMBA)-induced and nitromustine (NMU)-induced mammary tumours, and to block mammary tumour growth in ovariec-tomized rats treated with oestradiol.[19] In a small phase II clinical trial in women with metastatic breast cancer resistant to tamoxifen, none of the 14 patients showed an objective response to raloxifene with an oral application of 200 mg/day.[20] Currently, a dose of 300 mg/day is being investigated in chemotherapy and endocrine therapy-naive patients who have metastatic, oestrogen receptor-positive disease.

Droloxifene

Droloxifene is a new 3-hydroxy derivative of tamoxifen which, like toremifene, demonstrates no carcinogenic effects on the liver and other organs. It has a 10–60-fold higher binding affinity to the oestrogen receptor, compared with tamoxifen, but it shows lower oestrogenic and higher anti-oestrogenic effects in the rat uterus. In vitro studies showed a more potent growth inhibition in oestrogen receptor-positive cell

Table 17.2 Changes in bone metabolism, serum lipids and uterine oestrogenicity grade in patients being treated by placebo, two doses of raloxifene or oestrogen[18]

Variable	Placebo ($n = 64$)	Raloxifene 200 mg/day ($n = 60$)	Raloxifene 600 mg/day ($n = 63$)	Oestrogen 0.625 mg ($n = 64$)
Serum alkaline phosphatase (U/l)				
Baseline	75.7 (±2.6)*	75.6 (±2.5)*	71.8 (±2.7)*	74.3 (±2.5)*
Change	0.7 (±1.5)*	−5.7† (±1.1)*	−7.6† (±1.2)*	−4.7† (±1.4)*
Low-density lipoprotein cholesterol (mmol/l)				
Baseline	3.98 (±0.13)*	3.61† (±0.12)*	3.80 (±0.14)*	3.63† (±0.12)*
Change	−0.17 (±0.06)*	−0.38† (±0.08)*	−0.55† (±0.09)*	−0.45† (±0.07)*
Overall oestrogenic grade†				
	($n = 53$)	($n = 54$)	($n = 54$)	($n = 47$)
Baseline	0.11 (±0.04)*	0.09 (±0.05)*	0.13 (±0.06)*	0.21 (±0.08)*
Change	0.30 (±0.10)*	0.07† (±0.07)*	0.00† (±0.07)*	1.57† (±0.14)*

* Numbers in parentheses; median values.
† Statistically significant ($p < 0.05$) from placebo.
‡ Glandular shape, pseudostratification, nuclear to cytoplasm ratio and mitosis, stromal density, mitosis, metaplasias and tissue volume of uterus.

lines.[21] As the elimination half-life of droloxifene in humans is 25 hours, and 90% of this steady-state concentration of droloxifene can be achieved within 4 days, earlier clinical responses are expected than to tamoxifen (plateau concentrations of tamoxifen are achieved only after several weeks of oral dosing).

In a study of large doses, in 369 postmenopausal patients with hormone receptor-positive metastatic breast cancer, three different dosages of droloxifene (20, 40 and 100 mg/day orally) have been compared.[22] In 268 evaluable patients, the response rates of the 40 and 100 mg group were significantly higher than in the 20 mg group (47%, 44% and 30%, respectively; $p = 0.017$ and $p = 0.037$). Primary progressive disease was observed in 18%, 29% and 29%, respectively. The more favourable effect of a dosage of 40 mg was also obvious, when the time to progression was taken into consideration. In the 40 mg group, the patients progressed to a median of 8 months compared with 5 and 6 months in the 20 and 100 mg groups. However, this difference did not reach significant levels. Time to response was a median of 56 days, which was associated with a rapid relief of bone pain. This appears to be a shorter time than observed in historical tamoxifen data sets. Tolerability was generally good, and hot flushes and gastrointestinal disturbances were observed most frequently, with thromboembolism rarely. A slightly higher frequency of laboratory changes has been found in the 100 mg group.

Currently a trial comparing droloxifene and tamoxifen is under way.

ICI 182780

This compound represents the first candidate of a group of anti-oestrogens which, according to animal studies, have no agonist activity. It is a steroidal inhibitor with an alkylsulphinyl side chain in the 7α position. It is suspected that this side chain prevents dimerization of two oestrogen receptor molecules. This dimerization, which is induced by oestrogens or tamoxifen, is essential for the initiation of gene transcription and the oestrogen-specific response of the cell. It has also been shown that TAF1 and TAF2 are not activated by this group of anti-oestrogens.[23]

In animal studies, ICI 182780 fully blocks the uterotrophic action of oestradiol and reduces tibeal bone volume in intact rats, comparable to ovariectomy.[24] Co-administration leads to a dose-dependent inhibition.[25] Whereas mammary duct growth is promoted by partial agonist anti-oestrogens to the same extent as by oestradiol, pure antagonists have no effect and completely antagonize the effect of tamoxifen.[26]

So far there has been only one report on 19 postmenopausal patients with tamoxifen-resistant advanced breast cancer treated with ICI 182780. The compound was given as an intramuscular administration of a long-acting

Table 17.3 Correlation of response to ICI 182780 and previous response to tamoxifen[27]

Response to ICI 182780	Total no. of patients	Tamoxifen response of		
		NC	PR	Adjuvant
PR	7	2	1	4
NC	6	–	3	3
PD	6	2	2	2

PR, partial remission; NC, no change; PD, progressive disease formulation, at a dosage of 250 mg/month (the first four patients started with 100 mg for safety reasons). In 37% there was a partial remission and in 32% the disease was stabilized.[27] Median duration of response has not been obtained yet, but it will be over 18 months. In a case-control analysis, it could be demonstrated that this is significantly longer than in patients who are taking megestrol acetate. It is suspected that this prolonged activity of ICI 182780 is the result of its irreversible receptor binding. There was no apparent association of type, response and duration of treatment with tamoxifen and subsequent response to ICI 182780 (Table 17.3). Side effects have been very mild, such as blood-stained vaginal discharge and alteration of body odour. The frequency of hot flushes, vaginal dryness or altered libido has not changed after discontinuation of tamoxifen.

Further trials investigating this interesting new compound will start in the near future. Further pure anti-oestrogens under preclinical investigation are ICI 164384 and the non-steroidal ZM 189154.

NEW AROMATASE INHIBITORS

Background/mechanism of action

In postmenopausal women the main advantage of endocrine therapy is the interruption of oestrogen-induced proliferation of tumour cells. One means of achieving this in humans is to reduce oestrogen production. In post-menopausal women oestrogens are produced mainly in the adipose tissue, but also in the liver, muscle, hair follicle, and normal and cancerous glandular breast tissue, by the conversion of androstendione to oestrone and then to oestradiol. For this step of oestrogen synthesis, the function of an aromatase enzyme complex is critical and sets the pace (Figure 17.2). This step is found mainly in the ovaries in pre-menopausal women and in adipose tissue in postmenopausal women.

This enzyme complex consists of two different compounds:[28]

1. A specific aromatase P450 cytochrome, which binds the androgen and leads to the aromatic formation of a phenolic A ring of the steroid via a multistep sequence.

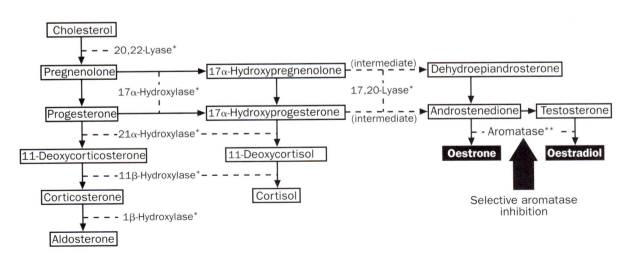

Figure 17.2 Biosynsthesis of oestrogens: different targets of selective** and non-selective* aromatase inhibitors.

2. An NADPH-dependent P450 cytochrome reductase, which transfers electrons from NADPH to the aromatase P450 cytochrome.

Aromatase inhibitors can suppress the aromatase enzyme complex and lead to decreased circulating oestrogen levels. The more specific the action of an aromatase inhibitor, the more marked is the oestrogen deprivation. Oestrogen levels in postmenopausal women are not controlled by feedback, unlike other hormone pathways. Low oestrogen levels do not stimulate excretion of gonadotrophin or of other hormones. Thus selective aromatase inhibitors can decrease oestrogens to below detectable levels.

Two different types of aromatase inhibitors are described, based on their mechanism of action (Figure 17.3).[29]

Type I

These are steroidal androstenedione derivates which are recognized as substrates by the aromatase cytochrome P450. They are processed through the normal catalytic mechanism to a product that binds covalently and irreversibly to the catalytic site of the enzyme, causing its definite functional loss. A resumption of oestrogen production is possible only via the synthesis of new aromatase molecules. Steroidal aromatase inhibitors include, for example, 4-hydroxyandrostenedione (formestane) and FCE 24304 (exemestane).

Type II

These agents are non-steroidal imidazoles which interfere reversibly with the cytochrome P450 reductase of the aromatase complex. The first aromatase inhibitor, aminoglutethimide, belongs to this type, although it also shows an inhibitory effect on other steroid hydroxylases because their cytochrome P450 prosthetic group is identical to that of the reductase. This results in considerable toxicity. Recently, a number of new, highly selective, non-steroidal, aromatase inhibitors have been synthesized. Adverse reactions are infrequent because of their selective inhibition of the cytochrome P450 reductase. The drugs that have been investigated most are anastrozole (ICI-D-1033), fadrozole and CGS 20267 (letrozole).

The molecular structure of the aromatase inhibitors and their classification is given in Figure 17.4. An overview of the efficacy of all aromatase inhibitors, estimated in relation to the inhibition constant of aminoglutethimide on human placental aromatase, is shown in Table 17.4.

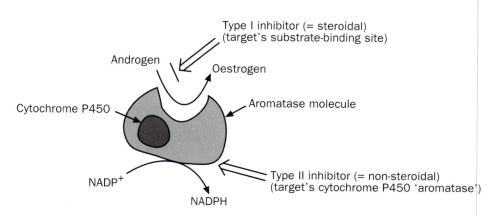

Figure 17.3 Working mechanism of aromatase inhibitors: difference between steroidal and non-steroidal substances.

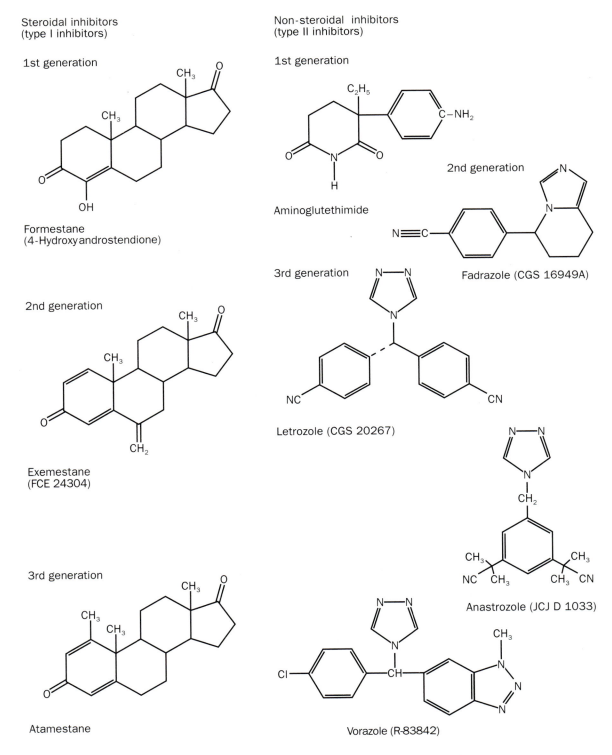

Steroidal inhibitors
(type I inhibitors)

1st generation

Formestane
(4-Hydroxyandrostendione)

2nd generation

Exemestane
(FCE 24304)

3rd generation

Atamestane

Non-steroidal inhibitors
(type II inhibitors)

1st generation

Aminoglutethimide

2nd generation

Fadrazole (CGS 16949A)

3rd generation

Letrozole (CGS 20267)

Anastrozole (JCJ D 1033)

Vorazole (R-83842)

Figure 17.4 Molecular structure of aromatase inhibitors (type I and type II inhibitors).

Table 17.4 Summary of aromatase inhibitors

Group	Substance	Aromatase inhibition	Dose schedule (mg/day p.o.)	Major toxicity
Non-steroidal				
Glutethimide	Aminoglutethimide	1	500	CNS, GI tract, allergic
Imidazoles	Fadrazole (CGS 16499A)	3000	2–4	GI tract
Triazoles	Anastrozole (Z D 1033)	400	1	Hot flushes, GI tract
	Letrozole (CGS 20267)	900	2.5	GI tract
	Vorazole (R-76713)	900	2.5	GI tract
Steroidal	Atamestane	7	500	GI tract
	Formestane	30	250 mg/14 days i.m.	Local reaction injection site, GI tract
	Exemestane (FCE 24304)	150	25	GI tract, hot flushes

GI, gastrointestinal; CNS, central nervous system.

Compounds

Aminoglutethimide

This drug was developed as an antiepileptic agent in 1966, but 8 years later Santen and co-workers demonstrated the inhibition of the non-gonadal oestrogen production in post-menopausal women.[30] This mechanism of action was first described as 'chemical adrenalectomy' after the frequently used surgical adrenalectomy.

Aminoglutethimide has proved to be effective in the treatment of metastatic breast cancer in postmenopausal women. Objective remissions are observed in about 30% and stabilization of disease in another 15%. This control of disease lasts for an average of 11 months.[31] The response rate is related to the detection of oestrogen receptors in the tumour tissue of the primary cancer and/or the metastasis.[32] In hormone receptor-positive disease, response rate increases up to 60%. In addition, the action of aminogluthetimide seems to be connected to the presence of aromatase in tumour tissue.[33]

However, aminogluthetimide does not specifically inhibit the aromatase; it also inhibits other enzymes involved in steroid biosynthesis, e.g. 11β-hydroxylase. This results, at least at doses over 750 mg, in a considerable number of adverse events, caused mostly by decreased cortisol levels. Therefore substitution of prednisone was recommended or, as shown in later trials, a dose reduction to 500 mg was possible without a reduction in effectiveness. The major aims of research were directed towards the synthesis of substances that specifically inhibited aromatases.

Fadrazole (CGS 16949 A)

This non-steroidal competitive aromatase inhibitor has also shown activity in postmenopausal women with oestrogen receptor-positive or unknown metastatic breast cancer. In a phase II study investigating doses of 1.0 mg or 2.0 mg twice daily, or 0.6 mg three times daily, in a total of 56 patients, response rates of 20% (four complete and seven partial responses) and stabilization in 50% were reached. The median time to treatment failure in the objective responders was 17 months and appears to be similar for those patients characterized as stable. Toxicity was minimal with mild orthostatic hypotension in one patient. There have been no significant biochemical or haematological changes. All three dose schedules produced identical clinical and endocrine effects.[34]

Table 17.5 Objective responses of fadrozole versus megestrol acetate in 683 patients of two prospective randomized trials[35]

	Response rates (%)			
	Fadrazole 2 mg		Megestrol acetate 160 mg	
	1st study	2nd study	1st study	2nd study
Complete response	2.1	2.7	4.3	2.7
Partial response	9.2	10.7	12.0	8.8
Stable disease	24.6	19.6	24.0	29.7
Progressive disease	64.1	64.1	62.7	58.8

There are now two randomized trials that compare fadrazole 1 mg twice daily with megestrol acetate 40 mg four times a day in a double-blind fashion. All patients needed to have prior treatment with tamoxifen. A total of 683 patients was included. Response rates are similar to those for other selective aromatase inhibitors (Table 17.5). Median time to treatment failure in the first trial was 116 and 114 days, and in the second trial 158 and 174 days, for fadrazole and megestrol acetate, respectively.[35]

These promising results have led to the investigation of this compound as first-line therapy in 176 patients. Preliminary data of this randomized trial, comparing fadrazole with tamoxifen, show a non-significant lower response rate for fadrazole (16%) and median time to progression (4.9 months) than for tamoxifen (24% and 8.3 months, respectively). Toxicity was more pronounced in the tamoxifen group.[36] However, definitive interpretation of these results has to be postponed.

Anastrozole (Arimidex)

This third-generation, non-steroidal, aromatase inhibitor was recently registered in the USA and Europe for the treatment of metastatic breast cancer. Anastrozole can be given orally with maximal plasma concentrations being reached after 2 hours. A single dose of 1 mg can suppress oestradiol levels in postmenopausal women to below detectable values.[37] As only a small amount is eliminated by the kidneys, no dose reduction is necessary in patients with renal failure.

In five phase I and II studies, toxicity was low for doses up to 60 mg. The only detectable alteration was an increase of luteinizing hormone (LH) and follicle-stimulating hormone (FSH) levels. In a European randomized phase III trial, including 378 patients who progressed after or during adjuvant or palliative treatment with anti-oestrogens, two doses of anastrozole (1 and 10 mg) have been compared with megestrol acetate 160 mg.[38] All the patients needed to have a good performance status (WHO grade

Table 17.6 Results of two randomized trials comparing two different doses of anastrozole with megestrol acetate[39]

Treatment	Anastrozole 1 mg	Anastrozole 10 mg	Megestrol acetate 160 mg
European study			
Patients	135	118	125
Median age (years)	64	66	64
Response rate* (%)	34	34	33
Median time to progression (months)	4.3	5.1	3.9
American study			
Patients	128	130	128
Median age (years)	65	66	66
Response rate* (%)	37	29	35
Median time to progression (months)	4.6	5.0	4.5

*Including complete and partial responses and stable disease.

0–2). Up to 40% of the patients had been previously treated with cytotoxic agents. Hormone receptors were detected in about 70% of all primary tumours. In this well-balanced study, no detectable difference could be found in response rates and median time to progression for the three groups. The same results were obtained by a confirmatory study conducted in the USA[39] (Table 17.6).

Hot flushes were reported in 13% and dryness of the vagina in 2% of the patients; this is comparable to the side effects observed during megestrol acetate treatment. Gastrointestinal symptoms, such as nausea, vomiting and diarrhoea, were mild and temporary in 29% of the patients treated with anastrozole. However, weight gain and oedema were observed significantly more often during megestrol acetate treatment (Table 17.7).

In future trials, anastrozole will be compared with tamoxifen in the palliative and adjuvant setting. In a recently started study, conducted by the German Adjuvant Breast Group (GABG), anastrozole is to be investigated as adjuvant therapy for postmenopausal node-negative and node-positive patients with hormone receptor-positive tumours. All patients will receive 2 years of tamoxifen and, thereafter, they are to be randomized to either a further 3 years of tamoxifen or to 3 years of anastrozole (ARNO-trial).

Letrozole (CGS 20267)

This non-steroidal aromatase inhibitor is under investigation in phase II and III trials. Recently 2.5 mg has been determined as the standard dose which is given orally on a daily basis. In three phase I trials, 58 patients with metastatic breast cancer have been treated and response rates of 33–48% have been achieved (including two complete responses). No patient was withdrawn from treatment for toxicity and the side effects, which were mostly mild, have been headache, constipation, heartburn, nausea and vomiting, and 'flu-like symptoms.[40–42]

In a recently published double-blind prospective trial two different doses of letrozole (0.5 mg once daily and 2.5 mg once daily) were

Table 17.7 Toxicity of anastrozole 1 mg daily compared with a standard dose of megestrol acetate 160 mg (data from two phase III trials)[39]

Signs and symptoms	Anastrozole (*n* = 262)	Megestrol acetate (*n* = 253)
	No. of patients (%)	No. of patients (%)
Weight gain	4 (1.5)	30 (11.9)
Oedema	19 (7.3)	35 (13.8)
Thromboembolic events	9 (3.4)	12 (4.7)
Gastrointestinal tract (nausea, vomiting, diarrhoea)	77 (29.4)	54 (21.3)
Hot flushes	33 (12.6)	35 (13.8)
Vaginal dryness	5 (1.9)	2 (0.8)

compared with megestrol acetate 160 mg once daily in advanced hormone receptor-positive breast cancer. All patients showed progression under anti-oestrogenic treatment. In this multi-centre study, 551 well-balanced patients were allocated to one of the three treatment arms. Oestrone and oestradiol were suppressed to a higher degree by letrozole than by megestrol acetate. Patients treated with letrozole 2.5 mg showed significantly better results than those treated with letrozole 0.5 mg or megestrol acetate, in respect of response rate, time to progression, time to treatment failure and time to death (Table 17.8). Letrozole was better tolerated than megestrol acetate, concerning cardio-vascular events and weight gain, whereas other side effects such as nausea, vomiting and arthralgia were more frequent. Discontinuation as a result of the treatment occurred significantly more often in the megestrol acetate group.[43]

Vorazole (R-83842)

This is another type II aromatase inhibitor that shows potential activity in metastatic breast cancer. In four phase II studies, including about 100 patients, a dose of 2.5 mg/day was given orally. Complete and partial remissions were observed in 26.5% of these postmenopausal women and stabilization of long-term disease occurred in another 30%. Responses lasted for 10–12 months. Toxicity was generally mild and rare with hot flushes, nausea and vomiting, pruritus and dry mouth.[44–47]

Table 17.8 Results of a double-blind randomized trial comparing two different dosages of letrozole and megestrol acetate[43]

	Letrozole 0.5 mg (n = 188) (%)	Letrozole 2.5 mg (n = 174) (%)	Megestrol acetate 160 mg (n = 189) (%)
All patients			
Complete response (CR)	3.2	6.9	4.2
Partial response (PR)	9.6	16.7	12.2
No change (NC)	12.8	9.8	15.3
Patients resistant to tamoxifen			
Responders with previous no response to therapeutic tamoxifen	6.7	28.6	15.4
Responders with previous relapse during adjuvant tamoxifen	7.7	14.0	16.4
Median duration of response (months):			
CR + PR	18.2	Not reached	18.0
NC > 6 months	17.7	17.5	12.3

Formestane

4-Hydroxyandrostenedione (formestane) represents the first highly selective aromatase inhibitor, which has become available for clinical use outside the USA. It belongs to the steroidal type and its inhibitory effect is 30 times that of aminogluthetimide. A dose of 250 mg has to be given fortnightly by intramuscular injection, because rapid glucuronidation at first-pass hepatic metabolism leads to inactivation of the drug. In early phase II trials an objective response rate of 19% was revealed on an intention to treat basis. Mainly soft tissue metastases and bone lesions responded to this therapy. The duration of response was between 10.5 and 13.8 months. The drug is safe and well tolerated with main side effects occurring at the injection site, with pain, induration and even sterile abscesses[48,49] (Table 17.9).

Little is known about the use of formestane in premenopausal patients. However, in one preliminary study, five premenopausal patients with advanced breast cancer were treated with formestane 500 mg i.m. weekly. No consistent fall in serum levels of oestradiol or obvious compensatory rise in gonadotrophins occurred and all five patients continued to menstruate during treatment. In all but one patient with stable disease, progressive disease was documented over the 8 weeks of treatment. The authors concluded that ovarian aromatase could not be efficiently inhibited at this dosage.[50] A further six premenopausal patients, who had a relapse after objective remission on goserelin, were treated with a combined formestane and goserelin regimen; four of them experienced a tumour response lasting for 8–24 months. In only one patient did the disease continue to progress. A significant further decrease in oestradiol levels could be detected (Figure 17.5).

Exemestane

This type I aromatase inhibitor binds covalently and irreversibly to the aromatase cytochrome P450. The induced inhibition of the aromatase is higher than that by formestane and it acts via the oral route.[51] In premenopausal women, a maximum suppression of plasma oestrogen levels to 28–39% of baseline levels was

Table 17.9 Side effects of formestane in postmenopausal women with advanced breast cancer: results of the German Study on 15 of 90 patients[49]

Symptoms[*]	Patients (%)
None	75 (83)
Systemic	10 (11)
Hot flushes	2
Constipation	2
Alopecia	2[†]
Pruritus	2
Urticaria (gluteal and legs)	1[†]
Peripheral oedema	1
Vaginal bleeding	1
'Feeling of sexlessness'	1[†]
Colpitis	1[†]
Emesis/vomiting	2
Sore throat	1
Exacerbation of existing exanthema	1[†]
Arthralgia	1[†]
Thrombophlebitis	1
Fatigue	1
Local	7 (8)
Pruritus	3
Local pain	4
Erythema	1

[*]Multiple symptoms possible.
[†]Treatment discontinued in three patients.

observed with a dose of 25 mg. In postmenopausal volunteers, this dose caused a suppression of about 40%, although there was evidence that exemestane metabolites interfered in the oestrogen assay at higher doses.[52]

In phase I–II trials doses ranged from 2.5 to 600 mg. The substance was well tolerated in most of the patients except for 3 of 165 (1.8%) in

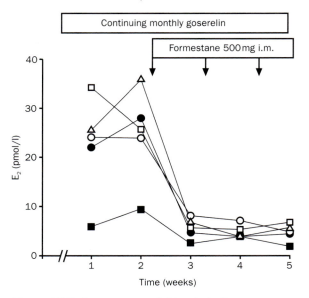

Figure 17.5 Serum oestradiol levels in five premenopausal breast cancer patients before and after the addition of formestane 500 mg i.m. weekly to ongoing monthly goserelin treatment.[50]

fatigue, nausea and vomiting (two patients), and mood change (one patient). The mild side effects were mainly hot flushes (22% in higher doses), nausea, dizziness and oedema. Androgenic effects such as hirsutism, alopecia, acne and voice deepening were observed only in doses above 100 mg (six patients; 9.3%) and were to some extent irreversible.[53]

About 100 patients could be evaluated for efficacy in metastatic breast cancer in the doses tested, from 2.5 to 600 mg. Interestingly there was a clear dose–response relationship of low (2.5–5 mg), intermediate (10–25 mg) and high (50–600 mg) doses. Response rates increased from 32% to 45% and 51%, and the median time to progression from 3.7 to 5.5 and 6.3 months (Table 17.10). However, it has been considered that, in the high-dose group, more patients with soft tissue disease were included. All patients have been heavily pre-treated with conventional hormone and cytotoxic treatment. In one trial responses were observed in 35% of a subgroup of patients with primary progression to aminoglutethimide.[54]

Recently, a multinational, double-blind, phase III study has started to compare exemestane at a dose of 25 mg with a conventional dose of megestrol acetate 160 mg. The dose was chosen as a compromise between efficacy and

whom the therapy was discontinued as a result of gastrointestinal disturbances. Grade III toxicity events have occasionally occurred, namely atrial fibrillation and heart failure (one patient),

Table 17.10 Efficacy of exemestane in heavily pre-treated patients with metastatic breast cancer: comparison of three dose groups[54]

	Dosage		
Best response	**2.5–5 mg**	**10–25 mg**	**50–600 mg**
	52 patients **n (%)**	**34 patients** **n (%)**	**80 patients** **n (%)**
CR + PR	6 (11.5)	7 (20.5)	22 (27.5)
CR + PR + NC ⩾6 months	17 (32.7)	19 (55.9)	34 (42.5)
Median time to progression (months)	4.0	6.2	6.9

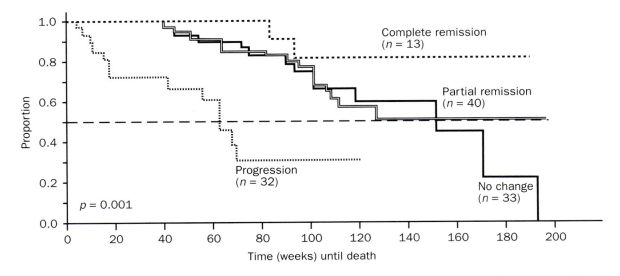

Figure 17.6 Overall survival of 118 premenopausal patients with advanced breast cancer after treatment with goserelin related to response to therapy.[60]

toxicity. All patients need to have had disease progression after previous tamoxifen treatment, but could have up to one palliative session of chemotherapy. It has been planned to recruit up to 1500 patients. Further investigations are under way on patients who have disease progression with non-steroidal aromatase inhibitors to see if a tumour response can be reached with exemestane, and whether, even after failure of low doses (25 mg), a response can be achieved with a dose of 100 mg.

Atamestane

This compound was investigated up to 1992 by Schering and has shown some activity in metastatic breast cancer resistant to tamoxifen. Out of 91 evaluable patients, 12 partial remissions were confirmed by an external review committee. As most of the patients had metastasis to the bone, objective response criteria such as recalcification were detected in only a few of these patients. This explains the large number of patients with stable disease (48%).

Further clinical studies have not, however, been carried out (AG Schering, personal communication).

The high potential shown by these new selective aromatase inhibitors cannot be interpreted as only an effect of oestrogen depletion. The role of an autonomous loop of oestrogen production by an aromatase in tumour cells has still not been elucidated. It can be speculated, however, that this aromatase is effectively inhibited by these new compounds, and this could lead to a potential activity in premenopausal women.

GONADOTROPHIN-RELEASING HORMONE ANALOGUES

Background

Oestrogen depletion in premenopausal women represents the first approach of endocrine manipulation in the treatment of breast cancer.

In 1896 George Beatson published the clinical responses to surgical removal of the ovaries in premenopausal women, after Schinzinger had theoretically suggested, in 1889, that castration could be used as a therapeutic procedure in advanced breast cancer.[55] The surgical and later the radiological elimination of ovarian function was a widely used treatment for metastatic disease until the development of cytotoxic drugs which replaced them both. Both these treatments were shown to be comparable and reached response rates of 21–37%.[56] Both approaches are, however, irreversible and represent major trauma, physically and emotionally, to the patients. With the introduction of gonadotrophin-releasing hormone (GnRH) analogues, an opportunity was provided to decrease circulating oestrogen concentrations without the need for irreversible surgery.[57]

Use of long-acting GnRH analogues overrides the normal pulsatory release of GnRH from the hypothalamus, and it is only this pulsatory release that leads to a pulsatile secretion of gonadotrophins, maintaining cyclical gonadal activity. Administration of GnRH therefore causes an initial stimulation of gonadotrophin release in the pituitary gland, followed by a fall in gonadotrophin secretion and a termination of ovarian function. This effect is maintained as long as GnRH analogues are given.[58]

As these polypeptides are usually degraded in the gastrointestinal tract, they have to be given by either an intranasal spray or subcutaneous injection. Recent formulations allow a monthly subcutaneous injection of a slow-releasing depot (goserelin, leuprorelin, triptorelin). These drugs are decapeptides with two amino acids of the original GNRH replaced.

Goserelin

In a meta-analysis (including a large German trial with 118 patients), in which the patients have been treated with goserelin, 333 patients could be

Table 17.11 Objective clinical response rate to goserelin depot by age of patient, histological grade and ER status[59]

Assessment	Classification		Objective response (%) (CR + PR)
Overall	Total assessed	228	36.4
Age (years)	<36	(37)	32.4
	36–40	(50)	38.0
	41–45	(77)	37.7
	>45	(64)	35.9
Tumour: degree of histological differentiation			
	High	(8)	50.0
	Medium	(85)	44.7
	Low	(69)	26.1
	Unknown	(66)	34.8
ER status			
	Positive	(102)	44.1
	Negative	(49)	30.6
	Unknown	(77)	29.9

evaluated for toxicity and endocrine response and 228 for efficacy. Sixty-six patients were either treated with a combination of goserelin and tamoxifen or had non-metastatic disease and were therefore excluded from efficacy analysis.[59,60]

After an initial rise above baseline, oestrogen levels were found to have decreased to below 40 pg/ml within 3 weeks of first use. In about half the patients one last menstruation occurred before complete suppression. The objective response rate was 36.4%, with a median time to response of 12 weeks (range 4–49) and a median duration of response of 44 weeks (range 4–160). Survival was similar in patients with remissions or stable diesease, however, patients with progressive disease during goserelin showed a significantly impaired outcome (Figure 17.6). The response rate was slightly better in patients with oestrogen receptor-positive tumours (44.1%) than in those with negative tumours (30.6%), but the rate was not influenced by the patient's age or tumour differentiation (Table 17.11). The response rate in visceral disease was between 24% and 28%. Primary progression was observed in 14%. Most of the observed adverse events were mild and mainly caused by the pharmacological action of goserelin (hot flushes, vaginal dryness, loss of libido and mood disturbances). Longer treatment can reduce bone mineral density. However, it is unclear to what extent this is of clinical relevance, whether, after termination of treatment, this loss can be regained, and whether the degree of bone mineral density reduction is a predictor for later osteoporosis.

Combination of goserelin with tamoxifen or other hormonal drugs provides an interesting approach. Young patients with medically induced menopause may become suitable for further endocrine manipulations. In one randomized trial in premenopausal patients, the primary combination of goserelin and tamoxifen was compared with a sequential treatment of tamoxifen and goserelin after disease progression occurred during goserelin treatment.[61] No clear differences could be observed between the two groups, but patients with bone metastasis seem to have an improved outcome, when both drugs are given primarily.

There is evidence that, even after disease progression with both hormones, further responses can be obtained if tamoxifen is replaced by an aromatase inhibitor or if a progestogen is used as a third treatment. This sequence of endocrine therapy, which is equivalent to what happens in postmenopausal patients, can be interrupted by chemotherapy if indicated clinically.[62] It is still unclear if the maintenance of the CnRh-analogue is of benefit during second or third-line therapy.

These promising results led to further investigation of GnRH analogues. So far four adjuvant therapy trials have evaluated goserelin in the primary setting in premenopausal women.

ZEBRA (Zoladex Early Breast Cancer Research Association) trial: This trial aims to recruit more than 1600 pre-/perimenopausal patients aged 50 years or less with stage II, node-positive breast cancer. After surgery, patients are randomized to receive either goserelin for 2 years or six cycles of CMF (cyclophosphamide, methotrexate and 5-fluorouracil) chemotherapy. Recruitment has been completed by the end of 1996 and the first results will be available in 1998.

Cancer Research Centre (CRC) Under 50s Study: This trial aims to recruit patients aged under 50 years, with stage I and II breast cancer. After surgery, patients can receive standard therapy (radiotherapy and/or chemotherapy), and are then randomized to receive goserelin or a combination of goserelin and tamoxifen or tamoxifen alone or no further therapy. The duration of treatment is 2 years. More than 2200 patients have already been recruited.

International Breast Cancer Study Group (IBCSG) IV Study: This trial aims to recruit 1200 pre-/perimenopausal patients with node-negative breast cancer. After surgery, patients are randomized to receive either goserelin (2 years) or six cycles of CMF or both (goserelin for only 1.5 years). About 750 patients have been included.

ECOG/Southwest Oncology Group (SWOG) Study: This trial recruited 1537 premenopausal patients with node-positive, receptor-positive breast cancer. After surgery, all patients received CAF (cyclophosphamide, doxorubicin [Adriamycin] and 5-fluorouracil) and were randomized to goserelin (5 years) or goserelin and tamoxifen (5 years) or no endocrine treatment. Recruitment has been completed.

The results of these trials will be available in the near future. Randomized trials comparing medical versus surgical ovariectomy have been launched; however, they had to be stopped as a result of insufficient recruitment. Only indirect comparisons such as meta-analysis can give a hint whether these treatment strategies are equipotential. Medical castration would mean that younger women can keep their full reproductive potential after adjuvant treatment, and this has a major impact on the complete recovery of the patient, because until now no clear negative effect of a pregnancy has been demonstrated after early stage breast cancer.

Experimental results of tumour growth inhibition and detection of GnRH receptors in human breast cancer tissues have also favoured the idea of the direct anti-tumour effect of GnRH analogues in postmenopausal breast cancer patients.[63] A number of small clinical studies failed to show efficacy in these patients. In a total of 250 pre-treated patients who had advanced disease, an overall response rate of only 7.5% was observed.[64]

Antiprogestins

Antiprogestins represent a group of compounds that have a new and promising approach to the treatment of hormone-dependent breast cancer. These compounds show a high affinity for the progesterone receptor and, to some extent, to the glucocorticoid receptor. They inhibit the progesterone-induced transformation of the endometrium and induce premature menstruation when administered during the late luteal phase. Follicular development and growth are inhibited.[65]

Whereas mifepristone has been investigated mainly for induction of early abortion, both mifepriston and onapristone (SHT 549 B, Schering), which have a weaker anti-glucocorticoid effect, haves been evaluated for the treatment of breast cancer.[66]

In in vitro and animal studies, onapristone induces terminal differentiation, induction of apoptosis and blockade of the tumour cell cycle with a reduction of cells in the S phase.[67] Its anti-tumour activity is as strong as, or even stronger than, that of tamoxifen or oophorectomy in hormone-dependent breast cancer in the rat and mouse. Although binding to a progesterone receptor is a prerequisite for the antiproliferative effects of onapristone, there is evidence that the mechanism of its anti-tumour effects does not depend on a classic antihormone mechanism.[68]

In one phase II trial, 118 postmenopausal patients with progressive breast cancer were given onapristone 100 mg/day orally. The duration of therapy was not predetermined. All patients had received at least one course of palliative or adjuvant endocrine therapy and had disease progression, with at least one measurable or evaluable lesion. Ninety patients were evaluated for efficacy and nine (10%) had an objective response (one complete and eight partial responses) with a median duration of 12 months. Thirty-eight patients (42%) had stable disease for at least 3 months (median duration 8 months) and 43 patients had disease progression at first. However, more than 50% of the patients had bony lesions in which it is difficult to determine response. This could explain the strikingly high rate of stable disease.

Subjective tolerance to the drug was good. The most frequent adverse events were nausea and headache, which in most cases were mild and transient. In several patients an elevation of liver enzymes was observed, although this was not clear cut. Seven patients dropped out as a result of possibly drug-related adverse events (Schering AG, personal communication).

Further investigations of onapristone have been stopped as a result of the unexplained elevation of liver enzymes. However, several new antiprogestins are being developed that have an even higher potency in tumour growth retardation. As a result of their new mechanism of action, combinations with other antihormones are of great interest.

CONCLUSION AND PERSPECTIVES

A broad field of possible indications for these new endocrine compounds can be forecast.

There is even an endeavour to reduce the extent of operative treatment further and to treat patients with hormones, for example, the use of GnRH analogues in premenopausal women instead of surgical oophorectomy or the sole use of tamoxifen in elderly women at low risk rather than axillary dissection or even breast cancer.

The value of simultaneous or sequential combinations of hormone plus hormone or hormone plus chemotherapy is more or less unknown for palliative and adjuvant treatment. Meta-analysis and indirect comparisons can cover the effect of a single biologically active regimen. Therefore, further trials, for example, those based on animal experiments, have to be designed to answer this question.

Tamoxifen has not only a documented anticancer activity, but also seems to maintain bone density and may reduce cardiac mortality in patients with long-term treatment. This was one of the reasons for two preventive tamoxifen trials in women at high risk of developing breast cancer. However, careful investigation of long-term side effects in connection with these studies has elucidated the carcinogenic potential of tamoxifen on the endometrium. This has encouraged a strengthening of the investigations into new anti-oestrogens that have no significant risk even as preventive agents, which could then replace tamoxifen in the future.

REFERENCES

1. Henderson IC. Endocrine therapy of metastatic breast cancer. In: *Breast Diseases* 2nd edn (Harris JR, Hellmann S, Henderson IC, Kinne DW, eds). Philadelphia: Lippincott, 1995:559–603.

2. Early Breast Cancer Trialist's Collaborative Group. Systemic treatment of early breast cancer by hormonal, cytotoxic, or immune therapy. *Lancet* 1992; **339**:1–15, 71–85.

3. Rose C. Endocrine therapy of advanced breast cancer. In: *Consensus Development in Cancer Therapy* 1: *Therapeutic Management of Metastatic Breast Cancer* (Kaufmann M, Henderson IC, Enghofer E, eds). Berlin: de Gruyter, 1989.

4. Fornander T, Rutqvist LE, Cedarmark B, et al. Adjuvant tamoxifen in early breast cancer: Occurrence of new primary cancer. *Lancet* 1989; **i**:117–20.

5. Draper MW, Flowers DE, Neild JA, Huster WJ, Zerbe RL. Antiestrogenic properties of raloxifene. *Pharmacology* 1995; **50**:209–17.

6. Gronemeyer H. Transcription activation by nuclear receptors. *J Recept Res* 1993; **13**:667–91.

7. Tzukerman MT, Estry A, Santiso-Mere D, et al. Human estrogen receptor transactivational capacity is determined by both cellular and promotor context and mediated by two functionally distinct intramolecular regions. *Mol Endocrinol* 1994; **8**:21–30.

8. Kangas L. Biochemical and pharmacological effects of toremifen metabolites. *Cancer Chemother Pharmacol* 1990; **27**:8–12.

9. Hayes DJ, Vogel CL and the 'Erbamont' Toremifene Phase II Study Group. A randomized comparison of tamoxifen and two separate doses of toremifene in postmenopausal patients with metastatic breast cancer. *European Congress on Clinical Oncology Paris*, Pergamon (Elsevier Science): Oxford, Abstract book, 1995.

10. Gershanowich M, Garin A, Baltina D, et al. and the Russian–Baltic Toremifene Phase III Study Group. Toremifene clinical phase III 'Russian–Baltic' study. *European Congress on Clinical Oncology Paris*. Pergamon (Elsevier Science): Abstract book, 1995.

11. Pyrhönen S and the 'Nordic' Toremifene Study Group in Finland, Hungary, Norway, Poland, Sweden and Czech Republic. Toremifene clinical phase III 'Nordic' study. *European Congress on Clinical Oncology Paris*, Pergamon (Elsevier Science): Oxford, Abstract book, 1995.

12. Bonneterre J, Review of the phase III studies of toremifene and tamoxifen in advanced breast cancer. *European Congress on Clinical Oncology Paris* Pergamon (Elsevier Science):, Abstract book, 1995.

13. Hard GC, Iatropoulos MJ, Jordan K, et al. Major difference in the hepatocarcinogenicity and DNA adduct forming ability between toremifene and tamoxifen in female Crl: CD (BR) rats. *Cancer Res* 1993; **53**:4534–41.

14. Gershanowich M, Moiseyenko M. Toremifene in the treatment of advanced renal cell carcinoma. *European Congress on Clinical Oncology Paris*, Pergamon (Elsevier Science): Oxford, Abstract book, 1995.

15. Raloxifene HCl (LY 139481): Clinical Investigator's Brochure. Eli Lilly & Co. July, 1995.

16. Black LJ, Jones CD, Falcone JF. Antagonism of estrogen action with a new benzothiophene derived antiestrogen. *Life Sci* 1983; **32**:1031–6.

17. Black LJ, Sato M, Rowley ER, et al. Raloxifene (LY 139481 HCl) prevents bone loss and reduces serum cholesterol without causing uterine hypertrophy in ovariectomized rats. *J Clin Invest* 1994; **93**:63–9.

18. Draper MW, Flowers DE, Huster WJ, Neild JA. Effects of raloxifene (LY 139481 HCL) on biochemical markers of bone and lipid metabolism in healthy postmenopausal women. In *Proceedings 1993. Fourth International Symposium on Osteoporosis and Consensus Development Conference* (Christiansen C, Riis B, eds). Aalborg, Denmark: Handelstrykkeriet, Aalburg Aps, 1993:119–21.

19. Raloxifene (LY 139481 C'HCl): Clinical Investigator's Brochure. Eli Lilly & Company July, 1995.

20. Buzdar AU, Marcus C, Homes F, et al. Phase 2 evaluation of LY 156758 in metastatic breast cancer. *Oncology* 1988; **45**:344–5.

21. Eppenberger U, Wosikowski K, Küng W. Pharmacologic and biologic properties of droloxifene, a new antiestrogen. *Am J Clin Oncol* 1991; **14** (suppl 2):5–14.

22. Rauschning W, Pritchard KI. Droloxifene, a new antiestrogen: its role in metastatic breast cancer. *Breast Canc Res Treat* 1994 **31**;83–94.

23. Wakeling AE. Use of pure antioestrogens to elucidate the mode of action of oestrogens. *Biochem Pharmacol* 1995; **49**:1545–9.

24. Gallaher A, Chambers TJ, Tobias JH. The estrogen antagonist ICI 182,780 reduces cancellous bone volume in female rats. *Endocrinology* 1993; **133**:2787–91.

25. Wakeling AE, Dukes M, Bowler J. A potent specific pure antiestrogen with clinical potential. *Cancer Res* 1991; **51**:3867–73.

26. Nicholson RI, Gotting KE, Gee J, Walker KJ. Actions of oestrogens and antioestrogens on rat mammary gland development: Relevance to breast cancer prevention. *J Steroid Biochem* 1988; **30**:95–103.

27. Howell A, DeFriend D, Robertson J, Blamey R, Walton P. Response to a specific antioestrogen (ICI 182780) in tamoxifen-resistant breast cancer. *Lancet* 1995; **345**:29–30.

28. Bossche HV, Moereels H, Koymans LMH. Aromatase inhibitors – mechanism for non-steroidal inhibitors. *Breast Cancer Res Treat* 1994; **30**:43–55.

29. Lonning PE, Kvinnsland S. Mechanism of action of aminoglutethimide as endocrine therapy of breast cancer. *Drugs* 1988; **35**:685–710.

30. Santen RJ, Manni A, Harvey H, Redmond C. Endocrine treatment of breast cancer in women. *Endocrine Rev* 1990; **11**:221–65.

31. Stuart-Harris RC, Smith IE. Aminoglutethimide in the treatment of advanced breast cancer. *Cancer Treat Rev* 1984; **11**:189–204.

32. Bhatnagar AS, Batzl Ch, Häusler A, Schieweck K. Pharmakologie der Aromatase Hemmstoffe. In: *Neue Aromatasehemmer-Konsequenzen für die Therapie des Mammakarzinoms* (Jonat W, ed.). Wehr: Ciba-Geigy, 1994:11–17.

33. Miller WR. Aromatase activity in breast tissue. *J Steroid Biochem Mol Biol* 1991; **39**:783–90.

34. Harvey HA, Lipton A, Santen RJ, et al. Phase I and phase II clinical trials of fadrazole hydrochloride in postmenopausal women with metastatic breast cancer. In: *Clinical Use of Aromatase Inhibitors. Current Data and Future Perspectives* (Robustelli della Cuna G, Manni A, Pannuti F, eds). Pavia: Edimes, 1994:155–9.

35. Buzdar AU, Smith R, Vogal C, et al. Fadrozole HCL (CGS-16949 A) versus megestrol acetate in postmenopausal patients with metastatic breast carcinoma: results of two randomized double blind controlled multi-institutional trials. *Cancer* 1996; **77**:2503–13.

36. Thurlimann B, Beretta K, Bacchi M, et al. First line fadrozole HCL (CGS-16949 A) versus tamoxifen in advanced breast cancer prospective randomized study SAKK 20/88 [abstract]. *Proc ASCO* 1995; **14**:A90.

37. Plourde PV, Dryoff M, Dukes M. Anastrozol, a potent and selective fourth generation aromatase inhibitor. *Breast Cancer Res Treat* 1994; **30**:103–11.

38. Jonat W, Howell A, Blomqvist C, et al., on behalf of the ARIMIDEX-Study Group, A randomized trial comparing two doses of the new selective aromatase inhibitor anastrozole (Arimidex) with megestrol acetate in postmenopausal patients with advanced breast cancer. *Eur J Cancer* 1996; **32A**:404–12.

39. Buzdar AU, Jonat W, Howell A, et al. Anastrozole (Arimidex), a potent and selective aromatase inhibitor, versus megestrol acetate (Megace) in postmenopausal women with advanced breast cancer: results of an overview of two phase III trials. *J Clin Oncol* 1996; **14**:2000–11.

40. Demers LM. Effects of fadrozole (CGS 16949 A) and letrozole (CGS 20267) on the inhibition of aromatase activity in breast cancer patients. *Breast Cancer Res Treat* 1994; **30**:95–102.

41. Iverson TJ, Smith IE, Ahern J, et al. Phase I study of the oral non-steroidal aromatase inhibitor (CGS 20267) in postmenopausal patients with advanced breast cancer. *Cancer Res* 1993; **53**:266–70.

42. Cocconi G, Bisagni G, Ceci G, et al. CGS 20267 a new oral aromatase inhibitor: phase I study in postmenopausal advanced breast cancer patients. Proceedings of the 8th NCI-EORTC Symposium on New Drugs in Cancer Therapy, March 15–18, 1994, Amsterdam [abstract]. *Ann Oncol* 1994; **5** (suppl 5):251.

43. Dombernowsky, P, Smith I, Falkson G, et al., for the Letrozole International Trial Group (AR/BC2). Double-blind trial in postmenopausal women with advanced breast cancer showing a dose-effect and superiority of 2.5 mg letrozole over megestrol acetate [abstract]. *Proc ASCO* 1996; **15**:A64.

44. Paradaens R, Piccart M, Nooji M, et al. Phase II study of Vorozole (R83842), a new non-steroidal aromatase inhibitor in advanced breast cancer. EORTC Breast Cancer Cooperative Group [abstract]. *Eur J Cancer* 1994; **30A** (suppl 2):22.

45. Goss PE, Clark R, Ambus U, et al. Phase II study of vorozole (R83842) a new aromatase inhibitor in postmenopausal women with advanced breast cancer [abstract]. *Proc ASCO* 1994; **13**:156.

46. Amoroso D, Boccardo F, Balestrero M, et al. Phase II study of vorozole as second line therapy in postmenopausal patients with advanced breast cancer: preliminary results of a multicentric trial [abstract]. *Ann Oncol* 1994; **5** (suppl 8):33.

47. Johnston SRD, Smith IE, Doody D. Phase II study of the oral aromatase inhibitor vorozole in human breast cancer [abstract]. *Eur J Cancer* 1994; **30A** (suppl 2):23.

48. Gross PE, Powles TJ, Dowsett M, et al. Treatment of advanced postmenopausal breast cancer with an aromatase inhibitor, 4-hydroxyandrostendione: phase II report. *Cancer Res* 1986; **46**:4823–6.

49. Höffken K, Jonat W, Possinger K. 4-Hydroxyandrostenedione in the treatment of advanced breast cancer. The German experience. In: *Clinical Use of Aromatase Inhibitors. Current Data and Future Perspectives* (Robustelli della Cuna G, Manni A, Pannuti F, eds). Pavia: Edimes, 1994:135–40.

50. Stein RC, Dowsett M, Hedley A, et al. The clinical and endocrine effects of 4-hydroxyandrostenedione alone and in combination with goserelin in premenopausal women with advanced breast cancer. *Br J Cancer* 1990; **62**:679–83.

51. Giudici D, Ornati G, Briatico G, et al. 6-Methylenadrosta-1,4-diene-3,17-dione (FCE 24304): a new irreversible aromatase inhibitor. *J Steroid Biochem* 1988; **30**:391–4.

52. Jeffry Evans TR, di Salle E, Ornati O, et al. Phase I single dose and endocrine study of exemestane (FCE 24304), a new aromatase inhibitor, in postmenopausal women. *Cancer Res* 1992; **52**:5933–9.

53. Exemestane. Investigator's brochure. Pharmacia, 1995.

54. Thürlimann B, Paredaens R, Roche M, et al. Exemestane in postmenopausal pretreated advanced breast cancer: a multicenter Phase-II study in patients with aminoglutethimide failure [abstract]. *Proc ESMO* 1994; **5** (suppl 8):144.

55. Beatson GT. On the treatment of inoperable cases of carcinoma of the mama: Suggestions for a new method of treatment with illustrative cases. *Lancet* 1896; **ii**:104–7.

56. Veronesi U, Franzo G, Galluzo D, et al. A reappraisal of oophorectomy in carcinoma of the breast. *Ann Surg* 1987; **205**:18–21.

57. Sandow J. Pharmacology of LH-RH agonists. In: *Pharmacology and Clinical Uses of Inhibitors of Hormone Secretion and Action* (Furr BJA, Wakeling AE, eds). London: Baillière Tindall, 1987:365–84.

58. Kaufmann M, Jonat W, Schachner-Wünschmann E, on behalf of the Cooperative German Zoladex Study Group. The Depot GnRH Analogue Goserelin (Zoladex) in the treatment of premenopausal patients with metastatic breast cancer – a 5 year experience and further endocrine therapies. *Onkologie* 1991; **14**:22–30.

59. Blamey RW, Jonat W, Kaufmann M, Bianco AR, Namer M. Goserelin Depot in the treatment of premenopausal advanced breast cancer. *Eur J Cancer* 1992; **28A**:810–14.

60. Kaufmann M, Jonat W, Kleeberg U, et al. Goserelin, a depot gonadotrophin-releasing hormone agonist in the treatment of premenopausal patients with metastatic breast cancer. *J Clin Oncol* 1989; **7**:1113–19.

61. Blamey RW, on behalf of the Zoladex Trial Group. Randomised trial comparing Zoladex with Nolvadex plus Zoladex in pre-menopausal advanced breast cancer. *Fourth International Congress on Anti-Cancer Chemotherapy*, Paris, 2–5 Feb. 1993, Abstract book, abstr. no. 3 (p. 58).

62. Kaufmann M, Jonat W, Schachner-Wiinschman E, Baster G. The depot GnRH analogue Goserelin in the treatment of premenopausal patients with metastatic breast cancer – a 5-year experience and further endocrine therapies. *Onkologie* 1991; **14**:22–30.

63. Kiesel L, Kaufmann M, Schmid H, Rabe T,

Klinga K, Runnbaum B. Gonadotrophic-releasing hormone receptors in breast cancer [abstract]. *J Cancer Res Clin Oncol* 1988; **114** (suppl):94.

64. Baumann KH, Kiesel L. Treatment of postmenopausal breast cancer. In: *Treatment with GnRH Analogs: Controversies and Perspectives.* (Filicori M, Flamigni C, eds). New York: Parthenon Publishing Group, 1995.

65. Puri CP. Induction of menstruation by anti-progesterone ZK 98.299 in cyclic bonnet monkeys. *Contraception* 1987; **4**:409–21.

66. Romieu G, Mandelonde T, Ulmann A, et al. The antiprogestin RU486 in advanced breast cancer: preliminary clinical trial. *Bulletin du Cancer* **74**:455–9.

67. Michna H, Schneider M, Nishino Y, et al. Progesterone antagonists block the growth of experimental mammary tumors in G0/G1. *Breast Cancer Res Treat* 1990; **17**:155–6.

68. Michna H, Schneider M, Nishino Y, et al. The antitumor mechanism of progesterone antagonists is a receptor mediated antiproliferative effect by induction of terminal cell death. *J Steroid Biochem* 1989; **34**:447–53.

18

The role of high-dose chemotherapy in breast cancer

Sjoerd Rodenhuis

CONTENTS • **High-dose regimens for breast cancer** • **Technical considerations** • **High-dose chemotherapy in stage IV breast cancer** • **High-dose therapy in the adjuvant setting** • **Prospects**

Although chemotherapy is often effective in stage IV breast cancer, most remissions induced by it are incomplete and the median remission duration does not usually exceed one year. This rather unsatisfactory state of affairs is caused by the phenomenon called drug resistance. A proportion of tumour cells may be resistant from the outset and may have a selective growth advantage during subsequent cycles of chemotherapy. In addition, the exposure to chemotherapy itself may induce drug resistance by a variety of mechanisms, several of which lead to collateral resistance to unrelated drugs as well. Strategies to overcome drug resistance have been clinically disappointing as a result of a variety of causes. One strategy, however, has met with a limited degree of success in a number of tumour types: dose escalation.

The existence of a dose–effect relationship for the chemotherapy of breast cancer has been recognized for many years. Clearly, the use of lower-than-standard doses* of chemotherapy is associated with lower remission rates and shorter remission durations, as has been shown in several randomized studies. The beneficial effect of higher-than-standard doses of chemotherapy has not been demonstrated as convincingly. Standard-dose chemotherapy has been designed to cause optimal efficacy in the presence of tolerable toxicity. As a result, substantial dose escalations lead to a significant increase in toxicity, hampering any large-scale studies of such a strategy. Only one type of organ toxicity, bone marrow suppression, can be effectively dealt with and bone marrow protection is expensive, cumbersome and not without risk. Other toxicities, such as mucositis, asthenia, damage to nerves or heart muscle, and many others quickly become dose limiting when doses of the best anti-breast cancer agents are escalated, even if only to a limited degree.

Nevertheless, a fairly large number of phase II studies has been published, in which the use of higher-than-standard chemotherapy doses has been explored. In most studies, haemopoietic growth factors, such as granulocyte colony-stimulating factor (G-CSF) or granulocyte–macrophage colony-stimulating factor (GM-CSF), have been employed to ameliorate bone marrow toxicity. In addition, most studies included

---

* The term 'standard-dose chemotherapy' is not well defined. For breast cancer, a 3-weekly intravenous administration of cyclophosphamide 500 mg/m², doxorubicin 50 mg/m² and fluorouracil 500 mg/m² is considered 'standard-dose' by many.

only relatively young patients with good performance status, to ensure that a higher level of toxicity would be tolerated. A third factor common to most of these studies is that a quantity called 'dose intensity' was escalated rather than the total (cumulative) dose or treatment duration.[1] Dose intensity is defined as the amount of drug delivered per unit time. Thus, escalation of dose intensity can be achieved by either increasing the dose of the drug(s) or decreasing the time between administrations.

The resulting phase I and phase II studies have shown that dose intensities of up to 1.5–2.0 times the standard can be achieved, employing growth factors in suitable young patients. Not unexpectedly, the increase in dose intensity comes at a price: neutropenic fevers, profound thrombocytopenia, mucositis and other toxicities are frequent. On the positive side, high remission rates of up to 90% have been reported in uncontrolled studies, but the durations of remission were similar to those seen after standard-dose chemotherapy and long-term remissions were exceptional. A small number of randomized studies have been reported, in both the adjuvant and the advanced disease setting, in which one group of patients received a modestly increased dose of chemotherapy. None of these studies has shown a survival benefit for the high-dose arm.

A substantial increase in chemotherapy dose clearly requires more supportive care than just the administration of a growth factor. Early experience with high-dose chemotherapy and autologous bone marrow transplantation has raised the hope that this treatment modality could achieve long-term survival for a proportion of patients. The recent advances in circulating blood progenitor cell harvest and transplantation[2] have greatly increased the feasibility of truly high-dose therapy and have reduced the risks involved. This has allowed two developments: the testing of the concept in large randomized multicentre studies and the conduct of new feasibility studies which explore the limits of dose escalation.

HIGH-DOSE REGIMENS FOR BREAST CANCER

Requirements

Ideally, a high-dose combination chemotherapy regimen for breast cancer should satisfy the following criteria:

- Each agent employed should have single-agent activity in breast cancer
- Each agent should have a steep dose–response curve at dose levels between the standard and that employed in the regimen
- The only (significant) toxicity at standard level of each of the agents employed should be bone marrow suppression, allowing substantial dose escalation before dose-limiting extramedullary toxicity occurs
- The extramedullary toxicities of the agents in the high-dose combination should not overlap
- The agents in the combination should not be subject to one of the types of multidrug resistance that could result from prior treatment with standard-dose chemotherapy (unless, of course, no prior chemotherapy has been given).

In practice, unfortunately, the best agents in the treatment of breast cancer are far from this theoretical ideal for high-dose regimens. Doxorubicin and the other anthracyclines cause severe mucositis and cardiac injury at high doses, and taxanes such as paclitaxel and docetaxel may cause severe neurotoxicity which is unpredictable at escalated doses because of their non-linear (saturation) pharmacokinetics. Despite these drawbacks, studies attempting to employ either of these drugs at escalated dosage have been reported or are in progress.

The group of drugs that comes closest to the requirements is that of the alkylating agents.[3,4] Essentially all alkylators, both classic and non-classic, have modest activity in untreated breast cancer. The effects of alkylating agents are unaffected by the currently known mechanisms of multidrug resistance, and they exhibit a log linear dose–effect relation in vitro. Acquired drug resistance to alkylating agents can be induced only with some difficulty in vitro, and its attainable level is much lower than that of anthracyclines or antimetabolites. Cross-resistance between alkylators is uncommon.

The published clinical studies of high-dose single agents and combinations in breast cancer have recently been reviewed.[5]

Multi-alkylator regimens

In view of the above, it is hardly surprising that most high-dose regimens are based on alkylating drugs. The most frequently used regimens in breast cancer (Table 18.1) are either variants of the CPB regimen (cyclophosphamide, cisplatin and carmustine/BCNU) or incorporate cyclophosphamide and thiotepa, often combined with carboplatin (CTCb). Other regimens have employed melphalan (L-PAM), etoposide or mitozantrone (see recent reviews[5,12]). Comparisons in terms of efficacy between the high-dose regimens reported in the literature cannot be made. There are no randomized studies and the patient groups treated are too different for meaningful retrospective analysis. Up to a point, however, toxicity can be compared, because extramedullary toxicity is more constant and does not depend on the type or extent of the primary tumour.

Table 18.1　High-dose regimens for breast cancer

Abbreviation	Regimen		Employed in
	Drugs	Dose (mg/m²)	
CPB[6]	Cyclophosphamide	5625	Adjuvant study and Randomized
	Carmustine (BCNU)	600	Intergroup study 0163
	Cisplatin	165	
CT[7,8]	Cyclophosphamide	6000–7500	Randomized Intergroup study 0121
	Thiotepa	675–800	
CTCb[9] ('STAMP V')	Cyclophosphamide	6000	Boston studies, Randomized
	Thiotepa	500	European studies
	Carboplatin	800	
CTC[10]	Cyclophosphamide	6000	Dutch national adjuvant study in
	Thiotepa	480	high-risk patients
	Carboplatin	1600	
MM[11]	Melphalan	140	Dutch study in complete responders with stage
	Mitozantrone	60	IV disease

From the literature.[6–11]

In general, the combination of cisplatin, carmustine and cyclophosphamide is associated with renal toxicity (as a result of the high-dose cisplatin) and with pulmonary toxicity caused by the nitrosourea derivative. The latter may increase the risk of radiation pneumonitis if radiotherapy of the chest wall is planned, as is often the case in breast cancer. Mucositis is usually mild or absent. CTCb-like regimens may cause mild mucositis for a few days, but renal failure and lung toxicity are absent. Both types of regimens allow discharge from the hospital as soon as the peripheral blood progenitor cell (PBPC) transplantation has taken place, provided that appropriate supportive care in the outpatient setting is available on a 24-hour basis, and that the patient has a place to stay near to the hospital. As neutropenic fevers are extremely common in the post-transplantation phase, many patients require parenteral antibiotics, which may dictate re-hospitalization in many settings. Ongoing studies focus on cost, morbidity and quality of life issues of 'outpatient transplantations' in comparison to the more usual clinical care.

Common toxicities of high-dose therapy

Nausea and vomiting are common during and after high-dose chemotherapy, despite the use of hydroxytryptamine HT_3-receptor blockers and high-dose dexamethasone. Diarrhoea and abdominal cramps are usually manageable with loperamide and spasmolytic agents, but at times require intravenous hydration or a somatostatin analogue. Most patients have at least one episode of neutropenic fever which is managed with broad-spectrum antibiotics. Frequently, no causative micro-organism is recovered. Some episodes are caused by Gram-positive bacteria – usually coagulase-negative staphylococci – which colonize the central venous access catheter. Other causes, including Gram-negative and fungal infections, have become much less frequent with prophylactic antibiotics and the relatively brief duration of absolute neutropenia associated with PBPC transplantation. Nevertheless, infection remains a major cause of morbidity and occasional mortality. Appropriate antibiotics should be used with care in the treatment and prophylaxis of infections.[13] Skin rashes, often ascribed to antibiotic hypersensitivity, are very frequent and commonly associated with fever. Although sometimes impressive in size and intensity, most are relatively benign and subside readily when the offending agent is discontinued.[14]

After PBPC transplantation, the neutrophil count begins to rise on day 8 or 9 after transplantation. The neutrophil recovery is hastened by the administration of G-CSF in this period, and virtually all patients have over $0.5 \times 10^9/l$ granulocytes by day 11 after transplantation. Platelet transfusion independence is reached in almost all patients by day 21 after transplantation. Most centres irradiate all blood products to be transfused in this period to prevent graft-versus-host disease.

In most respects, the supportive care required for PBPC transplantation in breast cancer resembles that given for the therapy of acute leukaemia. As a result of the rapid haemopoietic reconstitution after PBPC transplantation and the only minimal degree of mucositis induced by multiple alkylating agents, however, its associated morbidity and mortality may actually be lower.

TECHNICAL CONSIDERATIONS

Peripheral blood progenitor cell mobilization and harvest

Peripheral blood progenitor cells can be mobilized either by administration of a haemopoietic growth factor alone (usually G-CSF or GM-CSF), or by a combination of myelosuppressive chemotherapy and growth factor administration. The latter method is more common, because it allows the start or continuation of chemotherapy and probably yields a larger harvest than a growth factor alone. The specific type of chemotherapy used is of only minor importance. There appears, however, to be a dose–response relationship for the haematological growth factor. A typical mobilization regimen would be a standard course of cyclophosphamide, doxorubicin and fluoro-uracil on day 1, followed by daily administration of G-CSF (10 µg/kg body weight subcutaneously daily). Daily leukocytapheresis sessions begin when the white blood cell (WBC) count exceeds 3.0×10^9/l; they are continued (as is the G-CSF) until a sufficient number of PBPCs have been harvested.[14,15]

A variety of growth factors or combinations of growth factors has been used successfully to mobilize stem cells. Currently, G-CSF alone or in combination with chemotherapy is most widely used because of its low toxicity. This may change when thrombopoietin (rhTPO or 'megakaryocyte growth and development factor') becomes more widely available. It is possible that administration of rhTPO, together with G-CSF or other growth factors, may considerably enhance the yield of megakaryocyte progenitors during leukocytapheresis, leading to shorter times to platelet transfusion independence.

Size and quality of the graft

Following (sub)myeloablative therapy, reinfusion of autologous haemopoietic progenitor cells is required for (rapid) reconstitution of the bone marrow. Progenitor cells can be obtained either from the bone marrow or from the peripheral blood. Until recently, many centres used a combination of both sources. As it is now generally accepted that PBPC transplantations lead to sustained bone marrow recovery,[16] bone marrow transplantations have become uncommon in breast cancer and are even considered to be obsolete by many.

The question about what size of graft should be used for rapid and sustained bone marrow recovery is still a matter of debate. In the absence of an assay system for the human bone marrow stem cell, most investigators agree that the count of CD34$^+$ cells available is a reasonable, although imperfect, measure of graft size.[17] The absolute number of mononuclear cells is often misleading and should no longer be used. Colony-forming units (CFUs), particu-larly CFU-GMs, have been used extensively. The CFU-GM assay is, however, a non-standardized biological system and its results are highly variable between laboratories. Its prediction of recovery is no better than that of the CD34$^+$ count; it is laborious and takes 2 weeks before its results can be read. Consequently, the CFU-GM assay is no longer necessary for routine transplantations. Its main use is to check the vitality of the graft after cryopreservation and thawing. Laboratories with limited experience in the cryopreservation of the bulky PBPC harvests should routinely employ the CFU-GM assay as a quality control instrument after thawing.

Unfortunately, the flow-cytometric CD34$^+$ assays now routinely employed by most centres are also not well standardized. Although the degree of variation is certainly less than that of the CFUs, this may lead to important differences in results reported from different centres and it may even explain that some centres are unable to confirm the relationship between the number of CD34$^+$ cells reinfused and the time to bone marrow recovery observed by others. The following figures are used by the author's group: infusion of 8×10^6 CD34$^+$ cells/kg is probably optimal. It leads to platelet transfusion independence by day 14 after reinfusion in almost all patients. A reinfusion of 3×10^6 CD34$^+$ cells/kg is, in the author's experience, sufficient for rapid neutrophil recovery and sustained bone marrow recovery in all patients. Reinfusion of 1×10^6 CD34$^+$ cells/kg will result in rapid neutrophil recovery, but platelet recovery may be delayed and a patient has occasionally been seen with secondary bone marrow failure after receiving a graft smaller than 3×10^6 CD34$^+$ cells/kg.

Flow-cytometric subtyping of the CD34$^+$ cells harvested may provide additional information on the quality of the graft, which can be used to make a better prediction of the time to haemopoietic reconstitution.[18] This is of only minor importance where neutrophils are concerned, because neutrophil recovery is relatively invariant if G-CSF is employed after the transplantation. Platelet recovery is, however, more variable. This can be of clinical consequence, for example, in patients with poor platelet transfusion recoveries as a result of HLA sensitization, or when multiple high-dose courses are planned. Additional phenotyping of the mononuclear cells harvested may yield valuable information regarding the quality of the graft. For example, the number of CD34[+] cells that express L-selectin correlates well with the time to platelet transfusion independence.[19]

Presence of tumour cells in the graft

A much debated question is to what extent viable breast cancer cells circulate in the peripheral blood and whether or not PBPC collections are less likely to contain tumour cells than conventional bone marrow harvests. Viable breast cancer cells have occasionally been reported to have been cultured from peripheral blood samples and immunological methods can frequently detect cells with epithelial surface antigens in the blood or bone marrow of breast cancer patients (but not in the blood of healthy volunteers). The latter may or may not indicate the presence of breast cancer cells. Monocytes and macrophages can take up proteins of decaying cancer cells and can thus contain epithelial proteins. They can even present fragments of these proteins on their cell surface. To control for this and for related phenomena, either viable tumour cells must be cultured from the blood (a very difficult and cumbersome procedure), or the presence of mRNA coding for the pertinent antigens should be detectable in circulating cells. The conduct of appropriate control experiments has not yet been reported in a systematic fashion. Until that time, reports of significant numbers of tumour cells in PBPC collections, or even of mobilization of tumour cells by G-CSF,[20] should probably be viewed as inconclusive.

Despite all these uncertainties, several groups have attempted to remove tumour cells from bone marrow of peripheral stem cell preparations. In principle, this can be achieved by either positive selection for haemopoietic progenitor cells or elimination of cells that express epithelial surface antigens. The former method is usually based on the selection of CD34[+] cells employing monoclonal antibodies fixed to a column or to magnetic beads. This may allow enrichment of CD34[+] cells by one log or more, but it is often associated with significant loss of progenitor cells. Several methods and devices are currently the focus of early clinical studies. Methods that select and destroy cells with epithelial surface antigens, for instance employing antibodies and complement lysis, have been used as well. These should – in theory – be able to remove several logs of tumour cells, but a number of drawbacks are obvious. First, no reliable methods are available to detect very small proportions of tumour cells and the efficiency of the method cannot be determined. Second, PBPC collections usually contain very large numbers of cells (typically $100–500 \times 10^8$) and any purging attempts must be carried out in large volumes, requiring large amounts of expensive monoclonal antibodies. Finally, any attempts to purge the graft require extensive ex vivo manipulations, such as incubations with monoclonal antibodies and other proteins, washings, centrifugations, etc., which unavoidably decrease the number of vital progenitor cells in the graft.

There are, at present, no clinical data that indicate that graft purging is useful in breast cancer. Interestingly, a study of Myers et al[21] recently reported on 27 patients with breast cancer metastatic to bone marrow who underwent high-dose chemotherapy with PBPC transplantation. This group had the same median survival and time to progression as patients with negative bone marrows.[21] It is reasonable to assume that the large majority of relapses after PBPC transplantation stem from tumour cells not eradicated by the chemotherapy and that the available clinical studies lack the statistical power to identify a possible effect of tumour cell reinfusion.

HIGH-DOSE CHEMOTHERAPY IN STAGE IV BREAST CANCER

Early studies

Most of the information in the literature stems from phase I and II studies and from the American and European bone marrow transplant registries. Breast cancer is a remarkably polymorphic disease and there can be no doubt that the patients in these studies have been highly selected. As a result, it is difficult or impossible to generalize the findings.

An early landmark study was reported by Peters in 1988.[22] Twenty-two patients with metastatic breast cancer, none of whom had received chemotherapy previously, underwent high-dose therapy with cisplatin, carmustine and cyclophosphamide, followed by autologous bone marrow transplantation. No other chemotherapy was given. With a follow-up of 8, 9 and 11 years, three of these patients remain disease free and alive,[23] demonstrating that some patients can become long-term survivors with this treatment modality.

This impression is confirmed by other reports. Other conclusions drawn from non-randomized studies and from the data on some 2000 patients reported to the American and European bone marrow transplantation registries include:

- Patients with widely disseminated disease or patients who do not respond to standard-dose chemotherapy are unlikely to derive benefit from high-dose therapy
- Patients with extensive prior chemotherapy are unlikely to respond favourably to high-dose therapy
- Recurrences tend to occur in sites of previously bulky disease
- Patients who have a complete remission after standard-dose chemotherapy and who subsequently undergo high-dose therapy as late consolidation have an approximately 25% chance of achieving long-term survival.

A prospective multicentre study to confirm the last point was initiated in the Netherlands in 1989. Thirty advanced breast cancer patients, who had a rigorously documented complete remission within 6 months of initiating first-line chemotherapy, received a single course of high-dose melphalan and mitozantrone, followed by autologous bone marrow transplantation. With a median follow-up of 25 months, 17 patients remain disease free without further treatment at 13+ to 53+ months (Figure 18.1).[24] This and other studies appear to support the notion that a subgroup of patients with advanced breast cancer exists for whom long-term survival is achievable. It is, however, important to stress that long-term survivors also occur in patients who have received only conventionally dosed chemotherapy. A recent retrospective study of 1581 patients treated at the MD Anderson Cancer Center revealed that 49 of 263 patients (19%) who achieved a complete remission following doxorubicin-based chemotherapy continued to be in complete remission for over 5 years.[25]

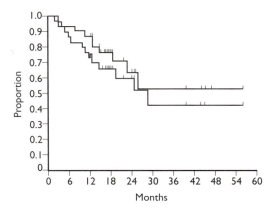

Figure 18.1 Event-free and overall survival after high-dose chemotherapy as consolidation of a complete remission of stage IV breast cancer: 30 patients, who had achieved a rigorously documented complete remission within 6 months of the beginning of chemotherapy for stage IV disease, underwent high-dose chemotherapy with melphalan and mitozantrone followed by autologous bone marrow transplantation. The upper and lower curves represent progression-free and overall survival, respectively. (Reprinted with permission from De Vries et al.[24])

Prognostic factors

A number of single-institution retrospective analyses have been published which focus on patient characteristics associated with long-term survival.[26,27] Reportedly, the most important characteristics are an objective response (preferably a complete remission) to standard-dose chemotherapy and the presence of only a single site or tissue of disease at the time of diagnosis. The presence of liver metastases has been reported to be an unfavourable factor, whereas a long disease-free interval between the first treatment of the primary breast cancer and the time at which metastases are diagnosed is a favourable factor.

In a retrospective analysis of 99 breast cancer patients who received high-dose chemotherapy as a consolidation, after having obtained at least a partial remission with standard-dose chemotherapy, Antman and co-workers reported that patients aged under 40 have a worse prognosis than older ones.[28] This finding was later confirmed by Ayash in a study of 62 patients, many of which may have been in the same database that had previously been studied by Antman.[29] In a multivariate analysis, however, age was no longer a significant factor (Table 18.2).

Most studies of high-dose therapy in advanced breast cancer include only patients with hormone-insensitive disease (operationally defined as tumours with a negative oestrogen-receptor assay or tumours that have

Table 18.2   Characteristics of advanced breast cancer patients benefiting from high-dose therapy as consolidation

Study	No. of patients	Patient characteristics	High-dose regimen	Significant prognostic factors (multivariate model)	p
Ayash[29]	62	1st relapse or stage IV	CTCb[a]	Single metastatic site[c]	0.002
				CR to induction chemotherapy	0.04
				DF interval[d] >24 months	0.066
Dunphy[30]	80	1st relapse Hormone insensitive	2 × CEP[b] (in 50% with Tx)	Liver involvement	0.001
				Soft-tissue involvement	0.039
				Prior adjuvant chemotherapy	0.028
Reed[31]	83	Metastatic Hormone insensitive	CTH[e]	DF interval >36 months	ND
				Absence of liver metastases	ND

All patients had advanced breast cancer and were either stable or responsive to a first line of induction chemotherapy.
[a] Cyclophosphamide, thiotepa and carboplatin (see Table 18.1).
[b] Cyclophosphamide 4.5–5.25 g/m^2, etoposide 750–1200 mg/m^2 and cisplatin 120–180 mg/m^2.
[c] Defined as spread to one visceral organ, bone or a discrete soft-tissue locus.
[d] Months between primary treatment and the diagnosis of metastatic disease.
[e] Cyclophosphamide 6 g/m^2, thiotepa 600 mg/m^2, hydroxyurea 18 g/m^2.

failed at least one line of endocrine treatment). As a result, the number of patients with hormone receptor-positive tumours available for analysis is small. Oestrogen-receptor positivity may, nevertheless, be associated with a lower long-term survival rate.[29] This would provide a second, independent reason to exclude patients from high-dose chemotherapy who have a fair chance of responding to endocrine therapy.

Analysis of failure patterns after high-dose therapy has shown that most relapses occur in sites of previously bulky disease. The control of these sites can be improved by radiotherapy after chemotherapy. This approach has been proposed for patients who are in complete remission after high-dose therapy, and who previously had fewer than three sites of disease, bulky disease or locoregional disease only.[32] There are indications that adjuvant radiotherapy in these situations may even have a beneficial effect on survival.

Another group of patients who may particularly benefit from high-dose therapy is made up of patients with metastatic disease that is resected, irradiated within a single field or presents as minimal bone marrow involvement. A recent report described 23 of these patients, 53% of whom were free of progression with a lead follow-up time of over 3.5 years after transplantation.[33]

Randomized studies

At the time of writing, data of only two randomized studies of high-dose chemotherapy had been either published in full or reported in abstract form.

The first study,[34] by Bezwoda et al from South Africa, compared six courses of 'standard-dose' cyclophosphamide 600 mg/m^2, mitozantrone 12 mg/m^2 and vincristine 2 mg (CNV) with two courses of a high-dose regimen incorporating cyclophosphamide 2400 mg/m^2, mitozantrone 45 mg/m^2 and etoposide 2500 mg/m^2 (HD-CNV). HD-CNV was administered on a single day and was followed by either autologous bone marrow transplantation or PBPC transplantation (Figure 18.2). All respon-

ders received 'maintenance therapy' with tamoxifen. A total of 90 patients with breast cancer, who had not previously received chemotherapy for advanced disease, were randomized. The two treatment arms were well balanced in terms of age, distribution of metastases and number of metastatic sites. Patients who had received HD-CNV had significantly more complete remissions (51% versus 4%), better response duration (median 80 vs 34 weeks) and overall survival (median 100 vs 45 weeks) than those who had received conventionally dosed chemotherapy. The follow-up of this study is still insufficient to determine whether long-term survival is more frequent in the high-dose group than in the standard-dose group. Seven patients in the high-dose group were disease free beyond 2 years, versus only one in the standard-dose group.

The results of the Bezwoda study are difficult to generalize. Both the conventional treatment and the high-dose regimen were developed for low cost and feasibility in the South African situation. Consequently, the 'standard' CNV arm of the trial would not be considered as 'standard' conventional treatment by most

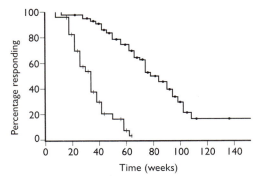

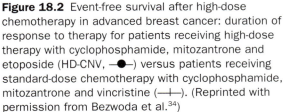

Figure 18.2 Event-free survival after high-dose chemotherapy in advanced breast cancer: duration of response to therapy for patients receiving high-dose therapy with cyclophosphamide, mitozantrone and etoposide (HD-CNV, —●—) versus patients receiving standard-dose chemotherapy with cyclophosphamide, mitozantrone and vincristine (—+—). (Reprinted with permission from Bezwoda et al.[34])

Western oncologists, and better results could possibly have been obtained if a more intensive, doxorubicin-based regimen had been selected as a control.

The second randomized study, of Peters and co-workers,[35] was conducted between 1988 and 1995. A total of 423 stage IV breast cancer patients who had hormone-refractory disease and no or only few bone metastases were entered. Treatment started with four cycles of doxorubicin, 5-fluorouracil methotrexate-based chemotherapy (AFM). Patients with progression or stable disease were taken out of the study. One hundred and ninety-three patients achieved a partial response and went on to high-dose therapy with the CPB regimen (cyclophosphamide, cisplatin and carmustine). The 98 patients who had achieved a complete remission were randomized to either 'immediate high-dose therapy' (IHD) or 'delayed high-dose therapy' (DHD). The IHD patients received CPB and the DHD patients received no further treatment until relapse, at which time CPB was administered.

The analysis of the randomized part of the study was done on an intention-to-treat basis. Not surprisingly, the disease-free survival of the IHD group was better than that of the DHD group: 0.9 and 0.3 years, respectively ($p = 0.008$). The overall survival was, however, significantly better for the DHD group (median 3.2 versus 1.9 years, $p = 0.04$). The partial remission patients who had received high-dose therapy did equally well (or poorly) as the patients in the IHD group.

This intriguing and somewhat confusing result argues against the common notion that high-dose therapy should be employed as early in the course of treatment as possible. Delay of high-dose therapy until relapse after complete remission may be the most effective strategy in terms of overall survival. Confirmation by independent studies of this counter-intuitive finding is now urgently required.

These two first randomized studies are encouraging in that both show failure-free survival and overall survival advantages for the high-dose chemotherapy arm. In both studies, however, the proportion of patients achieving long-term survival (if it exists) is very small at best. This underlines the need for further feasibility studies which aim to increase the dose intensity even further and which make optimal use of the novel agents that have recently been introduced in the clinic, either as part of the high-dose regimen or as a component of a remission–induction strategy. It also demonstrates the urgent requirement of new prognostic factors which may allow us to recognize the group of patients that may benefit from the high-dose approach.

Several further randomized studies in metastatic breast cancer are in progress, including a large US study (E-PBT01) for patients responding to standard-dose chemotherapy. For this group, 24 months of CMF maintenance chemotherapy is compared with high-dose chemotherapy with a CTCb regimen.

HIGH-DOSE THERAPY IN THE ADJUVANT SETTING

Experience with leukaemia and lymphoma, and also in breast cancer as described above, has shown that high-dose therapy has the best chance of achieving long-term survival when it can be administered at a time when there is little tumour bulk. Apparently, the treatment modality can sometimes deal effectively with micrometastatic disease. If this concept is valid, then high-dose chemotherapy could be of particular value in the adjuvant treatment of high-risk breast cancer.

Early studies

A number of relatively small and uncontrolled studies have been published which suggest that high-dose therapy with bone marrow support may be superior to conventional treatment. The largest and most publicized one is the study of Peters and co-workers,[36] in which 85 patients with 10 or more tumour-positive axillary nodes received four cycles of CAF followed by CPB with autologous bone marrow support (Figure 18.3). The event-free survival with a median follow-

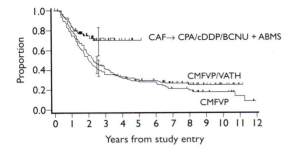

Figure 18.3 Event-free survival after adjuvant high-dose therapy: 85 patients with high-risk breast cancer (defined as having 10 or more involved axillary lymph nodes) were treated with CAF, followed by high-dose cyclophosphamide, cisplatin and carmustine, and autologous bone marrow transplantation (upper curve). The two lower curves represent the event-free survivals for similar patients selected from two trials using adjuvant CMFVP (CALGB 7581) or CMFVP/VATH (CALGB 8082). (Reprinted with permission from Peters et al.[36])

up of 2.5 years was 72%, which was significantly better than that of a matched control group (43%). The toxicity was, however, substantial. There were 12% toxic deaths, and almost a third of the patients experienced some degree of pulmonary toxicity, sometimes elicited by radiotherapy. The pulmonary toxicity was readily responsive to corticosteroids but occasionally required discontinuation of radiotherapy.

The findings of the Peters' study have essentially been confirmed by data from the American Bone Marrow Transplant Registry and from other uncontrolled studies. It is, however, important to realize that the patients on all of these studies had been highly selected and it is possible that similar results would have been obtained if the patients had received standard chemotherapy only. It has been argued that additional staging tests such as bone marrow examinations and computed tomography of brain and liver (as routinely done in many high-dose chemotherapy protocols) lead to exclusion of as many as 25% of otherwise eligible patients.[37] This may obviously lead to stage migration and complicates comparisons with historical controls even further.

High-dose sequential chemotherapy

A possibly important way to increase dose intensity further is the sequential administration of different agents in very high dose. In theory, high doses of single agents could overcome low-grade resistance. As every high-dose agent is employed only once, acquired resistance should not be a problem when non-cross-resistant drugs are used. The strategy also allows the completion of therapy in a very tight time frame, as has been shown in a study from Milan.[38] A total of 67 patients with high-risk breast cancer were entered onto a protocol which included high-dose cyclophosphamide, vincristine with high-dose methotrexate, cisplatin and high-dose melphalan (L-PAM), all administered sequentially within a period of 8 weeks. Circulating progenitor cells were harvested following the high-dose cyclophosphamide course, employing GM-CSF as a mobilizing growth factor, and were reinfused after the high-dose melphalan course.

This brief but very intensive therapy was given after surgery and before locoregional radiotherapy. It was well tolerated and the relapse-free and overall survival data compare favourably with the best results from conventional adjuvant studies. Specifically, the results were compared with those of the Milan Cancer Institute regimen of four cycles of doxorubicin followed by CMF,[39] which may be considered the 'best standard treatment' for high-risk disease published to date. With an overall survival and relapse-free survival at 5 years of 70% and 57%, respectively, high-dose sequential therapy appears to be more effective than the 60% and 40% reported for doxorubicin–CMF. A currently ongoing Italian randomized study that employs a slightly modified high-dose sequential regimen should provide a more definitive comparison by the end of the century.

Table 18.3 Three large ongoing randomized studies of high-dose chemotherapy in high-risk breast cancer

Trial	Patient selection	'Conventional' dose arm	'High-dose' arm
Intergroup 0163	Ten or more involved axillary lymph nodes	4 × CAF,[a] 1 × conventional CPB[b]	4 × CAF, 1 × high-dose CPB
Intergroup 0121	Ten or more involved axillary lymph nodes	6 × CAF	6 × CAF, 1 × CT
Dutch National Study	Four or more involved axillary lymph nodes	5 × FEC[c]	4 × FEC, 1 × CTC

[a] CAF, cyclophosphamide, doxorubicin and fluorouracil.
[b] CPB, cyclophosphamide, cisplatin and carmustine (see Table 18.1).
[c] FEC, fluorouracil, epirubicin and cyclophosphamide.

Randomized studies

Several randomized studies, both in the USA and in Europe, have been initiated to confirm the postulated survival advantage of high-dose adjuvant therapy (Table 18.3). As the time to relapse for high-risk breast cancer can be quite prolonged, the first interim analyses of these studies are not expected until 1999.

Interestingly, the two American intergroup studies of high-dose therapy in breast cancer recruit patients relatively slowly. In the first study, 120 centres collaborate and register some 150 patients per year, whereas the second was reported to register only 86 patients per year despite the collaboration of 155 centres.[40] This is markedly different in Europe, where the Dutch national study alone – a collaboration of only 10 centres – randomized a total of 410 patients in its first 32 months. Reportedly, American patients and American doctors have already accepted the advantage of high-dose adjuvant therapy over standard treatment, and it is difficult to find patients willing to be randomized. As only a very small proportion of eligible patients is randomized, the American studies may focus on a group of highly selected patients and the European data will be essential to confirm and generalize the American findings.[41]

Studies of adjuvant high-dose therapy in breast cancer should not only focus on long-term survival but also on cost–benefit analyses. Obviously, high-dose therapy is costly in terms of both health care costs and treatment-related morbidity, and a modest survival advantage over standard-dose therapy could easily be offset by an unexpected long-term toxicity. High doses of alkylating agents, for example, could conceivably induce a high frequency of second tumours or leukaemias, in analogy with the situation in Hodgkin's disease. Preliminary analyses of long-term survivors after high-dose therapy with bone marrow support suggest that this problem may be similar in size to that associated with chemotherapy for Hodgkin's disease, but these data have not been derived from patients who receive regimens as used for breast cancer.

Long-term toxicity after high-dose adjuvant therapy

The objective of adjuvant chemotherapy in breast cancer is cure and any irreversible toxicity after treatment completion may affect the quality of life of patients for many years. The main long-term toxicities include infertility and induction of premature menopause in nearly all patients, minor neuropathy and high-frequency hearing loss when cisplatin or carboplatin has been used, and residual organ toxicities that are not usually symptomatic. High-dose alkylating therapy is also likely to cause an excess of second tumours, but there is currently insufficient follow-up of long-term survivors of breast cancer after transplantation to study this question adequately.

A somewhat neglected long-term toxicity of high-dose therapy is central neurotoxicity, as can be detected employing neuropsychological tests. Every clinician knows that many post-transplantation patients report reduced exercise tolerance, concentration disturbances and sleep disorders, but it has been unclear whether these complaints were the result of the primary malignancy, the many months of standard-dose chemotherapy or the high-dose therapy. We have recently been able to study a series of high-risk breast cancer patients who had been randomized to undergo either high-dose therapy with PBPC transplantation, or standard therapy. It could be shown that patients who had undergone high-dose therapy had significantly more abnormalities at neuropsychological testing than patients who had received the identical treatment but not the high-dose therapy. The median time of testing was 2 years after the last chemotherapy, suggesting that all or part of the neuropsychological impairments may be irreversible.

PROSPECTS

High-dose chemotherapy with PBPC transplantation holds promise in breast cancer but cannot be regarded as standard therapy, not even for certain subgroups of patients, until the results of ongoing randomized studies become available.[42] The two studies in advanced breast cancer, one of which is only available in abstract form, require both longer follow-up and confirmation before generalizations can safely be made.

Multiple courses of high-dose therapy

The supportive care for patients receiving high-dose therapy is currently evolving rapidly. Haemopoietic growth factors and PBPC transplantation have only very recently been introduced in the clinic and have already revolutionized the practice of intensive chemotherapy. Stem cell factor and thrombopoietin have entered clinical studies, and the first successes of techniques such as ex vivo expansion of progenitor cells have been reported. In addition, important new agents for the treatment of breast cancer have recently been introduced, among which the taxanes paclitaxel and docetaxel, and the vinca alkaloid vinorelbine are the most prominent. Many of these innovations are so recent that they could not be incorporated in the pivotal randomized studies of high-dose therapy that are currently in progress. For example, multiple courses of high-dose therapy have become possible now that myelosuppression is no longer the dose-limiting factor. As all potentially curative chemotherapy at standard doses must be given repeatedly to obtain maximum effect, it is reasonable to assume that multiple courses of high-dose therapy could be better than a single one.

This concept has been addressed in a series of phase I and phase II studies (see Crown et al[43]). Perhaps the most extensive experience has been reported with double courses of CEP (cyclophosphamide, etoposide and cisplatin).[44] The feasibility of this approach has been demonstrated, but the dose of chemotherapy in a CEP course is not very high and certainly not myeloablative. In fact, it has been shown that two CEP courses can also be given with no bone marrow or stem cell support at all. Other double- or multiple-course strategies have been tested, but most of these avoided the use of two or more full-dose courses of alkylating agents. We have shown that two full-dose courses of cyclophosphamide, thiotepa and carboplatin (CTC) can be given within 5 weeks of each other, but that organ toxicity such as haemorrhagic cytistis or veno-occlusive disease of the liver may occur. Three subsequent CTC courses are too toxic and were associated with mortality from veno-occlusive disease and a late haemolytic uraemic syndrome.[45] It has become clear that there are limits to the cumulative dose of alkylating agents that can be delivered within a few months. Three CTC courses at 66% dose level can be delivered without excess toxicity and have turned out to be well tolerated.

Multiple courses of intermediate-dose therapy

Other variations on the theme of multiple courses of high-dose therapy have become possible by the finding that reinfusion of stimulated whole blood can also lead to rapid bone marrow recovery after high-dose therapy.[46] This approach may allow the administration of multiple cycles of intermediate-high dose therapy, perhaps four to six courses, as is common with standard-dose therapy. A distinct disadvantage of this approach is that the stimulated blood can be stored for only 3 days at 4°C, in order to prevent significant loss of vitality. As a result, the chemotherapy must be given at a possibly non-optimal point of time (for instance before the gastrointestinal toxicity has resolved or before platelet recovery is complete) and must be given as a bolus or short-term infusion, to allow sufficient time for clearance of the drug from the body. In addition, there is little time for adequate quality control (or even purging) of the graft. All these restrictions can be avoided conveniently by mobilizing PBPCs before high-dose therapy is started and by dividing the harvest in portions. Although attractive because of its simplicity and low costs, the stimulated whole blood procedure will probably be abandoned because a more versatile – albeit more expensive – alternative is readily available.

Gene therapy

A novel approach involving PBPC transplantation in breast cancer is gene therapy. It is now possible to introduce external functional genes into CD34$^+$ selected cells by several methods, most of which employ a retroviral vector (gene transduction). These methods have been pioneered to correct a rare immunodeficiency syndrome, in which the enzyme adenosine deaminase (ADA) is congenitally absent. In principle, similar methods could be used to insert a drug resistance gene into human stem cells. By transducing the *MDR1* gene, for example, which codes for the P-glycoprotein associated with multidrug resistance, the bone marrow of the recipient patient could be made resistant to a range of chemotherapeutic agents.

In practice, however, the gene transduction process is of very low efficiency. As a result, most – or even all – transduced cells are committed progenitor cells that have no self-renewal capacity. To arrive at a truly drug-resistant bone marrow, in vivo selection for the *MDR1*-transduced cells would be required. This could be done by repeated administration of one of the many agents that can be pumped out of the cell by P-glycoprotein, such as paclitaxel, doxorubicin, etoposide or vinca alkaloids. Clinical studies of this approach have been approved in both the USA and Europe. It is difficult to see, however, how the tumour to be treated could continue to be sensitive to *MDR1* drugs after repeated rounds of selection. Even if this were the case, *MDR1* drugs typically allow no or little dose escalation before extramedullary dose-limiting toxicity becomes prominent. Although gene therapy has the allure of novel and high-tech treatment, some experts believe that this clinical concept is not valid and its application is premature in the case of breast cancer.

REFERENCES

1. Livingston RB. Dose intensity and high dose therapy. Two different concepts. *Cancer* 1994; **74:** 1177–83.
2. Gianni AM, Siena S, Bregni M, et al. Granulocyte-macrophage colony-stimulating factor to harvest circulating haemopoietic stem cells for autotransplantation. *Lancet* 1989; **ii:** 580–5.
3. Frei III E, Teicher BA, Holden SA, Cathcart KNS, Wang Y. Preclinical studies and clinical correlation of the effect of alkylating dose. *Cancer Res* 1988; **48:**6417–23.

4. Frei III E, Antman K, Teicher B, Eder P, Schnipper L. Bone marrow autotransplantation for solid tumors – prospects. *J Clin Oncol* 1989; **7:**515–26.

5. Vahdat L, Antman KH. Dose-intensive therapy in breast cancer. In: *High-dose Cancer Therapy. Pharmacology, Hematopoietins, Stem Cells* (Armitage JO, Antman KH, eds). Baltimore: Williams & Wilkins, 1995:802–23.

6. Peters WP, Shpall EJ, Jones RB, et al. High-dose combination alkylating agents with bone marrow support as initial treatment for metastatic breast cancer. *J Clin Oncol* 1988; **6:**1368–76.

7. Williams SF, Bitran JD, Kaminer L, et al. A phase I–II study of bialkylator chemotherapy, high-dose thiotepa, and cyclosphosphamide with autologous bone marrow reinfusion in patients with advanced cancer. *J Clin Oncol* 1987; **5:**260–5.

8. Eder JP, Antman K, Elias A, et al. Cyclophosphamide and thiotepa with autologous bone marrow transplantation in patients with solid tumors. *J Natl Cancer Inst* 1988; **80:**1221–6

9. Elder JP, Elias A, Shea TC, et al A phase I–II study of cyclophosphamide, thiotepa and carboplatin with autologous bone marrow transplantation in solid tumor patients. *J Clin Oncol* 1990; **8:**1239–45.

10. Rodenhuis S, Baar JW, Schornagel JH, et al Feasibility and toxicity study of a high-dose chemotherapy regimen for autotransplantation incorporating carboplatin, thiotepa and cyclophosphamide. *Ann Oncol* 1992; **3:**855–60.

11. Mulder POM, Sleijfer DT, Willemse PHM, et al, High-dose cyclophosphamide or melphalan with escalating doses of mitoxantrone and autologous bone marrow transplantation for refractory solid tumors. *Cancer Res* 1989; **49:**4654–8.

12. Van der Wall E, Beijnen JH, Rodenhuis S. High-dose chemotherapy regiments for solid tumors. A review. *Cancer Treat Rev* 1995; **21:**105–32.

13. Holland HK, Saral R. Infectious diseases. In: *High-dose Cancer Therapy. Pharmacology, Hematopoietins, Stem Cells* (Armitage JO, Antman KH, eds). Baltimore: Williams & Wilkins, 1995:508–26.

14. Van der Wall, Nooijen WJ, Baars JW, et al. High-dose carboplatin, thiotepa and cyclophosphamide (CTC) with peripheral blood stem cell support in the adjuvant therapy of high-risk breast cancer: a practical approach. *Br J Cancer* 1995; **71:**857–62.

15. Elias AD, Ayash L, Anderson KC, et al. Mobilization of peripheral blood progenitor cells by chemotherapy and granulocyte–macrophage colony-stimulating factor for hematologic support after high-dose intensification for breast cancer. *Blood* 1992; **79:**3036–44.

16. Siena S, Bregni M, Di Nicola M, et al. Durability of hematopoiesis following autografting with peripheral blood hematopoietic progenitors. *Ann Oncol* 1994; **5:**935–41.

17. Van der Wall E, Richel DJ, Holtkamp MJ, et al. Bone marrow reconstitution after high-dose chemotherapy and autologous peripheral stem cell transplantation: correlation with graft size. *Ann Oncol* 1994; **5:**795–802.

18. Dercksen MW, Rodenhuis S, Dirkson MKA, et al. Subsets of CD34-positive cells and rapid hematopoietic recovery after peripheral blood stem cell transplantation. *J Clin Oncol* 1995; **13:**1922–32.

19. Dercksen MW, Gerritsen WR, Rodenhuis S, et al. Expression of adhesion molecules on DC34$^+$ cells: CD34$^+$ L-selectin$^+$ cells predict a rapid platelet recovery after peripheral blood stem cell transplantation. *Blood* 1995; **85:**3313–19.

20. Brugger W, Bross KL, Glatt M, Weber F, Mertelsmann, Kanz L. Mobilization of tumor cells and hematopoietic progenitor cells into peripheral blood of patients with solid tumors. *Blood* 1994; **83:**636–40.

21. Myers S, Mick R, Williams S. High-dose chemotherapy with autologous stem cell rescue in women with metastatic breast cancer with involved bone marrow: a role for peripheral blood progenitor cell transplant. *Bone Marrow Transpl* 1994; **13:**449–54.

22. Peters WP, Shpall EJ, Jones RB, et al. High-dose combination alkylating agents with bone marrow support as initial treatment for metastatic breast cancer. *J Clin Oncol* 1988; **6:**1368–76.

23. Peters WP. High-dose chemotherapy with autologous bone marrow transplantation for the treatment of breast cancer: Yes. In: *Important Advances in Oncology* (DeVita VT, Hellmann S, Rosenberg SA, eds). Philadelphia: Lippincott Co., 1995: 215–30.

24. De Vries EGE, Rodenhuis S, Schouten HC, et al. Phase II study of intensive chemotherapy with autologous bone marrow transplantation in patients in complete remission of disseminated breast cancer. *Breast Cancer Res Treat* 1996; **39:** 307–13.

25. Greenberg PAC, Hortobagyi GN, Smith TL, Ziegler LD, Frye DK, Buzdar AU. Long-term follow-up of patients with complete remission following combination chemotherapy for metastatic breast cancer. *J Clin Oncol* 1996; **14:** 2197–205.

26. Dunphy FR, Spitzer G, Rossiter Fornoff JE, et al. Factors predicting long-term survival for metastatic breast cancer patients treated with

high-dose chemotherapy and bone marrow support. *Cancer* 1994; **73**:2157–67.

27. Ayash LJ, Wheeler C, Fairclough D, et al. Prognostic factors for prolonged progression-free survival with high-dose chemotherapy with autologous stem-cell support for advanced breast cancer. *J Clin Oncol* 1995; **13**:2043–9.

28. Antman K, Ayash L, Elias A, et al. High-dose cyclophosphamide, thiotepa, and carboplatin with autologous bone marrow support in women with measurable advanced breast cancer responding to standard-dose chemotherapy: analysis by age. *J Natl Cancer Inst Monographs* 1994; **16**:91–4.

29. Ayash LJ, Wheeler C, Fairclough D, et al. Prognostic factors for prolonged progression-free survival with high-dose chemotherapy with autologous stem-cell support for advanced breast cancer. *J Clin Oncol* 1995; **13**:2043–9.

30. Dunphy FR, Spitzer G, Rossiter Fornoff JE, et al. Factors predicting long-term survival for metastatic breast cancer patients treated with high-dose chemotherapy and bone marrow support. *Cancer* 1994; **73**:2157–67.

31. Reed E, Tarantolo S, Cowles K, et al, Prognostic factors for patients with metastatic breast cancer treated with high-dose cyclohophamide, thiotepa, hydroxyurea and hematopoietic stem cell rescue. *Proc Am Soc Clin Oncol* 1995; **14**:123 [abstract].

32. Mundt AJ, Sibley GS, Williams S, et al. Patterns of failure of complete responders following high-dose chemotherapy and autologous bone marrow transplantation for metastatic breast cancer: implications for the use of adjuvant radiation therapy. *Int J Radiat Oncol Biol Phys* 1994; **30**:151–60.

33. Shpall EJ, Cagnoni P, Bearman SL, Purdy MP, Jones RB. High-dose therapy with autologous hematopoietic support for the treatment of high-risk breast cancer. *American Society of Clinical Oncology Educational Book*, 31st Annual Meeting May 20–23, Los Angeles, CA 1995:347–51.

34. Bezwoda WR, Seymour L, Dansey RD. High-dose chemotherapy with hematopoietic rescue as primary treatment for metastatic breast cancer: a randomized trial. *J Clin Oncol* 1995; **13**:2483–9.

35. Peters WP, Jones RB, Vredenburgh J, et al. A large, prospective, randomized trial of high-dose combination alkylating agents (CPB) with autologous cellular support (ABMS) as consolidation for patients with metastatic breast cancer achieving complete remission after intense doxorubicin-based induction therapy (AFM) [abstract 149]. *Proc Am Soc Clin Oncol* 1996; **15**:121.

36. Peters WP, Ross M, Vredenburg JJ, et al. High-dose chemotherapy and autologous bone marrow support as consolidation after standard-dose adjuvant therapy for high-risk breast cancer. *J Clin Oncol* 1993; **11**:1132–43.

37. Crump M, Goss PE, Prince M, Girouard C. Outcome of extensive evaluation before adjuvant therapy in women with breast cancer and 10 or more positive axillary lymph nodes. *J Clin Oncol* 1996; **14**:66–9.

38. Gianni AM, Siena S, Bregni M, et al. Efficacy, toxicity and applicability of high-dose sequential chemotherapy as adjuvant treatment in operable breast cancer with 10 or more axillary nodes involved – five-year results. *J Clin Oncol* 1997; in press.

39. Bonadonna G, Zambetti M, Valagussa P. Sequential or alternating doxorubicin and CMF regimens in breast cancer with more than three positive nodes. Ten-year results. *JAMA* 1995; **273**:542–7.

40. Smigel K. Women flock to ABMT for breast cancer without final proof. Phase III ABMT studies under way (news). *J Natl Cancer Inst* 1995; **87**:952–5.

41. Charlton BG. Randomized clinical trials: The worst kind of epidemiology? *Nature Medicine* 1995; **1**:1101–2.

42. Smith GA, Henderson IC. High-dose chemotherapy with autologous bone marrow transplantation (ABMT) for the treatment of breast cancer: the jury is still out. In: *Important Advances in Oncology* (DeVita VT, Hellmann S, Rosenberg SA, eds). Philadelphia: Lippincott Co., 1995: 201–14.

43. Crown J, Kritz A, Vahdat L, et al. Rapid administration of multiple cycles of high-dose myelosuppressive chemotherapy in patients with metastatic breast cancer. *J Clin Oncol* 1993; **11**: 1144–9.

44. Dunphy FR, Spitzer G, Buzdar AU, et al. Treatment of estrogen receptor-negative or hormonally refractory breast cancer with double high-dose chemotherapy intensification and bone marrow support. *J Clin Oncol* 1990; **8**: 1207–16.

45. Rodenhuis S, Westermann A, Holtkamp MJ, et al. Feasibility of multiple courses of high-dose cyclophosphamide, thiotepa and carboplatin for breast cancer or germ cell cancer. *J Clin Oncol* 1996; **14**:1473–83.

46. Pettengell R, Woll PJ, Thatcher N, Dexter TM, Testa NG. Multicycle dose-intensive chemotherapy supported by sequential reinfusion of hematopoietic progenitors in whole blood. *J Clin Oncol* 1995; **13**:148–56.

19

Current and future role of growth factors in the management of breast cancer

Sebastian Fetscher, Roland Mertelsmann

CONTENTS • **Standard-dose and high-dose chemotherapy** • **Experimental treatment modalities**

The clinical and preclinical use of growth factors has had a considerable impact on breast cancer management in the last decade. In this chapter we first assess the role of growth factors in optimizing breast cancer chemotherapy at different levels of dose intensity. Second, the importance of growth factors in supporting new forms of molecular cancer therapies is discussed. As breast cancer management is the focus of this chapter, the influence of paracrine and autocrine growth factor secretion in current experimental models of breast cancer pathogenesis[1] is discussed only where growth factor research has already led to clinically relevant or conceptually important therapeutic applications.

The most widely used class of growth factors in cancer therapy to date is the haemopoietic growth factors (HGFs).[2,3] Their well-documented ability to reduce the duration and severity of neutropenia and, more recently, other cytopenias after myelosuppressive chemotherapy has been applied in many clinical studies of HGF-supported, dose-intensified and high-dose chemotherapy.[4,5] As shown in the first section of this chapter, these developments have changed our current views of effective breast cancer treatment in both the high-risk primary and the metastatic setting.

In the second part of the chapter we deal with new modes of therapy that have not yet had an impact on the routine management of breast cancer.[6–8] So far, none of the immunological or genetic treatment strategies discussed in this section has been able to induce major remissions or survival benefits in a relevant number of patients with primary or metastatic breast cancer. We feel, however, that a discussion of these innovative therapies is important in the context of this textbook because this may give us an outlook into the management of cancer in the twenty-first century, when oncological therapies should become ever more individualized, tumour specific, less toxic and also more efficient with regard to long-term disease-free survival.

STANDARD-DOSE AND HIGH-DOSE CHEMOTHERAPY

In this section some of the biological characteristics of HGFs are introduced which have been most instrumental in supporting new modes of standard-dose (SDC) and high-dose chemotherapy (HDC) with haemopoietic stem cell transplantation (HSCT) for breast cancer. Thereafter, the guidelines for the use of HGF in cancer management are reviewed, which were issued by the American Society of Clinical Oncology (ASCO).[9,10] A brief overview of the role of HGFs in SDC and HDC of breast cancer follows and, last, different methods to reduce tumour cell contamination of peripheral stem cell harvests – including ex vivo expansion of autologous peripheral haemopoietic stem cells (HSC) – are discussed.

The role of SDC and HDC, with or without HGF support, has been analysed in part in previous chapters. To avoid repetitious discussion of the extensive and still controversial body of literature that exists about these topics, we focus on the specific relevance of HGFs for routine and experimental forms of SDC and HDC in breast cancer management.

Table 19.1 Cytokines involved in immunoregulation and haemopoietic blood cell development

Family	Molecules	Synonyms	Chromosomal localization	Molecular weight* (kilodaltons)
Growth factors	Multi-CSF	IL-3	5q23–q31	14–28
	GM-CSF	CSF-α	5q21–q32	14–35
	G-CSF	CSF-β	17q11–q22	18–22
	M-CSF	CSF-1	5q33	47–74
	EPO		7q11–q22	34–39
Interleukins	IL-1	Haemopoietin-1	2q14	31; 17
	IL-2	TCGF	4q26–q28	15
	IL-3	Multi-CSF	5q23–q31	14–28
	IL-4	BSF-1	5q	15–20
	IL-5	BCGF-II, TRF	5q	12–18
	IL-6	BSF-2	7q	24
	IL-7			
	IL-8			
	IL-9			
	IL-10			
	IL-11			
Interferons	IFN-α	Leukocyte IFN	9	18–20
	IFN-β	Fibroblast IFN	9	23
	IFN-γ	Immune IFN	12	20–25
Tumour necrosis factors	TNF-α	Cachexia	6	17
	TNF-β	Lymphotoxin	6	25
Others (examples)	PDGF	Platelet-derived growth factor		
	TGF-α	Transforming growth factor α		
	TGF-β	Transforming growth factor β		
	LIF	Leukaemia inhibitory factor		
	FGF	Fibroblast growth factors		
	SCF	Stem cell factor		

TCGF, T-cell growth factor; BSF, B-cell stimulatory factor; BCGF, B-cell growth factor; TRF, T-cell replacing factor; PDGF, platelet-derived growth factor; TGF, transforming growth factor.
*Variations in molecular weight are in most cases the result of different degrees of glycosylation.

Haemopoietic growth factors

HGFs are glycoprotein hormones of low molecular weight which regulate haemopoietic progenitor cell proliferation and differentiation, although they also act on the activation of mature blood cells and on cell survival. Their genes, chromosomal localizations and most associated receptor molecules have been identified; the recombinant proteins of these growth factors have revolutionized experimental and clinical haematology.[2-4] Among haemopoietic stimulatory hormones, the HGFs or colony-stimulating factors (CSFs) are the most important. They predominantly act on immature progenitor cells, but they also influence many functions of mature blood cells. In addition, they affect T cells, fibroblasts, macrophages and endothelial cells which represent the major natural cellular sources of HGF upon inflammatory stimuli or antigenic challenge.[3]

T-cell products, such as transforming growth factor β (TGFβ), interferon-γ (IFN-γ), or tumour necrosis factor α (TNF-α), are predominantly negative regulators of haemopoiesis, but act together with CSFs to form a 'cytokine network' that is constitutively important not only in haemopoiesis but also in immunoregulation.[2] An overview of the key features of the most important cytokines involved in immunoregulation and haemopoiesis is given in Table 19.1.

To date, the CSF family includes seven glycoproteins capable of directly stimulating colony formation of progenitor cells: granulocyte–macrophage colony-stimulating factor (GM-CSF), granulocyte colony-stimulating factor (G-CSF), macrophage colony-stimulating factor (M-CSF), interleukin-3 (multi-CSF or IL-3), interleukin-5 (IL-5), erythropoietin (EPO) and thrombopoietin (TPO). The major in vivo properties of EPO, G-CSF, GM-CSF and IL-3 are shown in Table 19.2. Some of the relevant biological and clinical data on GM-CSF and G-CSF – the two most widely used HGFs in breast cancer management – are reviewed here.

Granulocyte–macrophage colony-stimulating factor

GM-CSF is produced after activation by T cells, endothelial cells, fibroblasts and monocytes. GM-CSF receptors are expressed on mature neutrophils, monocytes and eosinophils. The in vitro biological activities of GM-CSF include the proliferation of neutrophil, macrophage and eosinophil colonies; together with IL-3 or EPO, it also acts on erythroid progenitors. GM-CSF also induces functional changes in mature target cells, such as enhanced phagocytic activity, stimulation of antibody-dependent cell-mediated cytotoxicity (ADCC) in macrophages, oxygen radical release and increased production of secondary cytokines.[3]

GM-CSF can be used in vivo as an adjunct to cytotoxic drug treatment, in marrow infiltration and in marrow failure. GM-CSF and G-CSF are used to treat myelosuppression after chemotherapy and for haemopoietic reconstitution after HSCT. They can shorten neutropenia, and reduce the incidence and severity of infections and other cytopenia-associated problems.[3,4,11]

GM-CSF-associated toxicity is tolerable, and side effects are usually mild, consisting of fever, bone pain and weakness. Another adverse effect is dyspnoea which is seen in occasional patients with elevated granulocyte counts; this effect might result from accumulation of activated neutrophils in the lung. GM-CSF is frequently used in breast cancer chemotherapy.[5,11,12] Both

	EPO	G-CSF	GM-CSF	IL-3
Neutropoiesis	0	+	+	+
Migration	0	+	−	?
Activation	0	+	+	?
Eosinopoiesis	0	0	+	+
Monopoiesis	0	0	+	+
Lymphopoiesis	0	0	0	+
Erythropoiesis	+	0	0	+
Thrombopoiesis	(+)	0	?	+

Table 19.2 In vivo properties of haemopoietins in clinical trials

+, stimulation; −, inhibition; 0, no effect; ?, not definitely documented.

major American randomized trials on the effects of HDC and HSCT in high-risk primary and metastatic breast cancer use subcutaneous GM-CSF for haemopoietic reconstitution at a dose of 5 μg/kg per day until an absolute neutrophil count (ANC) of $1 \times 10^9/1$ is achieved [South Western Oncologic Group (SWOG) protocols 9061 and 9412]. When G-CSF is used instead of GM-CSF, dose and target ANC are usually similar.

As is true for all HGFs in solid tumours, GM-CSF and G-CSF seem to have no intrinsic anticancer effects and no proven tumour growth-promoting effects (the more complex interplay of HGFs with leukaemias and lymphomas is not discussed here).

Recently, the role of growth factors in the promotion of local breast cancer recurrence was assessed by British investigators who raised the possibility that growth factors released by the healing wound after breast cancer surgery might promote growth of adjacent tumour cells bearing appropriate growth factor receptors.[13] However, the molecules involved in this form of tumour promotion belong almost exclusively to other classes of growth factor, such as insulin-like growth factor (IGF) or epidermal growth factor (EGF) and others.[1]

Therefore, and despite the occasionally documented low-level expression of GM-CSF or G-CSF receptors on tumour cells, this phenomenon does not seem to have biological relevance in post-surgical scar carcinomas or any other setting of breast cancer pathogenesis.[1,3] Long-term investigations on larger patient populations, with regard to these hypothetical side effects, are, however, not yet available.

Granulocyte colony-stimulating factor

G-CSF is produced by monocytes, endothelial cells and fibroblasts. In vitro, G-CSF induces granulocyte lineage-specific colony growth, acts synergistically with IL-3 to stimulate megakaryocyte and blast cell colonies, and causes functional activation of peripheral neutrophils, including enhancement of chemotaxis, ADCC

and expression of surface Fc receptors for immunoglobulins.[2,3]

The capacity of G-CSF to increase bone marrow cellularity and peripheral blood neutrophil counts in chemotherapy-induced neutropenia and after autologous bone marrow transplantation (ABMT) has been established.[5] Tolerance of G-CSF is very good, with only occasional occurrence of bone pain or mild fever. It is probably the best clinically tolerated of all the myeloid HGFs and is therefore widely used in breast cancer chemotherapy in both Europe and North America.

Guidelines for the use of growth factors

Recently, the American Society of Clinical Oncology (ASCO) has issued recommendations for the rational use of HGF in haematology and oncology.[9,10] Given the ongoing debate about proven and unproven indications for HGF use, referral to the ASCO guidelines is recommended for all physicians introducing HGFs into breast cancer therapy. For example, an accepted criterion of HGF use is an expected incidence of febrile neutropenia after myelosuppressive chemotherapy of over 40%; on the other hand, use, timing and dosage of HGFs for haemopoietic reconstitution after HDC and HSCT remain controversial.

Another example was given in a double-blind randomized study of the effect of GM-CSF on neutropenia after dose-intense chemotherapy with cyclophosphamide, etoposide and cisplatin.[14] Here, GM-CSF shortened neutropenia only after the first course of chemotherapy. Surprisingly, during subsequent treatments, platelet recovery was delayed and transfusion requirements increased in the GM-CSF group as compared with placebo. Although this study does not allow definitive conclusions as to the causes of such paradoxical and unwanted effects of HGF therapy, it underlines the ASCO recommendation that HGF administration should be compared with alternative forms of supportive care or placebo whenever possible.

Significant differences in infectious morbidity

and mortality, or cancer response and survival, have, however, been shown only in a minority of studies comparing HGFs and placebo.[3,5,9] Therefore, it might be argued that these endpoints are too crude to assess some of the more subtle, but still relevant, clinical benefits associated with HGF use. Much of the current debate about these issues will abate with the expected future reduction of HGF costs.

Side effects and other problems associated with the use of HGF

Pharmacological side effects of HGFs are generally mild, short-lived and reversible (bone pain, myalgia, arthralgia, rash, capillary leak syndrome). With appropriate dosage, timing and route of administration, contraindications to HGF therapy rarely arise. Neither tachyphylaxis nor significant antibody formation to HGFs has been observed with recombinant HGFs. A causal role of HGFs in the development of secondary leukaemias after chemotherapy has not been proved and is unlikely. 'Stem-cell exhaustion' by high-dose or long-term use of HGFs with chemotherapy is probably of more theoretical concern, but needs to be studied.[2]

Last, the inability of currently available HGFs to reduce thrombopenia after chemotherapy remains a problem; the use of GM-CSF and high-dose G-CSF may even be associated with a mild transient reduction in platelet counts. More rapid platelet recovery might be achieved by the combined use of early and late-acting HGF or by ex vivo expansion of megakaryocytic precursor cells. With the latest addition to the HGF family – the cMpl ligand or thrombopoietin (TPO) – this situation is, however, likely to change soon.[15] TPO has shown very promising activity in preclinical models and phase I human trials.

HGFs in standard-dose chemotherapy of breast cancer

The ability of HGFs to shorten chemotherapy-induced neutropenia has been used to increase the dose intensity of SDC in the adjuvant, neoadjuvant and metastatic settings.[5] Clinical results of HGF-supported chemotherapy, and the scientific rationale for the concept of dose intensity,[16] in the therapy of breast cancer have been discussed in previous chapters. Here a brief and therefore selective summary of the topic is given.

Neoadjuvant standard-dose chemotherapy
The role of HGF in dose-intensified neoadjuvant SDC of breast cancer has not yet been extensively explored. Randomized studies with different dose levels in this setting will be of interest because they offer the opportunity to assess treatment outcome by histological examination of surgical specimens (degree of necrosis etc.). Some oncologists believe that neoadjuvant chemotherapy will be part of the routine treatment of high-risk primary breast cancer in the future – the rationale for the earliest possible and most efficiently dosed systemic therapy in a disease that is systemic in most patients is obvious.

A recent report by French investigators demonstrated a significant reduction of infectious complications with the use of G-CSF over placebo in dose-intense neoadjuvant FEC (5-fluorouracil, epirubicin and cyclophosphamide) chemotherapy for inflammatory breast cancer; response rates were very encouraging.[17]

Adjuvant standard-dose chemotherapy
Most of the important studies demonstrating improved benefit of higher doses in the adjuvant chemotherapy of breast cancer have not yet made use of HGFs,[18–20] and larger randomized studies on the benefits of HGF-supported dose-intense SDC are unavailable.[5] The reasons for this are threefold: first, the degree of dose escalation made possible by HGFs in adjuvant SDC (1.5 to two-fold) may be insufficient to generate major additional benefits; second, the dose level demonstrated as responsible for most of the survival benefit in conventional adjuvant SDC may lie below the threshold that would make HGF use mandatory;[19] last, the next level of clinically relevant dose escalation

(five- to twentyfold) requires HGFs plus HSCT.[4] Accordingly, the main thrust of innovation in adjuvant chemotherapy has been towards true HDC with HSCT.[5]

Nevertheless, HGFs are able to make significant improvements in timely and complete dose delivery in patients with prolonged neutropenic episodes after non-HGF-supported adjuvant SDC;[21] furthermore, HGFs have been instrumental in developing intensive outpatient adjuvant SDC protocols.[22] Naturally, as in all studies of adjuvant chemotherapy in breast cancer,[19] a more definite assessment of the value of HGF-supported adjuvant SDC will require longer observation intervals.[18,20]

Standard-dose chemotherapy of metastatic disease

Standard-dose cytotoxic therapy has a negligible cure rate in stage IV breast cancer.[23] Of 12 randomized studies on the effects of different dose levels without HGFs, nine showed higher response rates in the dose-intensified arm and three a moderate improvement in short-term survival; the results of studies with HGF support were similar (reviewed in the literature[4,5]). Thus, without the advent of new agents that are highly active at lower dose levels, it seems very unlikely that HGF-supported SDC will have relevant impact on survival in metastatic breast cancer.

HGFs in high-dose chemotherapy of breast cancer

Peripheral blood stem cell transplantation (PBSCT) has largely replaced ABMT as haemopoietic support of choice after HDC.[4,5] HSCs harvested from peripheral blood after HGF application with or without prior chemotherapy offer some advantages:[2]

- Facilitation of autograft collection by leukapheresis and avoidance of general anaesthesia.
- Possibility of recruiting HSCs in patients with impaired marrow reserve as a result of myelofibrosis or pelvic irradiation.

- Possibly reduced risk of tumour cell graft contamination.
- Reduction of cytopenia-associated complications by accelerated haemopoietic engraftment after chemotherapy.

To achieve a maximum pre-transplantation response and optimal HSC harvests, HGF-supported intensive induction protocols are commonly used before HDC and HSCT. HGFs are also needed after the recruitment cycle before HSC harvest (some centres harvest HSCs in the steady state solely by administrating high doses of GM-CSF or G-CSF). Last, HGFs given after PBSCT may stimulate re-transfused HSCs and further accelerate haemopoietic recovery.[24] In sum, most of the advantages of PBSCT depend on the use of HGFs.

Neoadjuvant high-dose chemotherapy of breast cancer

HDC and HSCT in neoadjuvant chemotherapy of breast cancer are still experimental. As in SDC, randomized studies in this setting will be valuable because of histological outcome assessment. Should HDC and HSCT in the neoadjuvant setting prove to be efficient and safe, systemic and local, cytotoxic and surgical breast cancer therapy would enter a new phase. With a diminished amount of tumour left to be removed by surgery, breast cancer surgery would then undergo a major change comparable to the abandonment of radical mastectomy for breast-conserving surgical techniques.

Adjuvant high-dose chemotherapy of breast cancer

Adjuvant HDC of high-risk primary breast cancer is one of the most promising developments of the last decade. According to the non-randomized data published by Peters et al,[12] HDC and HSCT in stage IIA/IIB high-risk primary breast cancer with more than 10 positive axillary lymph nodes might improve 5-year survival rates from a historical figure of around 30 to 70%.

Based on these findings, patients with high-risk stage II breast cancer are increasingly treated with HDC and HSCT.[4] Furthermore, the efficacy of various HDC regimens in the adjuvant treatment of patients with more than four positive lymph nodes and in stage IIIA/IIIB breast cancer is being evaluated. As none of the ongoing randomized studies comparing adjuvant SDC and HDC in Europe and the USA has achieved sufficient recruitment or adequate follow-up, definitive conclusions about the ultimate role of HDC in the adjuvant management of high-risk primary breast cancer are not yet available. The results of the large-scale randomized SWOG trial 9061 are eagerly awaited.

High-dose chemotherapy of metastatic breast cancer

The situation here is similar, with the SWOG trial 9412 expected to report its first results in 1997. The only available randomized study comparing SDC and HDC with HSCT in metastatic disease by Bezwoda et al[25] has reinforced the hope, raised by the sentinel investigations of Peters, that this aggressive treatment modality might provide long-term disease-free survival for a select subgroup of stage IV patients.[4,5,12] Whether the use of multiple-cycle HDC will improve the results of single-cycle HDC with HSCT, without adding undue risks of toxicity, is unclear as yet.[26,27]

Tumour cell contamination of peripheral stem cell harvests

Co-mobilization of tumour cells during HSC recruitment has been documented repeatedly.[28–30] However, the incidence and importance of graft contamination in different entities vary. For example, malignant cells in the product of leukapheresis of patients with acute myeloid leukaemia, multiple myeloma or follicular lymphoma may play a significant role in relapse after HDC and HSCT. Conversely, the clinical consequences of cytokeratin-positive cells detected in the peripheral blood of patients with surgically removed high-risk primary breast cancer are unclear. On the other hand, circulating tumour cells in patients with active metastatic breast cancer may well contribute to

the high incidence of relapse after HDC and HSCT both at sites of previous disease and at new locations such as the lung, meninges or brain.[29] Investigations by the authors' group confirm that the risk of tumour cell mobilization with HSC recruitment is real, and may be particularly high in breast cancer patients with malignant bone marrow infiltration.[31]

In vivo tumour cell depletion

In the light of these findings, all breast cancer patients are treated with at least one cycle of tumour-reducing SDC before HSC collection after another cycle of chemotherapy. Using this approach, the number of circulating tumour cells before HSC harvest can be reduced by about 1 log.[31] This simple form of in vivo purging might be of particular importance in patients with marrow involvement.

Ex vivo tumour cell depletion

Ex vivo depletion of tumour cells by cytotoxic agents such as mafosfamide has been used in leukaemias and lymphomas with variable results. To date, this traditional form of negative selection has no established role in breast cancer autotransplantation. A recent investigation documented the stem-cell protective effects of amifostine in 4-HCC-purged bone marrow of patients with advanced metastatic breast cancer; a clear clinical benefit of 4-HCC purging was not, however, described.[30]

Positive selection of CD34+ cells

In this approach the product of leukapheresis is processed through any of a number of CD34+ cell concentrators, the most common being immunoadsorption columns. The yield of CD34+ cells varies from technique to technique and from patient to patient. Extensive previous chemo- or radiotherapy decreases the yield, an effect that can in most cases be overcome by the use of increased doses of HGFs during mobilization. The feasibility of positive selection of CD34+ cells and their efficacy to reconstitute haemopoiesis after HDC is well documented.[24] Using this procedure, contaminating tumour cells can be depleted by about 3 logs.[29–31]

The remaining question is therefore not whether positive CD34+ selection can be done, but whether and when it should be done. Given the costs of this procedure, prospective studies that assess the benefit of positive selection over no ex vivo manipulation of HSC are needed to clarify indications for use of this strategy.

The frequent presence of tumour cells in the marrow and blood of patients with metastatic breast cancer, as well as the high relapse rate of these patients after HDC and HSCT, indicate a suitable area of research.[29–32] A formal assessment of the risks and benefits of all in vivo and ex vivo purging strategies discussed in this section is, however, not yet available. Nevertheless, the unequivocal demonstration that even a few tumour cells in an autotransplant can contribute to relapse[33] mandates further investigations of tumour cell depletion.

Ex vivo expansion of peripheral stem cells

A further step towards reduced tumour cell contamination consists of the ex vivo expansion of HSCs. In the expansion approach recently published by the authors' group,[34] CD34+ cells were isolated and liquid cultures performed in the presence of a combination of stem cell factor (SCF), IL-1β, IL-6, IL-3 and EPO. Proliferation started at day 6 of culture with a maximum increase in cell numbers of up to 500-fold (median 420, range 150–980) at days 12–14. Ten patients with advanced malignancies were successfully transplanted with ex vivo expanded HSC, demonstrating that about 0.2×10^6 CD34+ cells/kg of unexpanded cells, transplanted after ex vivo expansion, can lead to a trilineage engraftment comparable to that observed after transplantation of 2×10^6 CD34+ cells.[34]

These data indicate that chemotherapy plus G-CSF-primed HSC can be expanded in vitro using a combination of HGFs. Apart from the beneficial effects on tumour cell contamination, this form of HSC manipulation has several other potentials:

- Expansion of CD34+ PBPC could further shorten or obviate cytapheresis.
- Partially committed post-progenitor cells of all three cell lines could be expanded, ex vivo, to accelerate a haemopoietic recovery to the point of completely avoiding cytopenia.
- High numbers of ex vivo expanded HSC could be used for repetitive cycles of HDC and HSCT after a single apheresis.
- Small samples of donor blood could be used as reservoirs of HSC for single or multiple allogeneic HSC recipients.
- Ex vivo expanded HSC might be an ideal target for gene therapeutic approaches such as the correction of inherited single-gene defects by gene transfer.

Given the early stage of this development, a number of questions remain, however. For once, ex vivo expanded CD34+ cells have not been used after aggressive myeloablative regimens such as busulphan/cyclophosphamide (BU/CY) or total body irradiation/cyclophosphamide (TBI/CY). Second, long-term haemopoietic stability after ex vivo HSCT has neither been reported nor proven by gene marking of manipulated stem cells. It is similarly unknown whether ex vivo expansion of HSC might limit the number of cell divisions that stem cells can undergo in vivo. Last, should ex vivo expansion come of age during the next decade, we will still have to determine appropriate indications for this elegant and, as yet, costly addition to our therapeutic armamentarium.

EXPERIMENTAL TREATMENT MODALITIES

The conventional forms of cancer treatment – surgery, chemotherapy and radiotherapy – suffer from the fact that, by and large, they are non-specific with regard to individual tumours or tumour cells. Therefore, more specific strategies, which take advantage of molecular differences between cancer cells and their normal counterparts, are increasingly investigated as an alternative mode of cancer therapy.

Paradoxically, although these new therapies are more specific, they have so far been less effective in eradicating cancer cells than, for example, most non-specific cytotoxic agents. The main reason for this is that most forms of molecular therapy only target one of the many peculiar properties of cancer cells, which then use escape mechanisms to overcome the specific attack. Furthermore, no 'core' component has been found common to all cancers or to all cancer cells in a given individual; this, if found, could be exploited with predictable success by molecular anticancer strategies. An overview of selected therapeutic strategies used in gene therapy of cancer is given in Table 19.3.

Therefore, immunological and genetic therapies have to face the considerable genetic heterogeneity and ingenuity of cancer cells. Breast cancer cells are particularly difficult in this regard, because they appear to have a special capacity for survival under adverse circumstances such as the stress of anticancer therapy. Of the many reasons for this complex phenomenon, the long natural history of breast cancer,

together with the attendant build-up of multiple genetic lesions and the limited immunological response elicited against breast cancer cells by the immune system, are probably the most therapeutically relevant.

Among solid tumours, the most immunogenic entities – malignant melanoma and renal cell carcinoma – have naturally been preferred objects of clinical investigation. Nevertheless, molecular alterations in breast cancer cells can be and have been used for immunological or genetic treatment strategies. Some of the currently pursued strategies in immunological and gene therapy are briefly described. Only a selected and limited overview of this rapidly expanding area of research can be given.

Monoclonal antibodies

Diagnostic use

Monoclonal antibodies (MABs) against the more preferentially expressed breast cancer antigens have been used to detect and tag tumour cells before surgery. In a recent study, the iodine-125 radiolabelled MABs B73.2 and FOC 23C5 (anti-carcinoembryonic antigen or CEA) were able to locate multicentric primary and axillary tumour involvement in 40% of patients with locally advanced breast cancer.[35] Monoclonal antibodies of this kind might improve the often poor accuracy of current breast cancer diagnostics, especially when more specific MABs should become available. By this technique, treatment decisions in conventional breast cancer therapy could be refined.

Therapeutic use

A number of trials assessing the therapeutic potential of MABs in breast cancer have been reported. Recent examples include the radiotherapeutic use of an iodine-131 labelled chimaeric-L6 MAB directed against a non-shed antigen,[36] interference with tumour growth by application of an antiepidermal growth factor MAB,[37] and use of MAB–toxin conjugates directed against the *c-erbB-2* receptor.[8] Objective responses of short duration, comparable to third-line chemotherapy regimens in metastatic

---

Table 19.3 Gene therapy for patients with cancer-Therapeutic strategies

Protection of drug-sensitive tissues by transferring genes rendering normal cells resistant to certain cytotoxic drugs

Modification of anticancer effector cells by transferring new biological properties, e.g. by transferring cytokine genes or new immunological specificity (e.g. various antigen receptors into cytotoxic cells)

Modification of cancer cells:
    Correction of aberrant gene function
    Introduction of drug-activating ('suicide') genes
    Enhancement of tumour cell immunogenicity ('tumour immunization')
    Gene marking ('genetic tagging')

Production of therapeutic proteins

breast cancer, have been observed with MAB therapies; the most notable recent example was therapy with anti-p185[HER2] monoclonal antibodies in patients with HER2/neu-overexpressing metastatic breast cancer.[38] The development of other and more efficient MABs and the combination of MAB therapies with other treatment modalities might improve the experimental status of this form of immune therapy in the management of breast cancer.

Gene transfer-mediated protection of drug-sensitive tissues

One indirect form of gene therapy is based on the protection of non-tumour cells by transferring the multidrug resistance gene (MDR) or genes for other detoxifying enzymes into HSCs. Preclinical data suggest that this approach allows for an increase in chemotherapy dose intensity without the expected increase in haemopoietic damage.[7,8]

Genetic modification of anticancer effector cells

A natural target of current trials in gene therapy has been non-specific, cytotoxic, anticancer effector cells. In experimental models, the killing properties of these cells can be enhanced by the transfer of cytokine genes.[7] The success of this method depends, however, on a pre-existent and potent anti-tumour response of the cancer-bearing organism; unfortunately, with few and incomplete exceptions,[39] this form of immunological clearance is not observed in breast cancer.

Generation of tumour-specific cytotoxic killer cells

The low specificity of immune effector cells can be increased by introducing genes which turn them into specific killer cells.[7] This can be achieved by transferring variant antigen receptors into effector cells, consisting of parts of an MAB molecule providing specificity and the intracellular part of a T-cell receptor molecule providing signal transduction. In preclinical models for c-erbB-2 in breast cancer, it has been shown that this approach can exhibit therapeutic efficacy in vitro and in vivo.[7,8]

Genetic modification of cancer cells

Instead of modifying anticancer cells, one can also modify the genetic set-up of cancer cells themselves. One method applied in this context is the correction of aberrant gene function. By site-specific recombination, the defective gene can be replaced or the defective gene function compensated for by insertion of a healthy gene. Another approach is to use anti-sense molecules to suppress the expression of a gene relevant for the cancer phenotype.[7,8]

Introduction of drug-activating ('suicide') genes

By insertion of drug-activating genes into cancer cells, the specificity of currently available chemotherapy agents could be enhanced. One way to achieve specific expression in cancer cells is to use promoters coupled to genes for drug-activating enzymes, to achieve selective or preferential expression in cancer cells. Drug-activating enzymes that have been studied in this context are thymidine kinase and cytosine deaminase. Possible promoters include those for α-fetoprotein in hepatoma or teratoma and c-erbB-2 in breast cancer.[7,8,32]

Immunization

As preclinical models have demonstrated that tumour immunization is more efficient in smaller tumours, minimal residual disease might be the preferred situation for immunotherapy. Accordingly, the situation after HDC with HSCT may be a suitable setting for immunization: here, maximal tumour reduction and an appropriately conditioned immunological environment could allow for the optimal induction and expansion of autoreactive cytotoxic T-lymphocyte (CTL) with tumour specificity.[7,40]

Enhancement of tumour cell immunogenicity

A large number of immunogenic tumour antigens recognized by T cells in human cancers have been described; a selected overview of antigens is given in Table 19.4. Tumour immunization is based on strategies to induce protective immunity, leading to tumour rejection and long-lasting specific anti-tumour immune responses. However, the limited effectiveness and duration of most spontaneous anti-tumour immune responses observed in humans indicate that, to achieve this goal, both tumour cell immunogenicity and immune effector mechanisms have to be therapeutically improved. Attempts to induce autologous graft-versus-host disease by administration of cyclosporin after HDC and ABMT of breast cancer have

---

Table 19.4 Tumour antigens recognized by T cells (examples)

Structurally abnormal proteins
    Mutated or abnormal overexpressed anti-/oncogenes (e.g. *ras*, *p53*)
    Breakpoint peptides (e.g. bcr/abl)

Abnormal expression of normal proteins
    MAGE family
    MART-1
    Tyrosinase
    Melan-A
    Carcinoembryonic antigen, α-fetoprotein

Other
    Restricted expression of normal proteins
    Idiotypes (T and B cells and lymphomas)
    CD30 (B cells, Hodgkin's cells)
    Prostate-specific antigen
    Viral gene products (e.g. Epstein–Barr virus, human papilloma virus)
    c-erb-B-2 in breast cancer

MAGE, melanoma associated antigens; MART, melanoma antigen recognized by autologous T-cells.

---

both been equally inefficient.[41] Furthermore, the development of vaccines requires identification of tumour-associated antigens expressed by all cancer cells and of efficient effector mechanisms for protective anti-tumour immunity; in addition, efficient ways to deliver the vaccine must be established. Given these restraints, the development of tumour cell immunization in breast cancer is still at an early stage.[7,8,39]

Cytokine-transfected fibroblasts

The efficacy of gene-modified tumour vaccines has, nevertheless, been investigated in several phase I/II trials.[7] Most studies analyse the potency of irradiated autologous or HLA-matched allogeneic tumour cells transfected with IL-2, IL-4, GM-CSF or IFN-α in melanoma or renal cell carcinoma patients, in whom systemic administration of cytokines as such occasionally leads to tumour responses. Given the difficulty of culturing and transfecting autologous tumour cells, some investigators propose the use of bystander cells as a source of cytokine production. Animal models suggest that 'paracrine' secretion of cytokines by gene-transfected fibroblasts, mixed with irradiated unmodified tumour cells, can induce anti-tumour immunity.[40]

Introduction of HLA genes into tumour cells

Another approach to enhancing tumour immunogenicity in vivo has been the introduction of histocompatibility genes into tumour cells. MHC class I molecules serve as restriction elements for cytotoxic T cells by presenting antigenic peptides derived from intracellularly degraded proteins. Tumour cells can escape recognition by the immune system through the loss or downregulation of MHC class I chain alleles or by the loss of functional β_2-microglobulin expression. The restoration of MHC class I expression by transfection of the missing α chain or β_2m gene could correct the antigen-presentation defect and lead to immunological recognition of tumour cells.[7]

Gene marking

Any piece of genetic information integrated into the cellular genome can serve as a tag for cancer or normal cells. One marker is the gene for neomycin phosphotransferase which can be used to select for cells resistant to neomycin as a result of the insertion of this gene.[32] This approach is applied in several current trials of breast cancer autotransplantation.[33,42] Engraftment of transplanted HSCs, as well as the fate of ex vivo cancer cells, can be followed with this technique. In relapse, tumour cells frequently carry the marker gene indicating failure of ex vivo purging techniques.

Ethical and regulatory aspects

Ethical concerns about these new forms of cancer management are widely voiced. However, committees in various countries have not found it necessary to introduce new ethical considerations for the use of MAB-mediated or somatic gene therapy. All new treatment strategies carry a risk and need to be evaluated in phase I, II and III trials, according to standard procedures. Although details about the approval process of new drugs differ between countries, the basic concept is the same world wide and has worked well so far. Potential risks, specific to gene therapy, include insertional mutagenesis and, when using recombinant viral vectors, infection by potentially pathogenic viruses. Also contamination by other pathogenic organisms or substances has to be considered as a possibility. Although none of these problems is very likely to occur, a detailed risk–benefit analysis and a protocol following the declaration of Helsinki guidelines should always be used in new forms of gene and immunotherapy.

Outlook

Gene therapy and immunotherapy of breast cancer are still in their infancy. Nevertheless, they will have a considerable impact on future treatment strategies in patients with breast cancer and other malignant and non-malignant diseases. At what point in time these therapies will become clinically relevant is difficult to predict. In most current trials we still define toxicity and biological endpoints such as the demonstration of specific cytotoxic killer cells after therapeutic intervention. But any progress made in this field will be important for the future expansion of these promising approaches either as adjuncts to currently established treatment modalities or as the advent of a new and independently effective generation of molecular cancer therapies.

REFERENCES

1. Ethier SP. Growth factor synthesis and human breast cancer progression. *J Natl Cancer Inst* 1995; **87**:964–73.

2. Brugger W, Kanz L, Mertelsmann R. Cell proliferation and differentiation and clinical application of hematopoietic growth factors. *Curr Opin Hematol* 1993; 214–20.

3. Lieschke GJ, Burgess AW. Granulocyte colony-stimulating factor and granulocyte–macrophage colony-stimulating factor. *N Engl J Med* 1992; **327**:28–35, 99–106.

4. Brockstein BE, Williams SF. High-dose chemotherapy with autologous stem-cell rescue for breast cancer. Yesterday, today and tomorrow. *Stem Cells* 1996; **14**:79–89.

5. Kröger N, Zschaber R, Krüger W, et al. Dose intensity in the chemotherapy of breast cancer. Results of clinical studies. *Onkologie* 1995; **18**: 419–28.

6. Mertelsmann R. Pilot study for the evaluation of T-cell mediated tumor immunotherapy by cytokine gene transfer in patients with malignant tumors. *J Mol Med* 1995; **73**:205–6.

7. Rosenthal FM, Mertelsmann R. Present strategies for gene therapy in cancer. *Onkologie* 1997; **20**:26–34.

8. Wels W, Moritz D, Schmidt M, et al. Biotechnological and gene therapeutic strategies in cancer treatment. *Gene* 1995; **159**:73–80.

9. American Society of Clinical Oncology. Recommendations for the use of hematopoietic colony-stimulating factors: Evidence-based clinical practise guidelines. *J Clin Oncol* 1994; **12**: 2471–508.

10. American Society of Clinical Oncology. Update

of recommendations for the use of hematopoietic colony-stimulating factors: Evidence-based clinical practise guidelines. *J Clin Oncol* 1996; **14:** 1957–60.

11. Gianni AM, Bregni M, Siena SM, et al. Recombinant human GM-CSF reduces hematologic toxicity and widens clinical applicability of high-dose cyclophosphamide treatment in breast cancer and Non Hodgkin's lymphoma. *J Clin Oncol* 1990; **8:**768–85.

12. Peters WP, Ross M, Vredenburg JJ, et al. High-dose chemotherapy and autologous bone marrow transplantation after standard-dose adjuvant chemotherapy for high-risk breast cancer. *J Clin Oncol* 1993; **11:**1132–43.

13. Reid SE, Scanlon EF, Kaufman MW, Murthy MS. Role of cytokines and growth factors in promoting the local recurrence of breast cancer. *Br J Surg* 1996; **83:**313–20.

14. Yao JC, Neidhart JA, Triozzi P, et al. Randomized placebo-controlled trial of granulocyte–macrophage colony-stimulating factor support for dose-intense cyclophosphamide, etoposide, and cisplatin. *Am J Hematol* 1996; **51:**289–95.

15. deSauvage FJ, Hass PE, Spencer SD, et al. Stimulation of megakaryocytopoiesis and thrombopoiesis by the c-Mpl ligand. *Nature* 1995; **369:**533–8.

16. Hryniuk W, Busch H. The importance of dose intensity in chemotherapy of metastatic breast cancer. *J Clin Oncol* 1984; **2:**1281–9.

17. Chevallier B, Chollet P, Meerouche Y, et al. Lenograstim prevents morbidity from intensive induction chemotherapy in the treatment of inflammatory breast cancer. *J Clin Oncol* 1995; **13:**1564–71.

18. Bonadonna G, Valagussa P, Moliterni A, Zambetti M, Brambilla C. Adjuvant cyclophosphamide, methotrexate, and fluorouracil in node-positive breast cancer. *N Engl J Med* 1995; **332:**901–6.

19. Early Breast Cancer Trialists' Collaborative Group. Systemic treatment of early breast cancer by hormonal, cytotoxic, or immune therapy. *Lancet* 1992; **339:**71–85.

20. Wood WC, Budman DR, Korzun AH, et al. Dose and dose intensity of adjuvant chemotherapy for stage II, node-positive breast cancer. *N Engl J Med* 1994; **330:**1253–9.

21. Ribas A, Albanell J, Bellmunt J, et al. Five-day course of granulocyte colony-stimulating factor with prolonged neutropenia after adjuvant chemotherapy for breast cancer is a safe and cost-effective schedule to maintain dose-intensity. *J Clin Oncol* 1996; **14:**1573–80.

22. Swain SM, Rowland J, Weinfurt K, et al. Intensive outpatient adjuvant therapy for breast cancer: results of dose-escalation and quality of life. *J Clin Oncol* 1996; **14:**1565–72.

23. Eddy DL. Treatment of metastatic breast cancer. *J Clin Oncol* 1992; **10:**657–70.

24. Shpall EJ, Jones RB, Bearman SI, et al. Transplantation of enriched CD-34-positive marrow into for breast cancer patients following high-dose chemotherapy: influence of CD-34-positive peripheral-blood progenitors and growth factors on engraftment. *J Clin Oncol* 1994; **12:**28–36.

25. Bezwoda WR, Seymour L, Dansey RD. High-dose chemotherapy with hematopoietic rescue for metastatic breast cancer: a randomized trial. *J Clin Oncol* 1995; **13:**2483–9.

26. Patrone F, Ballestrero A, Ferrando F, et al. Four-step high-dose sequential chemotherapy with double hematopoietic progenitor-cell rescue for metastatic breast cancer. *J Clin Oncol* 1995; **13:**840–6.

27. Rodenhuis S, Westermann A, Holtkamp MJ, et al. Feasibility of multiple courses of high-dose cyclophosphamide, thiothepa, and carboplatin for breast cancer and germ cell cancer. *J Clin Oncol* 1996; **14:**1473–83.

28. Ross AA, Cooper BW, Lazarus HM, et al. Detection and viability of tumor cells in peripheral blood stem cell collections from patients with breast cancer using immunocytochemical and clonogenic assay techniques. *Blood* 1993; **82:**2605–11.

29. Sharp JG, Kessinger A, Vaughan WP, et al. Detection and clinical significance of minimal tumor cell contamination of peripheral stem cell harvests. *Int J Cell Cloning* 1992; **10:**92–8.

30. Shpall EJ, Stemmer SM, Hami L, et al. Amifostine (WR-2721) shortens the engraftment period of 4-hydroxyperoxy-cyclophosphamide-purged bone marrow in breast cancer patients receiving high-dose chemotherapy with autologous bone marrow support. *Blood* 1994; **83:** 3132–7.

31. Brugger W, Bross K, Glatt M, et al. Mobilization of tumor cells and hemopoietic progenitor cells into peripheral blood of patients with solid tumors. *Blood* 1994; **83:**636–42.

32. O'Shaugnessy JA, Cowan KH, Wilson W, et al. Pilot study of high-dose ICE (ifosfamide, carbo-

platin, etoposide) and autologous bone marrow transplant (ABMT) with neo[R]-transduced bone marrow and peripheral blood stem cells in patients with metastatic breast cancer. *Human Gene Ther* 1993; **4**:331.

33. Brenner MK, Rill DR, Moen RC, et al. Gene marking to trace origin of relapse after autologous bone marrow transplantation. *Lancet* 1993; **341**:85–6.

34. Brugger W, Heimfeld S, Berenson RJ, Mertelsmann R, Kanz L. Transplantation of ex vivo expanded peripheral blood hematopoietic progenitor cells after high-dose chemotherapy in cancer patients. *N Engl J Med* 1995; **333**:283–7.

35. Percivale PL, Bertoglio S, Meszaros P, et al. Radioimmunoguided surgery after primary treatment of locally advanced breast cancer. *J Clin Oncol* 1996; **14**:1599–603.

36. DeNardo, Mirick GR, Kroger GR, et al. The biologic window for chimeric L6 radioimmunotherapy. *Cancer* 1994; **73**:1023–32.

37. Wu XP, Rubin PM, Fan Z, et al. Involvement of P27 (KIP1) in G(1) arrest mediated by an anti-epidermal growth factor receptor monoclonal antibody. *Oncogene* 1996; **12**:1397–403.

38. Baselga J, Tripathy D, Mendelsohn J, et al. Phase II study of weekly intravenous anti-p185[HER2] monoclonal antibody in patients with HER2/neu-overexpressing metastatic breast cancer. *J Clin Oncol* 1996; **14**:737–44.

39. Disis ML, Calenoff E, McLaughlin G, et al. Existent T-cell immunity and antibody immunity to HER-2/neu protein in patients with breast cancer. *Cancer Res* 1994; **54**:16–20.

40. Veelken H, Jesuiter H, Mackensen A, et al. Primary fibroblasts from adults as target cells for ex vivo transfection and gene therapy. *Human Gene Ther* 1994; **5**:1205–12.

41. Kennedy MJ, Vogelzang G, Beveridge RA, et al. A phase II trial of intravenous cyclosporine to induce graft-versus-host disease in women undergoing autologous bone marrow transplantation for breast cancer. *J Clin Oncol* 1993; **11**: 478–86.

42. Douer D, Levine A, Anderson WF, et al. High-dose chemotherapy and autologous bone marrow plus peripheral blood stem cells for patients with lymphoma or metastatic breast cancer – use of marker genes to investigate hematopoietic reconstitution in adults. *Human Gene Ther* 1996; **7**:669–84.

20

Breast cancer chemoprevention

Jenny Chang, Trevor Powles

CONTENTS • Experimental and clinical rationale for tamoxifen chemoprevention • Acute toxicity of tamoxifen • Safety of tamoxifen • Current tamoxifen chemoprevention trials • Other potential agents for chemoprevention • Future developments • Conclusions

The model of endocrine promotion of breast cancer, in which oestrogen is able to activate the development of a single transformed cell into a clinical cancer, offers a unique opportunity for the chemoprevention of a common and frequently fatal disease. Breast cancer affects about one in eight or one in nine North American women and one in thirteen European women. Mortality from breast cancer remains high despite advances in surgical techniques, screening mammography and adjuvant treatments. Epidemiological factors that confer an increased risk include early menarche, late menopause and delayed first pregnancy. These epidemiological data indicate that oestrogen may be an important factor in the endocrine promotion of clinical breast cancer from a single transformed cell. Experimental data have clearly shown that oestrogen is required for promotion of mammary tumours in rats and that this process can be blocked and tumours prevented by use of anti-oestrogenic interventions such as ovarian ablation or tamoxifen.[1]

The most readily identifiable 'high-risk' group consists of women with a positive family history. This risk is higher with increasing numbers of affected relatives, relatives diagnosed at an earlier age or relatives with bilateral breast cancer. Some women at a high risk of inheriting breast cancer are now identifiable by DNA analysis. The breast and ovarian cancer gene (*BRCA*1) and the familial site-specific breast cancer gene (*BRCA*2) have recently been identified. Women with *BRCA*1 mutations have a 65% lifetime risk of developing ovarian cancer and a 80% risk of breast cancer.[2,3] The involvement of endocrine promotion for cancer development in women with genetic mutations for breast cancer is currently unknown.

EXPERIMENTAL AND CLINICAL RATIONALE FOR TAMOXIFEN CHEMOPREVENTION

Tamoxifen is a non-steroidal triphenylethylene derivative with both oestrogenic and anti-oestrogenic activities; it has been shown to inhibit oestrogen-dependent proliferation of MCF-7 cancer cell lines in vitro and tumour growth in vivo.[4] Furthermore, in rats and mice it will inhibit promotion and development of mammary tumours.[1,5]

Tamoxifen has been in clinical use since 1971 for the treatment of more than five million women. It is effective in delaying response and prolonging survival in about

30% of women[6] and will prevent the development of about 40% of contralateral breast cancers in women who have received adjuvant tamoxifen for 2 or more years.[6,7] This has encouraged the use of tamoxifen as a possible chemopreventive agent for breast cancer in healthy women. However, its effective use for chemoprevention would depend on an acceptably low toxicity and a very high safety profile appropriate for long-term use in healthy women.

ACUTE TOXICITY OF TAMOXIFEN

Acute toxicity for tamoxifen in adjuvant trials has been reported as low. Similarly, in a pilot chemoprevention trial undertaken at the Royal Marsden Hospital, Surrey, UK, involving over 2000 healthy women randomized to receive either tamoxifen 20 mg/day or placebo, toxicity was found to be very low with a correspondingly high level of compliance for tamoxifen of 77% and placebo of 82% at 5 years.[8] The main side effects for tamoxifen versus placebo were a significant increase in hot flushes (34% versus 20%), mostly in premenopausal women, vaginal discharge (16% versus 4%) and menstrual irregularities (14% versus 9%).

SAFETY OF TAMOXIFEN

Serum cholesterol levels

Most studies with tamoxifen show a reduction in total plasma cholesterol by about 15–20% of pre-treatment values, and this is sustained throughout treatment.[9,10] These changes in plasma cholesterol are similar to those seen with the administration of hormone replacement therapy (HRT) and suggest that tamoxifen has an oestrogenic effect on cholesterol metabolism in the liver.[11] This may account for a reported 60% reduction in deaths from fatal myocardial infarction in an adjuvant breast cancer trial.[12]

Coagulation factors

Analysis of clotting factors in the Royal Marsden chemoprevention programme has shown a significant reduction in plasma fibrinogen, antithrombin III and cross-linked fibrinogen degradation products,[13] which should be associated with a decrease in thromboembolic disease. Although there has been a report of an increase in thromboembolism in one adjuvant trial,[14] the overview meta-analysis shows no evidence of an increase in thromboembolic or cardiovascular events and some trials have shown a trend for a decrease in acute non-cancer deaths for women on tamoxifen.[12]

Bone densities

Three randomized placebo-controlled trials conducted in predominantly postmenopausal women have shown that adjuvant tamoxifen given over 2 years is associated with an increase in bone mineral density (BMD).[15–17] A similar transient increase in BMD is also reported in the hip, the main site of clinical morbidity in postmenopausal women.[17] In contrast, in premenopausal women tamoxifen causes a significant but transient reduction in bone mineral density in the lumbar spine and hip during the first 2 years of medication.[17] These transient effects may have clinical implications and further long-term monitoring of women on tamoxifen is under way.

Gynaecological effects

Tamoxifen appears to have an oestrogenic effect on the endometrium in postmenopausal women, causing endometrial thickening with an increased risk of atypical hyperplasia and a possible increased risk of developing endometrial cancer. At a dose of 40 mg/day there is a reported sixfold increase in incidence of endometrial cancer,[18] whereas with a standard dose of 20 mg/day any increased risk is much less.[19–21] Use of transvaginal ultrasonography for screening for endometrial abnormalities in women on tamoxifen has shown an increased risk of endometrial hyperplasia, polyps and cysts in women with an endometrial thickening of over 8 mm.[22] However, the detection of endometrial atypical hyperplasia or cancer in this small screening series was low and may put in question the value of screening transvaginal ultrasonography in women on adjuvant tamoxifen or involved in chemoprevention trials.

Other cancers

Experimentally, tamoxifen is genotoxic and in some strains of rats low doses of the drug can cause liver cancers. High levels of stable DNA adducts have been detected by postlabelling with ^{32}P in rat livers, whereas in humans there is no apparent increase in adduct formation in liver or endometrial tissue obtained from women on tamoxifen.[23,24] In women treated for breast cancer, the clinical data at present indicate no evidence for increased risk of liver or other cancers (apart from cancer of the endometrium) in women receiving tamoxifen 20 mg/day. At 40 mg/day the Scandinavian adjuvant trials indicate a possible increase in the risk of gastrointestinal tumours.[25]

Miscellaneous effects

There have been sporadic case reports of eye problems associated with tamoxifen medication. Very high doses of tamoxifen (180 mg/ day or more) are associated with a characteristic retinopathy and keratopathy. At lower doses, one report indicated evidence of a non-specific retinopathy in four of 63 patients[26] that has not been confirmed in other controlled studies.[27]

Acute hepatic toxicity[28] and agranulocytosis have been reported as anecdotal events, the significance of which remains in doubt.[29]

In summary, tamoxifen is well tolerated with high compliance and few acute side effects. There are favourable effects on total plasma cholesterol and bone mineral densities in postmenopausal women. There is no definitive evidence for increase in thromboembolic events or

clotting abnormalities. There is probably a small absolute increase in the risk of endometrial cancer in postmenopausal women, not requiring special surveillance.

Overall, it would seem that the potential benefits of tamoxifen given to women at high risk of developing breast cancer far outweigh the potential risks in carefully controlled and monitored chemoprevention trials.

CURRENT TAMOXIFEN CHEMOPREVENTION TRIALS

Royal Marsden Pilot Trial

Before large-scale studies of tamoxifen prevention could be undertaken, a feasibility pilot trial was started at the Royal Marsden Hospital in 1986 to evaluate the logistic, ethical and clinical problems relating to the use of tamoxifen in healthy women. At that time, although there was considerable experience with the use of tamoxifen for treatment of breast cancer, its use in a prevention setting involving high-risk but healthy volunteers required more stringent monitoring. Results from this study indicate that compliance with tamoxifen was high, the side effects were low,[30] and that it was safe to extend the trial into multicentre international trials involving more than 20 000 healthy high-risk women.

NSABP Breast Cancer Prevention Trial

This study by the National Surgical Adjuvant Breast and Bowel Project (NSABP) was commenced in 1992 and planned to accrue 16 000 women. Currently, the study has recruited over 12 000 women who have a risk equivalent to a 60-year-old woman based on the Gail model,[31] which takes into account both genetic and nongenetic risk factors. A recent interim analysis showed that the registered patients had a higher risk profile than initially expected, and the targeted accrual was recalculated as 13 000 women.

Other national studies

The Italian trial based in the National Cancer Institute at Milan has limited the eligibility to healthy women not at special risk of breast cancer who have previously undergone hysterectomy. To date, about 4000 women have been enrolled into this study.

In the UK, over 1400 women at about three-fold risk of breast cancer have been recruited into a multicentre trial involving centres in the UK, Australia and Europe.

OTHER POTENTIAL AGENTS FOR CHEMOPREVENTION

Retinoids

Retinoids are natural and synthetic analogues of vitamin A. The clinical use of these agents was initially limited by their toxicity, in particular hepatic toxicity. The synthetic retinoid, fenretinide or N-(4-hydroxyphenyl)retinamide is better tolerated with few acute and long-term side effects. No skin or hepatic abnormalities have been observed in phase I studies. However, at a dose of 200 mg/day, about 50% of patients had impairment of dark adaptation which, however, can be moderated by incorporating a 3-day gap in medication at the end of each month. Fenretinide is currently under investigation to evaluate the possible reduction in contralateral new primaries in women with resected early stage breast cancer.[32,33] If found to be effective in preventing second primary cancers, fenretinide may then be considered as a chemopreventive agent in clinical trials involving healthy high-risk women.

Laboratory data with Sprague–Dawley rats has shown synergism between tamoxifen and fenretinide. This combination (tamoxifen 20 mg/day and fenretinide 100–400 mg/day for 27 days per month) is currently being investigated for its combined toxicity in previously untreated metastatic breast cancer patients.[34] Preliminary data indicate no significant renal, hepatic or haematological toxicity.

Gonadotrophin-releasing hormone agonists

The incidence of breast cancer is substantially reduced by oophorectomy.[35] Therefore, it is possible that luteinizing hormone-releasing hormone (LHRH) agonists in premenopausal high-risk women, used to inhibit ovarian oestrogen production to postmenopausal levels, may potentially reduce the risk of breast cancer. However, women receiving these agents may require low doses of oestrogens to offset long-term sequelae associated with oestrogen depletion, in particular accelerated bone loss and cardiovascular disease. It may be possible to give sufficiently low doses of oestrogen replacement to protect against bone loss and cardiovascular disease without losing any protective effect against breast cancer.[36] This type of regimen is complicated, likely to be difficult to give, and would only be necessary if tamoxifen is found to be ineffective in premenopausal women.

Diet

The effect of the quantity of fat in the diet and incidence of breast cancer is still controversial, although an overview analysis of over 10 000 women has shown a positive correlation between high unsaturated fat intake and breast cancer.[37] There would, however, be considerable methodological problems in setting up a trial of reduced fat intake, in particular difficulties in maintaining compliance in the intervention arm and a standard high-fat diet in the control arm.

FUTURE DEVELOPMENTS

Various synthetic analogues of tamoxifen, such as toremifene, droloxifene and raloxifene, have been shown not to be experimentally genotoxic[38] and are now in clinical development.

Of these agents, toremifene has been most extensively used for the treatment of breast cancer. Initial phase II studies indicate similar efficacy and toxicity to tamoxifen.[39] There are now several phase III studies under way evaluating toremifene for treatment of breast cancer and raloxifene is being evaluated as an agent that could be used in healthy women to prevent osteoporosis. The absence of experimental genotoxicity, together with their clinical and experimental effects on normal tissues, makes them attractive candidates after tamoxifen for feasibility testing in chemoprevention trials in healthy women.

CONCLUSIONS

In breast cancer chemoprevention, there are a number of possible agents which could be feasible for use. Tamoxifen has been the most extensively used for cancer treatment with advantages in terms of efficacy in established disease, low acute toxicity and low relative cost. Multicentre trials of tamoxifen chemoprevention are now under way involving over 20 000 women world wide.

Clinical trials of chemoprevention in healthy women are difficult and raise many controversial ethical issues. The recruitment of large numbers of women, together with the requirement that as little harm as possible should be done to volunteers, puts many constraints on the choice of intervention and trial design. Nevertheless, the theoretical possibility that a simple intervention could prevent a major disease encourages active clinical research into breast cancer chemoprevention. The efficacy of interventions such as tamoxifen as a chemopreventive agent for breast cancer can only be answered by long-term follow-up of these large multicentre clinical trials. Such efficacy, if proven, will encourage a new generation of trials aimed at reducing any risks, improving the chemopreventive effects and identifying those women likely to gain most benefit.

REFERENCES

1. Jordan VC. Effect of tamoxifen (ICI 46,474) on initiation and growth of DMBA-induced rat mammary carcinomata. *Eur J Cancer* 1976; **12**:419–24.

2. Miki Y, Swensen J, Shattuck-Eiden D, et al. A strong candidate gene for the breast and ovarian cancer susceptibility gene BRCA1. *Science* 1994; **266**:66.

3. Wooster R, Bignell G, Lancaster J, et al. Identification of the breast cancer susceptibility gene BRCA2. *Nature* 1995; **378**:789–92.

4. Lippman ME, Bolan G, Huff KK. The effects of androgens and antiandrogens on hormone-responsive human breast cancer in long-term tissue culture. *Cancer Res* 1976; **36**:4595–601.

5. Gottardis MM, Jordan VC. Antitumour actions of keoxifene and tamoxifen in the N-nitrosemethylurea-induced rat mammary carcinoma model. *Cancer Res* 1987; **47**:4020–4.

6. EBCTCG, Systemic treatment of early breast cancer by hormonal, cytotoxic, or immune therapy. *Lancet* 1992; **339**:1–15, 71–85.

7. Baum M, Houghton J, Riley D. Results of the Cancer Research Campaign Adjuvant Trial for perioperative cyclophosphamide and long-term tamoxifen in early breast cancer reported at the tenth year of follow-up. *Acta Oncol* 1992; **31**:251–7.

8. Powles TJ, Jones AJ, Ashley SE, et al. The Royal Marsden Hospital pilot tamoxifen chemoprevention trial. *Breast Cancer Res Treat* 1994; **31**:73–82.

9. Powles TJ, Tillyer C, Jones AJ, et al. Prevention of breast cancer with tamoxifen – an update on the Royal Marsden pilot programme. *Eur J Cancer* 1990; **26**:680–2.

10. Love RR, Newcomb PA, Wiebe DA, et al. Effects of tamoxifen therapy on lipid and lipoprotein levels in postmenopausal patients with node negative breast cancer. *J Natl Cancer Inst* 1990; **82**:1327–32.

11. Bush TL, Fried LP, Barratt-Connor. Cholesterol lipoproteins and coronary heart disease in women. *Clin Chem* 1988; **34**:B60–70.

12. McDonald CC, Stewart HJ. Fatal myocardial infarction in the Scottish adjuvant trial. The Scottish Breast Cancer Committee. *Br J Cancer* 1991; **303**:435–7.

13. Jones AL, Powles TJ, Treleaven J, et al. Haemostatic changes and thromboembolic risk during tamoxifen therapy in normal women. *Br J Cancer* 1992; **66**:744–7.

14. Fisher B, Costantino J, Redmond CK, et al. A randomised trial evaluating tamoxifen in the treatment of patients with node negative breast cancer who have estrogen receptor positive breast cancer. *N Engl J Med* 1989; **320**:479–84.

15. Love RR, Mazess RB, Barden HS, et al. Effects of tamoxifen on bone mineral density in post-menopausal women with breast cancer. *N Engl J Med* 1992; **326**:852–6.

16. Kristensen B, Ejiersten B, Dalgaard P, et al. Tamoxifen and bone metabolism in post-menopausal low-risk breast cancer patients: a randomised study. *J Clin Oncol* 1994; **12**:992–7.

17. Powles TJ, Hickish T, Kanis JA, et al. The effect of tamoxifen on bone mineral density measured by dual energy x-ray absorptiometry in healthy pre and postmenopausal women. *J Clin Oncol* 1996; **14**:78–84.

18. Fornander T, Rutquist LE, Cedermark B, et al. Adjuvant tamoxifen in early breast cancer: Occurrence of new primary cancers. *Lancet* 1989; **1**:117–20.

19. Van Leeuwen FE, Benraadt J, Coebergh JWW, et al. Risk of endometrial cancer after tamoxifen treatment of breast cancer. *Lancet* 1994; **343**:448–52.

20. Sasco AJ, Chaplain G, Amoros E, Saez S. Endometrial cancer following breast cancer: Effect of tamoxifen. *Epidemiology* 1996; **7**:9–13.

21. Cuenca RE, Giachino J, Arrendo MA, Hempling R, Edge SB. Endometrial carcinoma associated with breast carcinoma, low incidence with tamoxifen. *Cancer* 1996; **77**:2058–63.

22. Kedar RP, Bourne TH, Powles TJ, et al. Effects of tamoxifen on the uterus and ovaries of post-menopausal women in a randomised breast cancer prevention trial. *Lancet* 1994; **343**:1318–21.

23. Martin EA, Rich JR, White INH, et al. ^{32}P-Post labelled DNA adducts in liver obtained from women treated with tamoxifen. *Carcinogenesis* 1995; **16**:1651–4.

24. Carmichael PL, Ugwumadu AH, Neven P, Hewer AJ, Poon GK, Phillips DH. Lack of geno-toxicity of tamoxifen in human endometrium. *Cancer Res* 1996; **56**:1475–9.

25. Rutqvist LE, Johanson H, Signomklao UI, et al. Adjuvant tamoxifen for early stage breast cancer and second primary malignancies. *J Natl Cancer Inst* 1995; **87**:645–51.

26. Pavlidis N, Petris C, Briassoulis E, et al. Clear evidence that low-dose tamoxifen treatment can induce ocular toxicity. *Cancer* 1992; **69**:2961–4.

27. Longstaff S, Sigurdsson H, O'Keeffe M, et al. A controlled study of the ocular effects of tamoxifen in conventional dosage in the treatment of breast carcinoma. *Eur J Cancer Clin Oncol* 1989; **25**:1805–8.

28. Blackburn A, Amiel S, Millis R, Rubens R. Tamoxifen and liver damage. *Br Med J* 1984; **289**:288.

29. Ching CK, Smith PG, Long RG. Tamoxifen-associated hepatocellular damage and agranulocytosis. *Lancet* 1992; **339**:940.

30. Powles TJ, Hardy JR, Ashley SE. A pilot trial to evaluate the acute toxicity and feasibility of tamoxifen for prevention of breast cancer. *Br J Cancer* 1989; **60**:126–31.

31. Gail MH, Brintom LA, Byar DP, et al. Projecting individualised probabilities of developing breast cancer for white females who are examined annually. *J Natl Cancer Inst* 1989; **81**:1879–86.

32. Veronesi U, De Palo G, Costa A, et al. Chemoprevention of breast cancer with retinoids. *J Natl Cancer Inst* 1992; **12**:93–7.

33. Costa A, Formelli F, Chiesa F, et al. Prospects of chemoprevention of human cancers with the synthetic retinoid fenretinide. *Cancer Res* 1994; **54** (suppl):2032S–7S.

34. Costa A. Breast cancer chemoprevention. *Eur J Cancer* 1993; **29A**:589–92.

35. MacMahon B, Feinlieb M. Breast cancer in relation to nursing and menopausal history. *J Natl Cancer Inst* 1960; **24**:733–53.

36. Pike MC, Spicer DV. The chemoprevention of breast cancer by reducing sex steroid exposure: perspectives from epidemiology. *J Cell Biochem Suppl* 1993; **17S**:26–36.

37. Howe GR, Hirohata T, Hislop G, et al. Dietary factors and the risk of breast cancer: combined analysis of 12 case-control studies. *J Natl Cancer Inst* 1990; **82**:561–9.

38. Kanga L, Nieman AL, Blanco G, et al. A new triphenylethylene compound, Fc-1157a.II. Anti-tumour effect. *Cancer Chemother Pharmacol* 1986; **17**:109–13.

39. Valvaara R. Phase II trials with toremifene in advanced breast cancer. *Breast Cancer Res Treat* 1990; **16** (suppl):S31–5.

21

Routine treatment versus controlled trials

Gianni Bonadonna, A Massimo Gianni, Pinuccia Valagussa, Gabriel N Hortobagyi

Of all the arenas of cancer research open to clinical investigators, breast cancer has always represented one of the most appealing in which to challenge therapeutic problems. During the past few decades, this complex disease has served as a testing ground for ideas, terms, methods and strategies designed to achieve one single objective – cure. Innumerable therapeutic initiatives have been undertaken, some of which have exerted profound influence on current clinical practice. In the vast majority of cases, the relative merits of novel strategies were evaluated through prospective randomized trials. Through these trials, oncologists have established proper rules to assess therapeutic efficacy, and treatment outcome was also correlated to prognostic factors. Without the full appreciation that breast cancer treatment has progressed over time through different conceptual and technical phases, it is meaningless to attempt a critical analysis of the state of the art of the treatment of early breast cancer. This chapter will review the major advances brought about through controlled trials and discuss the future role of controlled trials in breast cancer.

MAJOR ACHIEVEMENTS FROM CONTROLLED TRIALS

Early breast cancer: understanding the complexity of the disease

The acceptance of the radical mastectomy, around the beginning of the twentieth century, as the treatment of choice for primary breast cancer served several useful purposes. On the one hand, it established a standard of care by which other treatments could be measured; on the other, it stimulated the systematic evaluation of treatment outcome and the assessment of the natural history of resectable breast cancer.

Up to about 30 years ago, treatment philosophy was dominated by the anatomical and mechanistic dogma of tumour cell dissemination.[1] At that time, effective therapy was concentrated on locoregional disease, and if the tumour was judged to be technically inoperable, the patient was referred for radiotherapy. For all those patients beyond the domain of surgery and radiotherapy, there were no treatment options because both specific and supportive therapy were in their infancy. Today, the situation is quite different. Thanks to acceptance of the concept that distant micrometastatic disease is present in many women presenting with apparently locoregional disease and to the agents available for women presenting with more advanced disease, all patients can be offered potentially curative or palliative therapy, regardless of age and clinical or pathological stage.

Refinements in the locoregional approach were undertaken around the 1950s. Proponents of more extensive surgery, the so-called extended and super-radical mastectomies, maintained that cancer spread centrifugally through the lymphatics. Therefore, *en bloc* dissection not only of the axillary chain, but also of the internal mammary and supraclavicular lymph nodes, could prevent tumour dissemination to distant sites. Opponents of extensive surgery argued, on the basis of observational data, that the more aggressive approach to breast cancer treatment was not necessarily better than less radical surgery followed by local and/or regional radiotherapy. As a result of the lack of randomized studies, until the early 1970s there was much discussion but few hard data to support either approach.

Since that time, several properly designed control studies have confirmed: that more aggressive surgery is unable to produce additional benefit beyond that produced by the classic Halsted procedure;[2] that breast-sparing procedures and modified radical mastectomy can produce similar disease-free and overall survival rates;[3,4] and that even the rates of isolated local recurrences are not significantly different with different surgical procedures.[5] Besides failing to confirm some aspects of the halstedian concept of surgery, these studies have opened new conceptual areas of breast cancer biology and lent clinical support to pioneering laboratory investigations[6] on the mode of spread of breast cancer.

Additional evaluations of two of the surgical trials[7,8] revealed that the prognosis is inversely related to the number of involved axillary nodes, patients with more than three positive nodes being at a very high risk of disease recurrence (about 85% during the first 10 years after surgery). Another finding of the surgical trials that a quarter of women with node-negative

breast cancer are also at risk of disease recurrence gave support to the hypothesis that occult micrometastases are already present at the time of diagnosis. These observations opened the era of adjuvant systemic treatments, which in turn have opened the era of prognostic determinants.

There is no doubt that the multidisciplinary strategy has served to highlight the complexity of breast cancer, namely the biological heterogeneity of the primary tumour.[9] Our understanding of the interactions between clinical and biological factors and how to construct probabilities for prognosis and treatment selection from these interactions remains incomplete. The number of prognostic variables available today and their degree of importance are subjects of great controversy. In addition, the use of different technical and statistical methodologies has hindered rather than facilitated the interpretation of the interrelationships of these prognostic factors. All of these caveats, as well as the results available on established and potentially useful indicators, have been elegantly summarized in Chapter 3.

Effectiveness of adjuvant systemic therapy in early breast cancer

The early biological hypothesis concerning micrometastatic disease and potential benefit from adjuvant systemic therapy was first tested in women with node-positive breast cancer through randomized trials of chemotherapy conducted by the National Surgical Adjuvant Breast and Bowel Project (NSABP) and the Milan Cancer Institute in the early 1970s.[10,11]

The publication of the early results of these two studies raised both hopes and controversies. In spite of numerous difficulties in coordinating efforts between medical and surgical departments, many research physicians accepted the message of the multidisciplinary approach and began to set up further prospective trials.

In 1977, the Nolvadex Adjuvant Trial Organization designed the first modern adjuvant trial of the anti-oestrogen tamoxifen in women with node-positive and node-negative breast cancer. This form of endocrine therapy achieved a moderately but significantly improved survival, compared with that achieved with locoregional treatment alone,[12] and was almost devoid of major side effects. Trials of adjuvant tamoxifen rapidly proliferated all over the world.

While efforts to improve treatment outcome further by using less empirical and more effective drug regimens were undertaken by major research centres, the medical community began to question the validity of adjuvant systemic treatment. A large group of physicians and health professionals maintained that adjuvant systemic treatment could at best delay disease recurrence but had no impact on survival.[13] This pessimistic view was essentially based on results from repetitive trials which were small and therefore lacked appropriate statistical power or delivered lower doses of chemotherapy, thus lowering the efficacy of the combinations without decreasing the frequency of the side effects.

It was only in 1985, when the Early Breast Cancer Trialists' Collaborative Group reported for the first time that adjuvant systemic treatments were indeed able to produce moderate but worthwhile reductions in the odds of disease recurrence and death, that this treatment modality gained favourable consideration. The findings were based on an overview of 61 adjuvant therapy trials. The results of this overview were published in 1988[14] and updated in 1992.[15] The results confirmed that highly significant reductions in the annual rates of both recurrence and death are produced by tamoxifen (25% and 17%, respectively; $p < 0.00001$) and by polychemotherapy (28% and 16%, respectively; $p < 0.00001$), regardless of age. Ovarian ablation can produce similar reductions, but only in patients younger than 50 years of age, whereas no reductions are achieved by ablation in women aged 50 years or older or by immunotherapy.

A brief note about overviews is warranted. The most important practical contribution of meta-analysis (or overview) is to focus attention on questions of clinical relevance by putting all available data in front of the clinical investigator. Separate evaluations of individual studies

can be misleading because they can create the impression of either no effect (owing to low statistical power) or positive effect (owing to selective reporting of promising results). The large amount of data available, however, does not obviate a critical evaluation of the individual trials that have contributed to the overview. Results from overviews rely heavily on 'arithmetic construct', which first calculates treatment differences within each trial separately and then accumulates these differences across all trials. The interpretation of results therefore requires an appreciation of the characteristics of the individual trials that are combined. Patient eligibility criteria, the nature of experimental and control therapies, dates of active accrual and follow-up time, and quality of the study are important. Combining studies that differ in these aspects may confuse rather than clarify, even if the mathematical criteria of the 'arithmetic construct' are satisfied. There are important examples of studies in which the terms 'treated group' and 'control group' are oversimplifications of the real nature of the therapies delivered. It does not make medical sense to include such individual trials in an overview, even if it makes arithmetic sense. Despite the above words of caution about the interpretation of results, however, there is no doubt that the results of the overview have made an important contribution to the treatment of early breast cancer.

It is important to clarify that the results of the overview are derived from studies designed and activated before 1985. As treatment regimens evolve, often for the better, the reported effects provide only lower limits as to what adjuvant treatment might now offer. Results from more recent studies as well as issues related to the two most commonly used adjuvant modalities, endocrine therapy and conventional chemotherapy, are described elsewhere in this book (see Chapters 8 and 7, respectively).

Trials of primary chemotherapy

Now that it has been established that the outcome of primary treatment is not related to the extent of surgery[5] and that in high-risk subsets systemic adjuvant therapy significantly lowers the risk of tumour recurrence and improves survival,[15] the use of primary chemotherapy (also called neoadjuvant or preoperative chemotherapy) has emerged as one of the next attractive approaches to explore.

The most significant advantage of primary chemotherapy appears to be the early elimination of metastatic microfoci of disease. In breast cancer, these metastases occur in most women harbouring large but resectable tumours.

Primary chemotherapy was first introduced in the multidisciplinary treatment of locally advanced breast cancer in 1973. The first studies undertaken by the Milan Cancer Institute[16] and by the University of Texas MD Anderson Cancer Center in Houston[17] were not classic randomized studies comparing locoregional treatment with or without primary chemotherapy. However, the results achieved with primary chemotherapy stimulated other research groups to adopt a similar treatment approach. Subsequent randomized studies demonstrated that, in locally advanced breast cancer, primary chemotherapy was able at least to produce disease-free and overall survival similar to those obtained after locoregional treatment followed by the same chemotherapy regimen delivered postoperatively (see Chapter 9). One positive effect of primary chemotherapy was that it made possible, in suitable patients, a breast-sparing approach with a reasonable risk of local recurrence.

In more recent years, a number of studies have tested primary chemotherapy in patients with resectable breast cancer. Most of these studies were prospective non-randomized trials; only a few were classic randomized trials comparing primary versus classic postoperative chemotherapy (see Chapter 6). Currently available findings, albeit with a median follow-up of no more than 5–6 years, suggest that primary chemotherapy is not detrimental, overall survival being, in at least two studies, better after this new approach than after classic adjuvant chemotherapy. One important finding from both randomized and non-randomized studies is that primary chemotherapy produces good tumour shrinkage, which results in a significant decrease in the proportion of women requiring mastectomy. This allows for the increased use of breast-saving procedures and thus potentially improves quality of life.

FROM CLINICAL TRIALS TO ROUTINE TREATMENT

In spite of the many years of intensive investigations, the complex biology of breast cancer is far from being understood. New drugs and novel technologies must still be tested in proper randomized studies to assess whether they can improve upon currently available results. Adequate evaluations of these studies will also be of help in improving our understanding of the biology of breast cancer.

It is estimated that about 185 700 new cases of female breast cancer were diagnosed in the USA alone during 1996,[18] yet only 75 000 patients world wide with operable breast cancer were accrued in the different randomized studies activated between the late 1950s and 1985. It is clear, therefore, that although even small improvements in the efficacy of treatment may represent tens of thousands of lives saved every year, overall mortality rates will not be influenced if improved treatments are given only to the small minority of patients enrolled in clinical trials.

Applicability of clinical trial results to the general population

The recently published data on the decrease in breast cancer mortality rates in the USA and various European countries are of historical importance. After decades of increasing mortality rates, there is today a clear trend in the opposite direction. This has undoubtedly been achieved through improved curability of the disease. Whether improved curability is the result of earlier detection or adequate forms of treatment is difficult to clarify and, to a certain extent, it is meaningless. New diagnostic tools that allow detection of minimal-risk breast cancers are important, but equally important are effective treatment modalities that can achieve cure in moderate- to high-risk patients.

Table 21.1 Actuarial disease-specific and overall survival after 7 years among women in British Columbia with newly diagnosed breast cancer

Year	Disease-specific survival (%)		Overall survival (%)	
	Age <50 years	Age 50–89 years	Age <50 years	Age 50–89 years
1974	65.2	63.2	64.8	56.0
1980	70.2	62.5	68.6	53.9
1984	76.3	70.4	74.6	58.3

Modified from Olivotto et al.[19]

In an attempt to determine whether the rate of survival among breast cancer patients had changed because of the introduction of adjuvant systemic therapy, investigators from British Columbia, Canada, evaluated breast cancer survival rates in their province.[19] In British Columbia a centralized cancer agency generates consensus recommendations on therapy and coordinates cancer treatment services. The different cohorts evaluated were: women diagnosed in 1974, when no adjuvant systemic therapy was recommended; women diagnosed in 1980, when adjuvant chemotherapy was recommended only for premenopausal women with node-positive disease; and women diagnosed in 1984, when adjuvant chemotherapy was also recommended for node-negative premenopausal patients with unfavourable indicators and tamoxifen was recommended for postmenopausal women with node-positive tumours or with high-risk node-negative cancers except when their tumours were negative for oestrogen receptors. Significant improvements were observed over the time period studied (Table 21.1). A 32% reduction in the risk of dying of breast cancer and a 28% reduction in the risk of dying of any cause within 7 years of diagnosis were observed among women aged under 50 years. The figures for women aged 50–89 years were 20% and 10%, respectively. The most compelling evidence that the observed improvements in survival can be attributed to the difference in treatment is that these improvements coincided with the introduction of recommendations that adjuvant systemic therapy be used in each age group. In fact, disease-specific survival remained unchanged among older women between 1974 and 1980, but improved in 1984, when tamoxifen began to be used in high-risk patients. In contrast, among premenopausal women, disease-specific survival began to improve between 1974 and 1980, when adjuvant chemotherapy was introduced for node-positive patients, and further improved in 1984, when adjuvant chemotherapy was introduced for high-risk node-negative women (Table 21.1). Although the possibility that other factors could have contributed to the reported survival improvement cannot be denied, these data are encouraging and indicate that the positive results of adjuvant trials can be replicated in the unselected general population.

Clinical trials and implications for routine treatment

Treatment recommendations depend on a wide range of considerations, of which trial results are only one part. Overviews, which provide readers with a large body of data on many individual studies, are less informative than single trials as far as detailed patient characteristics, treatment plans and side effects are concerned.

Therefore, when overviews provide definite answers, as in the case of the updated overview,[15] they can provide only general guidelines but not detailed recommendations to those concerned with treatment.

Individual studies, when carefully reported, describe in detail the population in which the treatment has been evaluated, the entire treatment plan, the therapeutic results, and the frequency and severity of early and late side effects. Oncologists can therefore derive adequate information from these studies to help choose the proper treatment for an individual patient.

It is generally accepted that all patients with node-positive breast cancer, except those with important coexistent morbidities, should receive adjuvant systemic treatment. Furthermore, many patients with node-negative breast cancer can be at high risk of disease relapse (e.g. those with invasive tumours >2 cm in diameter or with oestrogen receptor-negative or undifferentiated tumours), and these patients should also receive adjuvant systemic therapy. Once it has been determined that the benefit of adjuvant systemic therapy outweighs the risk, it is important to inform the patient accurately and openly about alternatives available. All patients younger than 50 years undoubtedly benefit from adjuvant chemotherapy, but the impact of anti-oestrogens or other new hormonal treatments in this age group still needs to be clarified. For older patients, the definition of the risk category is important. Patients in the low-risk category who have oestrogen receptor-positive tumours can be treated with tamoxifen; patients at high risk of recurrence can be treated with conventional chemotherapy with or without the addition of tamoxifen. Regardless of the patient's age and risk category, high-dose chemotherapy still remains experimental.

Another important question is the use of primary chemotherapy in the management of resectable breast cancer. Although available randomized studies have shown that disease-free and overall survival rates after primary chemotherapy are at least equivalent to those observed after classic postoperative systemic treatments, only large well-designed trials with newer effective regimens will demonstrate the worthiness of this approach. Nevertheless, present results confirm that primary chemotherapy can produce significant tumour regression in the great majority of tumours, with a reasonable risk of local recurrence in women subjected to conservative surgery. Consequently, women who have large tumours not suitable for primary conservative surgery can be treated with primary chemotherapy. It is of note that prognosis for these patients is usually poor and, after mastectomy, patients are generally treated with adjuvant systemic therapy. Attempts at reducing the primary tumour to enable a breast-conserving procedure can be an attractive option for women who are concerned about body integrity.

COMMENT

Multidisciplinary treatment of breast cancer has expanded rapidly during the past quarter of a century. There is no doubt that clinical and scientific efforts have brought about important improvements in the prognosis of breast cancer. If the improved cure rate is the result of advances in treatment strategy, then it must be quantified and compared with the cure rate with conventional therapy. In spite of their known limitations,[20] randomized clinical trials remain today the only method for properly assessing the relative merits of new treatment modalities. Actually, randomized clinical trials have produced magnificent scientific achievement when they have been properly conceived and conducted. However, too often trials have been regarded as a panacea for all types of intellectual challenges in clinical management, and repetitive trials lacking sound biological hypotheses and methodology have distracted clinicians from the art of medicine.

Although large well-designed trials are still required to answer important questions, should we expect a specifically designed randomized study for all clinical situations upon which we can rely without too much controversy, dissension or doubt? If we really believe in the results achieved so far in the treatment of early breast cancer, then these therapies must be applied fully to suitable patients in the attempt to bring about a further decrease in tumour mortality from breast cancer. Unfortunately, analysis of practice patterns suggests that even the diagnostic therapeutic progress that has been amply documented by clinical trials is not translated rapidly and fully into community practice.[21] Full implementation of accepted recommendations for screening, primary local therapy and adjuvant systemic treatments should improve disease-free and overall survival figures further. The widespread information on therapeutic results has helped to increase public awareness of the degree of risk and the options available to prevent this risk. Probably, greater public awareness of the strategy of choice for well-selected clinical situations could promote a more rapid adoption of effective therapies and result in cure in a larger proportion of women with breast cancer.

REFERENCES

1. Fisher B. Personal contributions to progress in breast cancer research and treatment. *Semin Oncol* 1996; **23**:414–27.
2. Veronesi U, Valagussa P. Inefficacy of internal mammary node dissection in breast cancer surgery. *Cancer* 1981; **47**:170–5.
3. Fisher B, Redmond C, Poisson R, et al. Eight-year results of a randomized clinical trial comparing total mastectomy and lumpectomy with or without irradiation in the treatment of breast cancer. *N Engl J Med* 1980; **320**:822–8.
4. Veronesi U, Banfi A, Salvadori B, et al. Breast conservation is the treatment of choice in small breast cancer: long-term results of a randomized trial. *Eur J Cancer* 1990; **26**:668–70.
5. Early Breast Cancer Trialists' Collaborative Group. Effect of radiotherapy and surgery in early breast cancer. An overview of the randomized trials. *N Engl J Med* 1995; **333**:1444–55.
6. Fisher B, Fisher ER. The interrelationship of hematogenous and lymphatic tumor cell dissemination. *Surg Gynecol Obstet* 1966; **122**:791–8.
7. Fisher B, Ravdin RG, Ausman RK, et al. Surgical adjuvant chemotherapy in cancer of the breast: results of a decade of cooperative investigation. *Ann Surg* 1968; **168**:337–56.
8. Valagussa P, Bonadonna G, Veronesi U. Patterns of relapse and survival following radical mastectomy. Analysis of 716 consecutive patients. *Cancer* 1978; **41**:1170–8.
9. Heppner GH. Tumor heterogeneity. *Cancer Res* 1984; **44**:2259–65.
10. Fisher B, Carbone P, Economou SG, et al. L-Phenylalanine mustard (L-PAM) in the management of primary breast cancer: a report of early findings. *N Engl J Med* 1975; **292**:117–22.
11. Bonadonna G, Brusamolino E, Valagussa P, et al. Combination chemotherapy as an adjuvant treatment in operable breast cancer. *N Engl J Med* 1976; **294**:405–10.
12. Nolvadex Adjuvant Trial Organization. Controlled trial of tamoxifen as adjuvant agent in management of early breast cancer: Interim analysis at four years. *Lancet* 1983; **i**:257–61.
13. Bailar JC III, Smith EM. Progress against cancer? *N Engl J Med* 1986; **314**:1226–32.
14. Early Breast Cancer Trialists' Collaborative Group. Effects of adjuvant tamoxifen and cytotoxic therapy on mortality in early breast cancer: an overview of 61 randomized trials among 28,896 women. *N Engl J Med* 1988; **319**:1681–92.
15. Early Breast Cancer Trialists' Collaborative Group. Systemic treatment of early breast cancer by hormonal, cytotoxic, or immune therapy. 133 randomised trials involving 31000 recurrences and 24000 deaths among 75000 women. *Lancet* 1992; **339**:1–15, 71–85.
16. Bonadonna G, De Lena M, Brambilla C, et al. Combination chemotherapy and combined modality in disseminated and locally advanced breast cancer. In: *Breast Cancer: Progress in Clinical and Biological Research* (Montague ACV, Stonesifer GL, Lewison EF, eds). New York: Alan Liss, 1977:437–58.
17. Hortobagyi GN, Blumenschein GR, Spanos W, et al. Multimodal treatment of locoregionally advanced breast cancer. *Cancer* 1983; **51**:763–8.
18. Parker SL, Tong T, Bolden S, Wingo PA. Cancer Statistics 1996. *CA Cancer J Clin* 1996; **46**:5–27.
19. Olivotto IA, Bajdik CD, Plenderleith IH, et al. Adjuvant systemic therapy and survival after breast cancer. *N Engl J Med* 1994; **330**:805–10.
20. Feinstein AR. An additional basic-science for clinical medicine. *Ann Intern Med* 1983; **99**:393–7, 544–50.
21. Hand R, Sener S, Imperato J, et al. Hospital variables associated with quality of care for breast cancer patients. *JAMA* 1991; **266**:3429–32.

Index